Hospice Ethics

HOSPICE ETHICS

Policy and Practice in Palliative Care

Edited by Timothy W. Kirk

and

Bruce Jennings

OXFORD
UNIVERSITY PRESS

OXFORD
UNIVERSITY PRESS

Oxford University Press is a department of the University of
Oxford. It furthers the University's objective of excellence in research,
scholarship, and education by publishing worldwide.

Oxford   New York
Auckland   Cape Town   Dar es Salaam   Hong Kong   Karachi
Kuala Lumpur   Madrid   Melbourne   Mexico City   Nairobi
New Delhi   Shanghai   Taipei   Toronto

With offices in
Argentina   Austria   Brazil   Chile   Czech Republic   France   Greece
Guatemala   Hungary   Italy   Japan   Poland   Portugal   Singapore
South Korea   Switzerland   Thailand   Turkey   Ukraine   Vietnam

Oxford is a registered trademark of Oxford University Press
in the UK and certain other countries.

Published in the United States of America by
Oxford University Press
198 Madison Avenue, New York, NY 10016

Library of Congress Cataloging-in-Publication Data
Hospice ethics : policy and practice in palliative care / edited by
Timothy W. Kirk and Bruce Jennings.
p. ; cm.
Includes bibliographical references.
ISBN 978-0-19-994383-8 (pbk. : alk. paper)—ISBN 978-0-19-994494-1 (hbk : alk. paper)
I. Kirk, Timothy W., editor.   II. Jennings, Bruce, 1949–editor.
[DNLM: 1. Hospice Care—ethics.   2. Terminal Care—ethics. WB 310]
R726
179.7—dc23
2014007912

9 8 7 6 5 4 3 2 1
Printed in the United States of America
on acid-free paper

CONTENTS

CONTRIBUTORS

Terry Altilio, MSW, LCSW, is social work coordinator in the Department of Pain Medicine and Palliative Care at Beth Israel Medical Center in New York, NY. She teaches pain and symptom management and ethics in the postgraduate end-of-life certificate programs at New York University Silver School of Social Work and Smith College School of Social Work. Together with Shirley Otis-Green, she is coeditor of the *Oxford Textbook of Palliative Social Work.*

Jennifer Ballentine, MA, is executive director of the Life Quality Institute and President of The Iris Project, an end-of-life consulting and education initiative. Formerly, she was director of programs for the Colorado Center for Hospice & Palliative Care. She serves on the education committee of the National Hospice & Palliative Care Organization, the palliative care task-force of the Center for Improving Value in Health Care, and on the board of directors of the Colorado Healthcare Ethics Forum.

Joy Buck, RN, PhD, is associate professor in the West Virginia University School of Nursing with secondary appointments in the School of Medicine and the School of Public Health. Dr. Buck's research is focused on the history of hospice and palliative care and the intersection of policy, culture, and health outcomes in chronic and advanced illness.

Courtney S. Campbell, PhD, is a member of the board of directors of Benton Hospice Service in Corvallis, OR, and is the chair of the Benton Hospice ethics committee. He is the Hundere Professor for Religion and Culture at Oregon State University, where he has authored several articles on hospice philosophy and physician-assisted death.

Nessa Coyle, RN, ACHPN, PhD, FAAN, is former director of the Supportive Care Program of the Pain and Palliative Care Service at Memorial Sloan-Kettering Cancer Center in New York, NY. She retired in 2012 after 40 years of service and continues as a volunteer member of the Center's ethics committee and clinical consultation team and as a facilitator in the communication skills laboratory. Together with Betty Ferrell, she is coauthor of *The Nature of Suffering and the Goals of Nursing* and coeditor of the *Oxford Textbook of Palliative Care Nursing*.

Pamela Dalinis, RN-BC, BSN, MA, is senior associate director for education in the Division of Accreditation and Certification Operations of The Joint Commission. She has served on the board of directors of the Hospice and Palliative Nurses Association and on the ethics committee of the National Hospice and Palliative Care Organization. Together with Craig M. Klugman, she is coeditor of *Ethical Issues in Rural Health Care*.

Tara Friedman, MD, FAAHPM, is national medical director of Palliative Medical Associates. She serves on the board of directors of the American Academy of Hospice and Palliative Medicine; is past chair of the ethics committee for VITAS Innovative Hospice Care, Philadelphia; and is an active member of the ethics committee at Hahnemann University Hospital in Philadelphia, PA.

Muriel R. Gillick, MD, provides palliative care consultations for Harvard Vanguard Medical Associates, a multispecialty group practice in the Boston area. She conducts scholarly work on health policy and ethical issues near the end of life at the Harvard Pilgrim Health Care Institute and is clinical professor of population medicine at Harvard Medical School.

Joan Harrold, MD, MPH, FACP, FAAHPM, is medical director and vice president of medical services at Hospice & Community Care. She has served on the boards of directors of the American Academy of Hospice and Palliative Medicine and the Pennsylvania Hospice Network, and she serves on the ethics committees of two local hospitals. Together with Joanne Lynn, she is coauthor of *Handbook for Mortals: Guidance for People Facing Serious Illness*.

Bruce Jennings, MA, is director of bioethics at the Center for Humans and Nature, a private, nonpartisan research and educational institute that studies philosophical, ethical, and policy questions concerning environmental and health issues. He holds faculty appointments in public health at Yale University and the New York Medical College and is senior advisor and fellow at The Hastings Center, where he served as executive director from 1991 to 1999. Together with Nancy Berlinger and Susan M. Wolf, he is coauthor of *The Hastings Center Guidelines for Decisions on Life-Sustaining Treatment and Care Near the End of Life*.

Timothy W. Kirk, PhD, serves as ethics consultant for VNSNY Hospice & Palliative Care, chair of the ethics advisory council of the National Hospice and Palliative Care Organization, and assistant professor of philosophy at the City University of New York, York College.

Marcia Levetown, MD, FAAHPM, is regional medical director for VITAS Innovative Hospice Care and an independent educator and consultant specializing in health care communication, ethics, and palliative care. She serves on the ethics committee of the American Board of Pediatrics and is past chairperson of the American Academy of Pediatrics section on hospice and palliative care. Together with Brian S. Carter and Sara E. Friebert, she is coeditor of *Palliative Care for Infants, Children, and Adolescents: A Practical Handbook.*

Jean Munn, PhD, MSW, is a John A. Hartford Faculty Scholar who focuses on social work involvement at the end of life in long-term care. She is associate professor in the College of Social Work and assistant professor in the College of Medicine at Florida State University in Tallahassee, FL.

Stacy Orloff, EdD, LCSW, ACHP-SW, is vice president of palliative care and community programs at Suncoast Hospice in Clearwater, FL. She serves on the executive board of the Social Work Hospice & Palliative Care Network, and she chairs Florida's Partners in Care: Together for Kids steering committee.

Patrick T. Smith, PhD, is ethics coordinator for Angela Hospice in Livonia, MI, and assistant professor of philosophy and theology at Gordon-Conwell Theological Seminary in Roxbury, MA. He is a board member of the Hospice and Palliative Care Association of Michigan. He also serves on the ethics advisory councils of the National Hospice and Palliative Care Organization and Boston Children's Hospital, and the Community Ethics Committee sponsored by the Harvard Ethics Leadership Group.

R. Timothy Tobin, RPh, BS, is palliative care pharmacist for Providence Hospice & Home Care of Snohomish County in Everett, WA. He serves on the hospice ethics committee and on the steering committee of the National Council of Hospice and Palliative Professionals Pharmacist Section.

Sheryl Zimmerman, PhD, is Kenan Distinguished Professor and associate dean of the School of Social Work; adjunct professor at the School of Public Health; and codirector for the Program on Aging, Disability, and Long-Term Care, Cecil G. Sheps Center for Health Services Research, University of North Carolina at Chapel Hill. Her scholarship focuses on quality of life, quality of dying, and quality of care for people receiving long-term care.

Introduction

TIMOTHY W. KIRK AND BRUCE JENNINGS

Since passage of the Medicare hospice benefit in 1982, the number of patients in the United States served each year by hospice has grown by a factor of 15: from fewer than 100,000 in 1982 to over 1.65 million in 2011 (NHPCO, 2012a, 2012c). Indeed, by 2011, 44% of all deaths in the United States occurred while the individuals who died were receiving hospice care (NHPCO, 2012c). Similarly, the number of US hospice programs has also grown significantly, from under 1,300 in 1982 to over 5,300 in 2011 (NHPCO, 2012b). Despite the high rate of growth and wide reach of hospice care, relatively little has been written about the ethics of a practice and model of care that attends to the dying experience of almost half of all Americans. Many hospice leaders and researchers recognize the importance of having a broad-ranging and robust discussion of the ethical issues arising in hospice care as practiced in the United States. This book seeks to stimulate and contribute to that discussion.

Although much has been written about end-of-life decision making in the hospital, an ever-increasing proportion of end-of-life care is delivered to patients in the home, and within the particular care environment of hospice. This migration (return, really) to dying in the home reflects a long-standing and widespread preference in society and among the elderly. As it has taken place, hospice professionals and programs have been faced with a broader array of terminal illnesses, cultural values and traditions, and patient and family values than ever before. Originally designed as a model of care for terminally ill cancer patients, US hospice organizations now care for patients whose illnesses are highly variable in progression and whose treatment plans include many medical options. The ethical framework that has served hospice for the past 50 years—a framework that is holistic and inter-disciplinary; centered on the dying person in relationship with family and others; and marked by the values of relief from suffering, commitment to presence and nonabandonment, and quality of the life lived in and through the dying process—remains the foundation on which to build. Nonetheless, this framework will need to be supplemented and refined if hospice is to ful-fill this changing social mission. The values embedded in the hospice model of care need to be made explicit so that the resonances and dissonances between those values and the values of patients, families, and communities served by hospice organizations can be explored and discussed. We believe that the time is right for a book that makes those implicit values explicit and begins that process of exploration, providing a new educational resource for giving care, and learning to give care, at the end of life.

In the United States, "hospice care" and "palliative care" have distinct histories and practice environments. In this book, we have chosen to focus on the former. This was a deliberate choice, reflecting our considered con-clusion that the ethical issues embedded in the organization and delivery of care present themselves differently in the two models of care. With a significant majority of patients receiving care in the home, hospice care is delivered through largely autonomous interdisciplinary care teams, often headed by nurses, who are the primary coordinators of clinical care for patients who are terminally ill. As of 2014, most palliative care teams func-tion as consultation services in hospital environments, often comingled with pain and symptom management services and largely staffed by phy-sicians and nurse practitioners, serving patients in all phases of the life span. So, while some chapters will apply especially well to the experience of giving and receiving both kinds of care, readers will find the material most squarely focused on hospice care.

Thirteen new chapters, commissioned specifically for this volume and written by 17 hospice experts, are centered around four themes, each devoted to an aspect of the intersection of ethics and hospice care. These themes are as follows: the hospice philosophy, the interdisciplinary team approach to care, organizational and policy issues in hospice, and ethical ideals and the future of hospice care. The authors presented here are pro-fessionals and scholars of long experience and have the ability to articulate, explain, and respond to ethically significant phenomena that—while not always unique to hospice care—arise in especially poignant and complex ways when caring for patients enrolled in hospice. As a whole, the book is the first comprehensive collection devoted to analyzing distinctive ethical issues arising in the delivery of hospice care and designed to promote best ethical practices for hospice care professionals.

SECTION I: HOSPICE: THE EMERGENCE OF A PHILOSOPHY OF CARE

The first section orients readers historically and philosophically to hospice care as it has come to be delivered in the United States. The chapters explain the intersection of economics, medicine, politics, and a certain philosophy about the care of the dying that came together as hospice care emerged in the 1960s and 1970s. The implicit ethical framework as the movement coalesced and grew is articulated and analyzed.

Joy Buck opens with a chapter tracing the history of hospice in the United States. Drawing upon her original archival and oral history research, the author explains how the rise of nursing—as an academic discipline and scholarly practice profession distinct from medicine—intersected with economic and political forces in the 1970s and 1980s to shape the development and growth of hospice care in the United States.

In his chapter, Timothy Kirk uses the context of Buck's work to articulate the philosophical framework at the heart of hospice care, a framework that was well established by the founder of the modern hospice movement, Cicely Saunders. Kirk uncovers an ethical framework embedded in the hospice philosophy of care and explains that framework as one which seeks to restore and respect the moral agency of dying patients and their families. As such, he claims that hospice is an inherently moral practice and argues that its moral nature would benefit from further exploration and critique.

SECTION II: THE INTERDISCIPLINARY TEAM: ETHICAL OPPORTUNITIES AND CHALLENGES

The second section of the book focuses on the ethical possibilities and limitations arising from the interdisciplinary team (IDT) at the core of all hospice care delivery. A product of both the hospice philosophy of care and regulatory mandates, the IDT is one of the hallmark components of hospice care. The structure and function of the IDT is at the heart of many of the most important ethical issues in hospice, and the chapters in this section explore how different roles on the team, and the health of the team itself, can dramatically impact the care experience for providers, patients, and families in ways that are ethically significant.

Timothy Tobin opens Section II with an exploration of the increasingly important role of specialist pharmacists on the hospice IDT in Chapter 3. Traditionally, nurses, social workers, spiritual care providers, and physicians have constituted the core members of the IDT. However, Tobin argues persuasively that access to a pharmacist specializing in hospice and palliative care, and ongoing, reciprocal consultation between that pharmacist and the IDT are crucial to a hospice organization fulfilling its mission to treat symptom distress and address the suffering of patients and families. Tobin also reveals ways that pharmacist participation on ethics committees can open up important opportunities for reflection and potentially lower the risk for moral distress in pharmacists, whose "behind the scenes" role may give the inaccurate impression that they are somehow immune to ethical challenges or unable to act on ethical opportunities.

Joan Harrold presents a portrait of the role of medical director that is today far different from the part-time, volunteer physician whom many hospice providers remember filling that role from the 1970s into the 1990s. Changes in regulatory requirements, an increasingly heterogeneous illness distribution among hospice patients, and the evolution of hospice and palliative medicine as an academic medical subspecialty recognized by the American Board of Medical Specialties have all contributed to changes in the complexity and focus of the role of hospice medical director. This analysis draws on Harrold's own clinical and administrative experience as well as the peer-reviewed literature to identify ethical challenges and opportunities in the medical director's relationships with patients, IDT colleagues, and hospice administrators.

Section II closes with a chapter proposing an integral role for individual and collective reflection and deliberation in hospice teams. Drawing on many decades of teamwork in palliative care, Nessa Coyle and Terry Altilio adapt models of reflection and deliberation from multiple literatures and connect them to the stresses that can arise during extended interdisciplinary efforts to address complex suffering at the end of life. In so doing, the authors remind readers that ethics is not simply about addressing disagreements or discerning right from wrong. Creating moments of stillness and introspection, allowing teams to identify and explore resonances and dissonances within the team and between the team and those it serves, are ways of bringing the values, hopes, and fears of team members from the background into the foreground so they can be discussed, explored, and addressed. The authors also suggest that engaging in a process like the one they put forward promises to play an important role in detecting and addressing moral distress. Doing so, according to Coyle and Altilio, is one way to ensure that teams are thriving in a way that allows them to relieve—rather than add to—the suffering of patients and families in hospice care.

SECTION III: ORGANIZATIONAL AND POLICY ETHICS IN HOSPICE

The health and functioning of the IDT and the nature of ethical dilemmas that arise in clinical practice are directly impacted by the organizational, policy, and regulatory systems in which hospice operates. With those systems becoming increasingly complex and influential, the chapters in Section III explore the dynamic interaction between hospice organizations and the environments in which they offer care, uncovering multiple layers of interconnectedness that inform hospice ethics.

Marcia Levetown and Stacy Orloff explain the cultural, social, organizational, and regulatory barriers to giving and receiving high-quality pediatric hospice care. Offering a nuanced analysis of the many intersections of these layers of influence, the authors demonstrate systems-level impediments to pursuing excellence in hospice care of children and their families. In so doing, they identify openings for change at multiple levels that would empower individual clinicians, care organizations, and communities, allowing them to better honor ethical obligations to reduce distress and improve quality of life for children, families, and clinicians in pediatric end-of-life care.

Hospice care is family-centered care. Patrick Smith addresses this familiar mantra, explaining what it means and exploring the ways in which it troubles assumptions in traditional approaches to health care ethics. Unpacking the complexity of discerning ethical obligations to not only patients but also their family members, and analyzing the conceptual strain of considering those obligations when family members are simultaneously receiving care from hospice providers and giving care to their loved ones, Smith argues that a commitment to family-centered care is one of the hallmark challenges distinguishing traditional health care ethics from a more distinctly "hospice ethics."

While the great majority of hospice care in the United States is delivered in patient homes, patients whose symptom management needs cannot be adequately addressed in the home become eligible for inpatient hospice care. As with any shift in care environment, the ways in which ethical issues present themselves—and the most effective ways of addressing those issues—also shift. Exploring the hospice inpatient environment through the lens of clinical and organizational ethics, Tara Friedman reveals the multiple layers of complexity that arise when hospices open dedicated inpatient units, especially if those units inhabit leased space within hospitals or other health care facilities that have different philosophies and goals of care. While such arrangements often make sense from a business point of view—allowing hospices to purchase housekeeping, security, meal, and pharmacy services already onsite—Friedman highlights areas of potential tension and suggests ways of addressing them via some basic tenets of preventative ethics.

Historically, the hospice model of care has favored patients living in private homes who have loved ones available to be informal caregivers. A side effect of this model, however, is that patients who live in residential facilities—including assisted living and long-term care facilities—have not had the same access to hospice care at the end of life as those living in private residences. Drawing on many years of their own research on end-of-life care in residential facilities, Jean Munn and Sheryl Zimmerman open by offering readers a powerful overview of the long-term care landscape in the United States. They proceed to identify four critical points in the lives of residents where the intersection of hospice and long-term care can align or misalign in ways that powerfully impact residents' ability to receive timely, high-quality hospice care. Following this analysis, they propose an innovative fusion of hospice and long-term care that, they argue, could close current gaps such that residents' access to hospice care improves and hospice providers' expertise is more seamlessly integrated into facility-based care.

Whether in the home, in a facility, or on an inpatient unit, few questions are likely to rouse the passion of hospice health care providers as predictably as whether hospice patients should be offered the option of resuscitation. Muriel Gillick provides a thoughtful and balanced explanation and critique of the arguments and perspectives on all sides of the issue. While her chapter ends with a position familiar to many hospice care providers, the journey the author takes to reach that position incorporates important regulatory requirements, outcomes research, and robust ethical reasoning in an attempt to address both patient and provider rights in the context of the hospice philosophy of care.

"Hospice," claims a familiar refrain, "neither hastens nor prolongs death." However, in four US states (Oregon, Washington, Montana, and Vermont), hospice patients have the option of seeking the assistance of physicians in hastening their deaths. In states where aid in dying is legal, Courtney Campbell has done research on hospice policies in this environment. His study of how hospices do (or do not) engage and support patients who pursue the aid-in-dying option—or, just ask about doing so—offers readers important empirical information in what is often a discussion driven more by rhetoric than data. After presenting his findings, Campbell offers a carefully crafted conceptual framework through which he recommends hospice organizations in all states collectively examine the ways in which their policies addressing this and related phenomena reflect clearly articulated organizational values; offer concrete, well-justified guidance to hospice caregivers; and honor basic ethical obligations to patients and their families at the end of life.

Policy review and development is one of the traditional tasks of health care ethics committees. However, it is not known how many hospice organizations have their own ethics committees, what such committees look like, and what role they play in those organizations. Indeed, as Jennifer Ballentine and Pamela Dalinis highlight, it is not even clear whether the traditional model of health care ethics committees, a model developed by and for acute care hospitals, is an effective way for hospices to address the ethically significant aspects of their clinical and operational practices. After reviewing the scant data available on how hospices address ethics, Ballentine and Dalinis propose guidelines for hospice ethics committees that seek to create spaces within organizations wherein questions of value, obligation, and rights can be asked in a manner informed by the basic philosophical tenets of hospice care and integrated into the daily lives of hospice employees and those whose lives they touch.

SECTION IV: ETHICS AND THE FUTURE OF HOSPICE

In the final section, Bruce Jennings draws together several themes from the preceding chapters and contextualizes the discussion of hospice ethics by exploring ways in which the philosophy, structure, and delivery of hospice care can be refined and expanded as an ethical model for care across the life span. Drawing upon his collaborative work with colleagues that resulted in an influential 2003 study of hospice policy, *Access to Hospice Care: Expanding Boundaries, Overcoming Barriers*, Jennings finds in the hospice philosophy, its model of health care delivery, and the social movement supporting hospice fruitful points of departure for a more general reform of long-term care and chronic illness care in an aging society. Begun as a refuge of hospitality and protection for terminal cancer patients and their families, hospice today, the author argues, holds the key to a vastly improved long-term and chronic care system in the future. The next stage in the development of hospice and palliative care can lead the way toward an ethical institutional and public policy response to the inevitable challenges of frailty and vulnerability in an aging society.

Picking up where Kirk left off in his essay at the beginning of the volume, Jennings reminds us that the internal moral structure of hospice is deeply affected by the larger social, cultural, and political milieu in which hospice care is practiced. Moreover, such influence can be reciprocal: The philosophical commitments of hospice can radiate outward into the communities served by hospice organizations.

The hallmarks of hospice—its genuinely interdisciplinary model of care that evolved out of a desire to holistically address suffering and support the moral agency of dying persons and their families; its commitment to treating not just the disease but persons' experience of illness—that have proven their worth in care near the end of life must now move upstream into earlier stages of those progressive, incurable, and debilitating chronic conditions that now dominate the landscape of American morbidity and mortality. Here is a vision in which hospice ethics can extend beyond the delivery of hospice care, helping us think individually and collectively about what it means to have a good birthing experience, a good dying experience, and pursue a good and meaningful life in whatever time we have between the two. It is a vision to which this volume is dedicated.

ACKNOWLEDGMENTS

The creation of a volume of original essays by a group of expert authors is both a privilege and a difficult task. While those who made this volume possible are too numerous to mention, the editors wish to acknowledge some without whose assistance this book would not be possible.

First, and foremost, our contributing authors have offered not just their written contributions but their expertise, good will, and patience during a process that took far longer than we estimated. Their generosity and forbearance have been exemplary of the qualities that make for good colleagues, and we thank them. Our editors at Oxford University Press, Peter Ohlin and Lucy Randall, have offered their expert support and advice throughout the creation of the book, for which we are grateful. Anonymous reviewers have given very helpful suggestions and critiques at several stages of the project, many of which have improved the quality of the final product.

Tim Kirk wishes to thank colleagues at VNSNY Hospice and Palliative Care and the National Hospice and Palliative Care Organization, many of whom have reviewed chapters, suggested content to be included in the book, and helped identify experts to review and contribute to the project. Particularly helpful and supportive along the way have been Randi Seigel, Daniel Cogan, and E. Willis Partington at VNSNY and Jon Radulovic at NHPCO.

Bruce Jennings wishes to acknowledge and thank the remarkably caring and thoughtful colleagues from whom he has learned about hospice and end-of-life care at The Hastings Center, the National Hospice Work Group, the National Hospice and Palliative Care Organization, and the Hospice Foundation of America. In particular, he would like to acknowledge his coauthors on two publications closely related to this book: Nancy Berlinger and Susan M. Wolf, with whom he worked on *The Hastings Center Guidelines for Decisions on Life-Sustaining Treatment and Care Near the End of Life* (Oxford University Press, 2013); and True Ryndes, Carol D'Onofrio, and Mary Ann Baily, with whom he worked on *Access to Hospice Care: Expanding Boundaries, Overcoming Barriers.*

REFERENCES

Jennings, B., Ryndes, T., D'Onofrio, C., & Baily, M. A. (2003). Access to hospice care: Expanding boundaries, overcoming barriers. *Hastings Center Report, 33*(2, Suppl.), S3–S60. Retrieved April 2014, from http://www.thehastingscenter.org/Publications/SpecialReports/Detail.aspx?id=1352.

National Hospice & Palliative Care Organization (NHPCO). (2012a). *Growth in U.S. hospice programs, 1974 to 2011.* Retrieved April 2014, from http://www.nhpco.org/sites/default/files/public/Statistics_Research/NHPCO_growth_patients_providers_2011.pdf.

National Hospice & Palliative Care Organization (NHPCO). (2012b). *Patients served by hospice in the U.S., 1984 to 2011.* Retrieved April 2014, from http://www.nhpco.org/sites/default/files/public/Statistics_Research/NHPCO_growth_patients_providers_2011.pdf.

National Hospice & Palliative Care Organization (NHPCO). (2012c). *NHPCO facts and figures: Hospice care in America* (2012 Ed.). Alexandria, VA: NHPCO.

Hospice: The Emergence of a Philosophy of Care

CHAPTER 1

"From Rites to Rights of Passage"

Ideals, Politics, and the Evolution of the American

Hospice Movement

JOY BUCK

Hospice is many things. Hospice is home care with inpatient back-up facilities...pain control...skilled nursing...a doctor and a clergyman coming to your home...But most of all, hospice is the humanization of our health care system.

—Senator Edward Kennedy, National Hospice Organization (NHO) Meeting, Nov. 8, 1978

Another example is Medicare and Medicaid—programs with worthy goals but whose costs have increased...Waste and fraud are serious problems...the time has come to control the uncontrollable.

—President Ronald Reagan, State of the Union Address, 1982

The issues of medical beneficence, quality of life, and respect for the sanctity of life have been described in medical and philosophical writings since the earliest documented history. The central questions remain constant through history, but advances in scientific knowledge and technology continually reframe our understanding of both the questions and answers. In mid-20th-century America, when the hospice movement began, ethical debates centered on questions about an individual's right to self-determination, the rights of surrogates acting on behalf of others, determinations of the quality and futility of life, the conditions under which one might choose to end life, and protections for those who helped them die in the manner they chose (Webb, 1997). In the United States, hospice began as a humane alternative to standard care for persons in the late stages of cancer. When the formalized hospice programs were being developed, they were viewed as either a moral imperative to transform cancer care or an anathema to the cure imperative, a "one-way escalator toward death," and a threat to persons with disabilities. Nevertheless, due to a combination of social, political, and economic forces, hospice was catapulted onto the political agenda for reform at unprecedented speed. Less than 10 years after the first state-certified hospice home care program began operations in 1974, hospice became an entitlement under the Medicare program in 1982.

Translating the hospice ideal into a reimbursable model of care, without changing its nature, proved to be a challenge, and serious issues remain. Today, palliative care enthusiasts point to the limitations of hospice when calling for reimbursement for their emergent medical subspecialty. Yet are these limitations attributable to the hospice concept itself or its operationalization within the constraints of the American system? This first chapter seeks to answer this question by examining the processes by which the hospice philosophy of care was translated into the Medicare hospice benefit and the subsequent impact of this translation on contemporary hospice care.

Historical research methods provide a useful social distancing mechanism that allows the scrutiny of events outside of the temporal bias in which the events evolved (Lynaugh & Reverby, 1987). This brief history raises questions of how ideals and boundaries about health care are created in a market-oriented society and in turn how health care innovations are shaped as they are institutionalized. In doing so, it offers a cautionary tale that is particularly germane to contemporary discourse surrounding the ethos, ethics, and future of hospice and palliative care.

POLICY AND CONTEMPORARY HOSPICE CARE

Kathy, a nurse colleague, was 46 years old when she had her first heart attack and was permanently disabled by a stroke she suffered during heart bypass surgery. For the next 8 years, Kathy was plagued by endless fatigue, breathlessness, and pain—all constant reminders that her heart was slowly but steadily failing her. Unable to work, she lost her health insurance. Her escalating medical bills depleted her savings soon thereafter. Collectors repossessed her car when she could no longer pay her bills. Even reading, her one last pleasure, was taken away as she went blind due to complications of diabetes. By the time Kathy was referred to hospice at the age of 54, she was living in poverty and tethered by disability to a trailer that, like her fragile health, was crumbling around her.

Once in hospice, Kathy's quality of life improved dramatically. The nurses taught her how to use medications and relaxation techniques to manage her symptoms more effectively. The social worker facilitated family meetings to help Kathy and her loved ones make sense of their difficult past and uncertain future. The nursing assistant helped her with household chores, allowing Kathy to conserve her energy for outings with her favorite hospice volunteer. Kathy benefitted from hospice for 2 years before she was discharged because she had far outlived her predicted life expectancy. Over the next 2 months, she was read-mitted to the hospital four times before she was transferred to the only available "Medicaid" nursing home bed in a neighboring county. The nurses would not give her the morphine that eased her breathing; they thought that it would kill her. The nursing home staff avoided her. Her family did not have transporta-tion and could not visit. Kathy died a month after admission, in a room at the end of the hall, alone, frightened, and struggling as she took her last breath. (Anonymous, personal communication, June 21, 2009)[1]

American hospice programs provide services to over 1.2 million peo-ple annually, and Kathy is just one of the 212,000 people who were dis-charged from hospice alive in 2008 (National Hospice and Palliative Care Organization [NHPCO], 2009). The majority of these "live discharges" were women with a noncancer diagnosis such as heart failure. Others who are "sick enough to die" and might well benefit from hospice are not eli-gible because they do not fit neatly into the Medicare eligibility criteria. This is especially true for people with advanced dementia. For example, in December 2001, an 84-year-old woman called an ambulance in panic after her husband collapsed in front of her eyes. Two days later, the cardiolo-gist told her that he was dying. She and her husband were referred to and admitted to a local hospice program. She was told 24 hours later that his admission was denied; he did not fit eligibility criteria for persons with noncancer diagnoses. He died 2 days later in the hospital. The woman was Florence Wald, an American nurse who is known to many as the American "hospice midwife" (F. Wald, personal communication, July 21, 2001). She and her beloved husband, Henry, were cofounders of the very hospice that he was denied access to. While the cruel irony of this scenario is obvious, the compassionate care they received in the hospital is testimony to the significant changes that came about, in part, as a result of their advocacy and that of their compatriots.

To best understand the complexities associated with past and present health care reforms, it is instructive to revisit transitions in the manner and location of dying during the 20th century as a prelude to the American hospice movement. During the 20th century, a combination of sociopolitical factors influenced the cause, manner, and location of dying. At the beginning of the century, the leading causes of death were acute infectious diseases, such as pneumonia, influenza, tuberculosis, and infant diarrhea, or accidents. Over half of the recorded deaths were among children under the age of 15, and it was rare for a family not to have buried at least one child (Lerner, 1970). This changed when public health measures, sanitation, and the pasteurization and refrigeration of food dramatically decreased mortality rates during pregnancy, infancy, and childhood. Improved and widespread use of asepsis techniques significantly decreased surgical mortality rates.

While these advances were cause for celebration, they also led to growth in the number of Americans living with chronic illness. By the early 1940s, the percentage of American deaths caused by chronic diseases had increased from 24.4% to 61.2% (Backer, Hannon, & Russell, 1982). In 1936, one person in six had chronic debilitating diseases, more than 70% of whom were under the age of 55, and the poor were disproportionately affected (Technical Committee on Medical Care, Interdepartmental Committee to Coordinate Health and Welfare Activities, 1938). The nation's 1950 census revealed that the elderly population, those aged 65 and older, had grown from 3 million in 1900 to 12 million in 1950, or from 4% to 8% of the total population (Social Security Administration, 2003). The elderly were sicker, hospitalized more often, and were more prone to untoward effects of medical and surgical interventions. The once "quick or sudden death" associated with infectious diseases and accidents was being supplanted by the "lingering death" that accompanied the newfound longevity.

Until the early 1900s, most dying persons were cared for at their home by family members, the vast majority of whom were women (Walsh, 1929). For those with financial means, private nurses were hired to care for the dying person. Those without the resources to remain at home, financial or familial, or whose conditions were such that the family could not care for them either languished in the streets or were sent to almshouses or asylums until they died. Beginning in the late 19th century, a number of homes opened in the British Isles and America to provide specialized care for the hopelessly ill poor. Most though not all of these homes were founded and operated by religious groups. Although there were denominational differences in their approach to care for the dying, they were united in their dedication to serve the poorest of the poor (Humphreys, 2001).

THE ROLE OF THE STATE IN AND THE STATE OF HEALTH CARE

The medicalization of dying and the professionalization of care of the dying in the United States were directly linked to the pervasive role of government in the configuration, financing, and oversight of the American health care system. Immediately following World War II, there was a significant American political expansion, economic prosperity, and corresponding advances in health care technology and medical research. Concurrent with the medical expansion, there was also a shortage of health care professionals. Congress passed legislation that provided the funds for traineeship grants, medical specialization, and the emergence of medical research centers. The resultant increase in the number of hospital beds and capacity for "lifesaving" was in part due to other changes in society such as the mobility of the population, the transference of the extended family to the nuclear family, and women's work outside the home. Federal funding also fueled the growth of the National Institutes of Health (NIH), the National Institute of Mental Health (NIMH), and the National Cancer Institute (NCI). By 1947, the NIH, which had been created in 1930 with a budget of less than $50,000, had become the nation's major center for medical research with a budget of more than $8 million (Feldstein, 1996).

CANCER, TECHNOLOGY, AND THE QUEST FOR CURE

By the mid-20th century, cancer was the second leading cause of death in the United States, and the cure rate continued to be low. For the most part, chemotherapy and radiation were considered to be temporary or palliative treatments that had disabling side effects associated with their use. The preferred method of treatment was surgery, and cancer surgeons commonly believed that in order to cure cancer, tumors must be excised in a manner so radical that the "diseased area is removed widely, irrespective of the deformity which is produced" (Raven, 1949, p. 262). Even when the results of a National Cancer Institute study indicated that there was no difference in the 5- and 10-year survival rates for breast cancer patients whether a radical or simple mastectomy was performed, advocates of radical surgeries vehemently held their position (Haagensen, 1947).

After World War II, chemotherapy and radiation became viable treatment options, but they were highly toxic and produced severe nausea, vomiting, and pain, none of which were well managed by physicians and nurses. As advances in the use of radiation, radioactive isotopes, and chemotherapy continued throughout the 1960s, cancer care became more specialized, fragmented, and depersonalized. Persons with cancer became research subjects who were treated by a variety of cancer specialists who were not known to them. When combined with other factors such as the curative medical milieu and the increased use of and research funding for experimental treatments and surgeries, this dual role posed an ethical dilemma, and patients were often subjugated to continued treatment long after any hope of cure or remission of the disease was possible (Coser, 1962, p. 76).

INSTITUTIONAL CARE FOR THE DYING

By the end of the 1960s, more than 60% of deaths in the United States were caused by cancer and complications of debilitating chronic disease, and 61% of those deaths occurred in institutions (Backer, Hannon, & Russell, 1982; Lerner, 1970). Research funded by the US Public Health Service Division of Nursing revealed that communication about prognoses was virtually nonexistent and persons often died in a room at the end of the hall, in pain, and alone. Physicians rarely discussed terminal prognoses, maintaining that it was in the patient's best interest not to speak about it, and nurses and families joined the conspiracy of silence (Duff & Hollingshead, 1968; Glaser & Strauss, 1965). The impact of this philosophy was significant. In one study, more than 50% of the hospitalized patients expressed fear and anxiety, often related to the response of physicians and nurses to their concerns. Patients reported that they overheard nurses talking in the halls about other patients, often with graphic details about the horrors of disease (Duff & Hollingshead, 1968). Despite advances in cancer treatment, little was done to alleviate the suffering that persons with cancer experienced. For example, a 22-year-old man was diagnosed with advanced cancer after having surgery at a local hospital. Neither the family nor the physician told him his diagnosis, and he was referred to a cancer hospital for further surgery and treatment. During the last months of his life he suffered terribly. In his mother's words: "He lived for eleven months after that—never once out of pain, never once feeling good, and, in the end, telling us that he was more afraid of living than dying...He was more or less treated as a research specimen for the remainder of his life...In the eleven months that he lasted, Flip had not a day without pain and most of his pain was created by doctors continuing in their efforts to help him" (Josephs, 1971, p. 31). These conditions also had severe implications for staff on units where the death rate was high (Klagsbrun, 1969). It was within this context that the modern hospice concept emerged as a viable option and an ethical imperative for reform (Buck, 2007b).

BIRTH OF THE AMERICAN HOSPICE MOVEMENT

Dame Cicely Saunders is the acknowledged founder of the international hospice movement. Her commitment to care of terminally ill cancer patients evolved from her work at St. Luke's Home for the Dying Poor and St. Joseph's Hospice as a nurse, as a medical almoner (social worker), and finally as a physician. In the late 1950s, she began corresponding with American leaders in cancer care about the "cancer problem" in the United States. In 1963, she made her first of many visits to North America and gave lectures about her work at St. Joseph's Hospice. She shared compelling stories about terminally ill cancer patients who came to St. Joseph's expressing feelings of guilt, failure, and rejection. In the words of a woman with breast cancer: "I knew I needed attention. They [previous hospital] never asked me back. They didn't see me, I didn't have any treatment, no pills or medicine or anything. I was so ill. When I came here everywhere I was in agony" (Saunders, 1966, p. 3). To illustrate the benefits of hospice, Saunders showed slides of patients on admission and again during the last days of their lives looking comfortable, alert, and active. Her vision for St. Christopher's, the hospice she was building, was "a community . . . a common giving of people who share the cost of being vulnerable" (Saunders, 1971, p. 8). This philosophy blurred the boundaries of how health professionals and patients existed in relationship to each other.

Saunders was motivated by her deep religious conviction and profound experiences with dying patients, as well as the euthanasia movement in England, which she and many other physicians adamantly opposed (Kemp, 2002; Weikart, 2004). So fervent was she to advance hospice as an alternative to euthanasia that the first article she wrote for a series on terminal care that was published in *Nursing Times* was devoted to the "problem of euthanasia" (Saunders, 1959). The essay drew from public discourse of "mercy killing" to address two questions: "Is euthanasia morally right?" and "Is there really no other way of relieving distress of patients in the terminal stages of cancer?" Drawing on her Christian belief in transcendence, she argued that euthanasia was morally wrong because it deprived patients of an opportunity to "grow in patience and courage right up to their last moments" (Saunders, 1959, p. 960).

Saunders's passion for hospice particularly resonated with Florence Wald, who was dean of the Yale School of Nursing when she first heard Saunders speak in 1963. Wald was a self-proclaimed idealist and Saunders's conceptualization of hospice and the centrality of nursing within it resonated with her. Hospice offered her a vehicle by which she could forge significant reforms with medicine and nursing as equals at the helm. Wald maintained correspondence with Saunders and invited her back to the United States for a visiting professorship in nursing in 1966. This visit culminated with an Institute on Care for the Dying that brought together imminent leaders, scholars, and clinicians in the emerging field of thanatology. Reverend Edward Dobihal, an evangelistic Methodist minister and chaplain at Yale-New Haven Medical Center with a background in pastoral counseling and bereavement, was one of the attendees. Together, Wald and Dobihal and other like-minded individuals launched a multidisciplinary effort to transplant Saunders's vision of hospice to American soil (Buck, 2007; E. Dobihal, personal communication, July 20, 2001; F. Wald, personal communication, July 21, 2001).

By 1968, Wald had stepped down as dean and obtained funding from the Division of Nursing and the American Nurses Foundation to conduct two interdisciplinary research studies that were pivotal to the initiation of the hospice movement in Connecticut. The research notebooks from both of these studies provide a rare and detailed account of how the group negotiated their personal spheres of influence, as well as professional and disciplinary boundaries, as they began caring for and advocating on behalf of terminally ill patients within the existing system. The studies served to coalesce and crystallize the growing group's vision for the creation of their hospice and revealed that nurses, younger physicians, students, and others not firmly entrenched in the curative professional paradigm were the most likely to follow their lead. In 1971, Hospice, Inc. was founded and a rapidly expanding group of nurses, clergy, and community leaders was steadily gaining financial and community support to build their "St. Christopher's in the Field" (Buck, 2007b, 2010).

NAVIGATING THE CONNECTICUT MEDICAL SYSTEM

The unfettered idealism of Hospice, Inc.'s founders and their dedication to social justice cannot be overstated. In Wald's words: "During the course of our original research in 1968-1971, we were as apt to meet at vigils for peace, meetings in the black ghettoes of New Haven on behalf of their civil rights as we were in corridors, clinics and meeting rooms of the medical center" (Wald, 1986). They uniformly believed that humane terminal care was a basic human right. While they were committed to the hospice ideal, each viewed what that care should entail and who should direct it through slightly different personal and disciplinary lenses.

Between March and May 1971, the newly founded Hospice, Inc. steering committee expended a considerable amount of time and energy developing a statement of philosophy and underlying assumptions about hospice care. The group quickly agreed on three assumptions of hospice. First, hospice was a "total community" that included staff, patients, and their families. Care would be directed by the expressed desires of patient and family about how "they wished to be served." Second, the hospice facility would be physically structured to maximize socialization and community participation. Unlike St. Christopher's "open ward," adaptations in the environmental design would be made to accommodate the "American routine and expectations" for privacy and autonomy. Third, professional roles would be blurred to allow team members to "substitute" for each other and "call on each other for help" (Hospice, Inc., 1971, p. 3). Wald and Saunders agreed that nurses were central to hospice, because they were omnipresent and responsible for blending various approaches in the care of patients and their families. As such, Wald reasoned, the hospice would be a nursing facility. Other disciplines, such as the hospice chaplain, social worker, and physician, would then be brought in when necessary to make recommendations about care as consultants to the nurse (St. Christopher's Hospice, 1971). A fourth assumption, concerning the role of religion, resulted in a debate over whether the religious underpinning of hospice care should be implicit or explicit. The question of how to integrate this spiritual component of care was vexing to the American group for two primary reasons: their perceptions of the federal government's grant requirements for the separation of church and state and the demographics of the religiously plural steering committee. The group struggled to find the proper language that would accommodate myriad faiths and personal philosophies (Hospice, Inc., pp. 4–7; St. Christopher's Hospice, 1971).

While the steering committee's collective idealism fueled their efforts, pragmatic issues such as funding and organizational structure were paramount. Unlike Saunders, who chose to remain independent of the British National Health Service, Hospice, Inc. tested the waters for integration early in the planning stages. To do so, they needed to redefine hospice as a patient care model that was "distinctly different from care in nursing homes or hospitals" so they would not be seen as duplicating services or competing with existing programs (Dobihal, 1971, pp. 1–3). Navigating the turbulent waters of the Connecticut medical system in an era of shifting political agendas for health care reform proved to be no small feat.

HOME HEALTH VERSUS HOME HOSPICE

The early hospice movement in Connecticut began in an era of cooperation with local visiting nurses associations (VNAs). Before the advent of Medicare, VNAs were the primary providers of home care in the United States. Jane Keeler, then executive director of the South Central Connecticut VNA, joined Wald in her quest due to her concerns over the many elderly patients who were being discharged from the hospitals "sicker and quicker" during this era of deinstitutionalization. In 1970, 37.6% of all nursing visits were illness focused; by 1980, that percentage rose to 99.2% (Daubert, 1981; E. A. Daubert, personal communication, July 13, 2002). Medicare eligibility criteria defined which patients received particular services under specific conditions. Patients were required to need "skilled nursing" as defined by Medicare to be eligible for up to 100 home care nursing visits planned and "supervised" by the patient's physician. Surprisingly, physicians did not receive reimbursement for supervision. While hospitals were not required to be Medicare certified to receive payment for services rendered, VNAs were. The requisite paperwork and governmental oversight associated with this certification and billing were extensive. In fact, whereas one VNA reported that in 1965, one person handled all of the reimbursement issues, by 1967, 15 administrative staff members were dealing "exclusively with Medicare detail" (Rauch, 1967, p. 1).

Unlike VNAs, who had to contend with the particulars and peculiarities of the formal reimbursement streams, when Hospice Inc.'s home care program began operations in 1974, it was funded through charitable contributions and grants from private foundations. Even though Dr. Sylvia Lack, the British physician who trained under Saunders and was the group's first medical director, was frustrated by having to deal with the American system and its regulatory requirements for licensure, they still had relative freedom to provide services attuned to the needs of individual patients and families. The same held true when they applied for and were the only group selected by the National Cancer Institute for Hospice Demonstration Project funding (Lack & Buckingham, 1978).

Hospice, Inc. had been successful in securing funding to support their early home care program and facility planning. Yet financial concerns were omnipresent, the program's viability once the National Cancer Institute demonstration project ended was in question, and there was considerable debate about how soon to integrate into the existing system of health care financing. Its financial woes were compounded by relative naiveté about nascent changes in federal and state health planning legislation, which presented a whole new set of regulatory hoops to jump through to move forward. It soon became clear, at least to some, that they needed help in navigating the turbulent waters of the Connecticut medical system in an era of shifting political agendas for health care reform. Dennis Rezendes fit the bill and was retained as a consultant to the board in 1973 and as the executive director in 1974. Rezendes had a bachelor's degree in public administration, and this politically astute entrepreneur possessed the skills, knowledge, and contacts to help the hospice board deal with regulatory agencies and obtain licensure (Buck, 2007b).

Between 1974 and 1978, Hospice, Inc. went through a critical transition. Rezendes carved out a niche for hospice in the increasingly competitive home health care marketplace. In 1976, he achieved a political victory for state legislation that liberalized Medicaid eligibility criteria for home care for terminally ill patients. Financial backing for the facility was secured, and in 1978, he patented the term "hospice" and secured legislation that designated hospice as a distinct type of health care provider *and* health care facility under Connecticut state law. That same year Rezendes joined forces with Don Gaetz and Hugh Westbrook, two hospice entrepreneurs from Wisconsin and Florida, to form the National Hospice Organization (NHO) and the National Hospice Education Project (NHEP) (Beresford & Connor, 1999; Buck, 2007b). Their mission was to both create and corner the market for hospice at the national level, and standardization of hospice was a critical element of their potential success.

MEDICARE AND THE POLITICIZATION OF THE HOSPICE IDEAL

By the time Rezendes took the helm of Hospice, Inc. from Wald, new hospices were rapidly opening across the country. Similar to Hospice, Inc., they were voluntary initiatives that developed in accordance with the worldview of their founders and the environments in which they evolved. There were three basic models of hospice organization structures and variations in the type and configuration of services among them (Mor, Greer, & Kastenbaum, 1988). Hospital-based hospice programs typically consisted of administrative staff, a medical and nursing director, staff nurses, a social worker, and a minister. Home hospice programs were usually affiliated with urban/suburban VNAs, and were staffed almost entirely by nurses, with aides and homemakers providing the bulk of personal care to patients. Most had small volunteer programs and the majority of patients had in-home family caregivers. Independent hospices, such as Hospice, Inc., evolved from community-based volunteer efforts to reform care of the dying. Most relied on charitable giving and funding from foundations to hire program coordinators and develop formal relationships with local VNAs and hospitals (Mor et al., 1988, pp. 17–18). For the most part, volunteer nurses provided nursing services. Because many of these volunteers had full-time jobs in other clinical settings, they typically were only able to see two hospice patients per day (Mor et al., 1988, p. 190). By the time the NHO was founded, hospice was looming large on the national political radar screen as a promising terminal care reform. A Government Accounting Office study of hospice requested by key Senate leaders identified 59 organizations that considered themselves to be "providing at least one" hospice-type service and another 73 organizations were in various stages of planning. The study further revealed a wide variability of the configuration, type, and quality of services provided by hospices across the nation. Only one state, Connecticut, had regulations specific to hospice licensure (US General Accounting Office, 1979). Although the National Cancer Institute Demonstration projects that began in 1974 provided baseline data by which to evaluate hospice's potential, serious national program planning required a more comprehensive analysis prior to nationalization. At this juncture, the Robert Wood Johnson Foundation (RWJF) joined forces with the newly formed Health Care Finance Administration (HCFA) and the John A. Hartford Foundation to fund a comprehensive study of the cost and efficacy of hospice care, the National Hospice Study (NHS). At the time the NHS was initiated, it was the largest health services research study undertaken anywhere to evaluate the impact of hospice care on terminally ill patients and their families (Marx, Blendon, & Aiken, 1978).

Two hundred fifty hospice programs responded when the call for proposals for the NHS or HCFA waiver, as it was called, was issued. HCFA selected 26 of the 40 participating sites for the waiver program. The waiver program provided funding for hospice services that were not already covered under Medicare (Chun, 1978). HCFA was particularly interested in how the organizations would respond to the availability of special funding for care provision. In particular, they wanted to know whether the additional funding would stimulate the provision of "unnecessary" services. To obtain cost data, hospices that relied on volunteers had to hire full-time nurses to increase their productivity. As often happens in research projects of this magnitude, there were delays in its implementation. Data collection began in 1980, and the final report was completed in 1984 (Mor, 1988).

The NHO had the support of powerful Congressional leaders, many of whom believed that hospice was a possible answer to the "problem of long-term care" for the elderly. By the end of the 1970s, nursing home scandals were widely publicized, and projections about the continued growth of a chronically ill aging population and escalating costs of long-term care permeated the popular press. In this era of deinstitutionalization, home care was central to debates surrounding the cost and quality of long-term care for the elderly. The Congressional Budget Office (CBO) recommended liberalizing the "skilled care" and "home bound" requirements under Medicare. Nevertheless, legislators continued to emphasize deinstitutionalization, privatization, and the use of market-based and other strategies to constrain and control Medicare and Medicaid expenditures.

NURSING THE MEDICARE HOSPICE BENEFIT

Nurses were dominant players in the development of hospice in America and intricately involved with the development of the Medicare hospice benefit. For example, Mary Taverna, a nurse from California and executive director of Hospice of Marin, another early modern hospice program in the San Francisco Bay area, was a strong supporter of legislation creating the benefit and worked with the NHO leaders to secure its passage. In discussing the early years of hospice with her, she explained that stable reimbursement streams were critical to the organizational viability of her hospice, and the same was true of many other hospice programs (M. Taverna, personal communication, March 29, 2007). Maryanne Fello, RN, MS, the first executive director of Forbes Hospice in Pittsburgh, Pennsylvania, provided Congressional testimony at a public hearing held by Republican Senator John Heinz in early 1982. When she was finished, Senator Heinz (R-PA) asked her whether she understood how the legislation might impact hospice care provision. She responded: "I am willing to take the risk" (M. Fello, personal communication, July 16, 2007). Heinz, a powerful political leader at the time, agreed to champion the legislation in the Senate, despite the conservative Reagan administration, which was eager to rein in the Medicare program.

Madalon O'Rawe Amenta, RN, Dr.P.H, was director of education and research at Forbes Hospice, founded the Pennsylvania Hospice Network, and served on the NHO's research committee from 1979 to 1983 (M. O. Amenta, personal communication, July 17, 2007). She also coauthored *Nursing Care of the Terminally Ill*, one of the first comprehensive texts of its kind (Amenta & Bohnet, 1986). She was particularly concerned about how political concessions required to gain the support of conservative legislators would impact hospice care provision (M. O. Amenta, personal communication, July 17, 2007). She raised critical questions about the potential impact of several of the provisions, particularly the expansion of the scope of hospice care to include individuals who were in the terminal stages of *all* diseases, not just cancer.

Political debates leading to the eventual passage of the Medicare hospice benefit in 1982 were heated and protracted. NHO had the support of powerful Congressional leaders, many of whom believed that hospice was a possible answer to the "problem of long-term care" for the elderly. Home care was central to debates surrounding the cost and quality of long-term care for the elderly, a growing problem. The political question at hand was whether Congress should liberalize the "skilled care" and "home bound" requirements under Medicare as the Congressional Budget Office (CBO) recommended or provide reimbursement for hospice under Medicare. Political discourse that accompanied the "home health versus home hospice" debate was particularly harsh in regard to the proprietary agencies; allegations of fraud and abuse resounded in the halls of Congress (Benjamin, 1993; Buck, 2007a; Buhler-Wilkerson, 2001). Nevertheless, the newly elected President Ronald Reagan introduced a new type of federalism that relied heavily on deinstitutionalization, privatization, and the use of market-based strategies to contain costs. During this era of retrenchment and reform, the prospects for new entitlement programs looked grim.

In the months leading up to a vote on the hospice legislation, the hospice benefit debates continued with compelling arguments for and against it introduced by legislators, the administration, the home health and insurance industries, and the NHO. Congressional testimony reveals that the home health and hospice industries' representatives were aligned in their support for the liberalization of Medicare home care requirements and argued for the elimination of stringent eligibility criteria. There were, however, differences of opinion about how these reforms should be enacted. The debates were framed by four major constituencies: (1) the NHO, which supported the bill; (2) the home health industry, which believed the hospice benefit would result in duplication of services and increased competition that could threaten its financial viability; (3) legislators, who were divided on the issue for a variety of political and economic reasons; and (4) the Reagan administration, which argued against it because of its desire to reform Medicare and the lack of conclusive cost data on hospice. Despite the lack of "hard cold data" and intense lobbying by hospitals, the home health, nursing home, and insurance industries against the bill, Congress enacted the Medicare hospice benefit in July 1982.

Many celebrated the passage of the legislation, but it was not the panacea some had hoped for. The benefit, while promising to expand access to hospice, also offered the opportunity for legislators to mold hospice into the prevailing template for reform in an era of retrenchment and the dawn of managed care. Within this context, tensions between competing social, political, and economic forces created a contradictory benefit that both increased and decreased access to hospice services. As the Medicare hospice rules were promulgated, capitated payment rates were set for comprehensive core services, and although volunteer and bereavement services were mandated, reimbursement to cover the cost of providing these services was not incorporated in the rate. Eligibility criteria required that a patient be in the last 6 months of life, abandon all intensive treatment, and forfeit traditional Medicare benefits. In essence, this provision forced the patient to choose between curative treatment and death, and it left the physician with the difficult task of predicting exactly when that death would occur. Hospice was responsible for providing comprehensive services associated with the "terminal diagnosis" but not coexisting diagnoses, thereby splitting the person into the living and dying components. Whereas Medicare traditionally reimbursed for home care on a fee-for-service basis, the benefit provided the opportunity for legislators to experiment with managed home care, transferring accountability for cost-effectiveness to the patient and the provider. The benefit also included a reimbursement mechanism and financial incentives for proprietary hospices, an entity that did not exist at the time.

As regulatory debates raged in Washington, the hospice movement itself was deeply divided. Many hospice advocates celebrated passage of the Medicare hospice benefit. Still others were concerned about how governmental involvement in hospice would shape care provision or might threaten the organizational viability of smaller hospices unable to contend with the bureaucratic maze associated with it. As hospice leaders advocated for increased per diem reimbursement rates and liberalization of the hospice benefit eligibility criteria, divisions emerged within the hospice movement that reflected philosophical differences among its various factions. New national organizations were formed in an effort to balance the NHO leaders' power within the political arena. This was accompanied by the rapid emergence of the professional specialty organizations in medicine and nursing.

CONSTRUCTING THE HOSPICE NURSES ASSOCIATION

Prior to the creation of the Hospice and Palliative Nurses Association, the NHO—now the National Hospice and Palliative Care Organization

(NHPCO)—had been the most dominant organization in the standardization of hospice care across the burgeoning industry. Many nurses, however, were more concerned about the day-to-day clinical practice of hospice nursing and its potential as a new nursing specialty. In 1986, the same year that the ANA Councils of Community Health Nurses and Medical Surgical Nurses offered to partially fund a task force to help "define the dimensions of practice and develop standards for hospice nursing care," the Michigan Hospice Nurses Association was incorporated (Amenta, 2001, p. 128). That same year, the Hospice Nurses Association, A National Organization (HNA) was formed. The addition of "A National Organization" reflected the optimism of the organization's founders. The HNA leaders were committed to developing standards for quality assurance, professional advocacy, and in negotiating interprofessional and disciplinary dynamics. As important, at least to some of the early founders, the organization provided an opportunity to network, give and receive peer support, and to gain and exercise a political voice ("Minutes of the organizational meeting of the Hospice Nurses Association," 1986).

Much of the HNA's early organizational structure was developed by California hospice nurses, who had expertise in clinical practice, administration, and in managing educational conferences. Educational conferences offered the opportunity to collect nurses together for a legitimate purpose to further define the scope of hospice nursing and to set standards for its provision. The first HNA meeting was held on September 19, 1986, at the home of Dorothy Caruso-Herman, RN, and attended by 19 founding members. The minutes reflect that the organization had 60 members, each paying $25.00 in dues to the organization. In addition, the group had seed money from the Hospice Organization of Southern California that they could use for holding the Third Annual Western Hospice Nurses Conference ("Minutes of the organizational meeting of the Hospice Nurses Association," 1986).

The group was resourceful and highly motivated. The vast majority of the founding members used their personal funds to attend meetings, which were typically held at Caruso-Herman's home. They quickly developed bylaws and assigned responsibility for specified organizational tasks. Of greatest interest to the group was the development of a newsletter. To help offset the cost for its distribution, members were asked to bring 10 self-addressed stamped envelopes to their next meeting. The strong commitment to personal investment in the organization continued throughout the early years of its development.

In January 1987, the board of directors ballot reflected the scope and expertise of the candidates. For example, Janice Brown, BSN, MS,

M.Div., was the director of ministry development for the St. Joseph Health System in Michigan; she had a background in research and writing on assertiveness in nurses. Dorothy Caruso-Herman was an independent consultant on hospice, death and dying, and sexuality and facilitated bereavement support groups. Each of the 19 individuals on the ballot had entrepreneurial spirits and had served in leadership positions within their organizations and states ("Minutes of the Hospice Nurses Association," 1987).

By June 1988, HNA had 168 members from 26 states and the District of Columbia. The organizational structure consisted of the usual officers and chairpersons of the standing committees, which included membership, bylaws, newsletter, standards, historian, education/research, ways and means, and three members at large. The organization was designated as an approved provider for nursing continuing education credits in the state of California and the standards tool "Quality Assurance for Hospice Patient Care" had been developed. Riding on the coattails of the larger hospice movement, the group quickly gained national recognition. In the spring of 1989, a representative from the National Institute of Nursing Research invited a member of the group to participate in a conference about nursing's role in the HIV epidemic. In 1990, First Lady Barbara Bush held a luncheon in honor of National Nursing Day, and a representative of the organization attended. That same year the summer issue of *FANFARE*, the HNA newsletter, reported board discussions about certification, and a survey was distributed to the membership. They received 1,550 responses from all 50 states, 91% of which favored developing a certification in hospice nursing (Amenta, 2001, pp. 130–132). Yet there were comments that indicated that all hospice nursing required was "compassion, common sense, and good nursing skills," reflecting the beliefs of some that hospice was just good nursing. The vast majority of the nurses preferred that the certification exam be administered by the HNA (Amenta, 2001, p. 132).

Once initiated, the certification process not only served to improve the knowledge base of certified hospice nurses and provide an air of credibility to the new specialty; it also served to further the visibility of the organization. By 1994, the year that the first certification exam was given and the HNA and Academy of Hospice Physicians cosponsored their first joint Clinical Hospice Care/Palliative Medicine conference in San Francisco, more than 500 candidates sat for the certification exam and 482 passed. Impressed by the manner in which the HNA had developed the certification process, the Academy of Hospice Physicians asked for advice about setting up their certification process and exam. Thus, the HNA not only influenced the practice of hospice nursing but also provided a framework and guidance for physician colleagues to follow suit. The growth of specialty groups in nursing and medicine reflects the enormous growth in American hospices, stimulated, in large part, by the availability of formalized reimbursement streams linked to passage of the Medicare hospice benefit.

HOSPICE AND ITS TRANSFORMATION

Between 1986 and 1996, hospice was steadily integrated into the American medical system. In 1985, the Consolidated Omnibus Budget Reconciliation Act (COBRA) allowed for reimbursement for hospice under Medicaid programs, and the benefit became available to the military in 1991 (TRICARE, 2008). The provisions contained in the Medicare hospice benefit served as a template for reimbursement for hospice under these programs. By the mid-1990s, most commercial health insurance policies typically covered comprehensive hospice services, including nursing, social work, therapies, personal care, medications, and medical supplies and equipment, and there was considerable variability among the programs.

There is little question that hospices are vitally important to the provision of quality palliative care in the United States. Nevertheless, in 2008, a report on the benefit noted the significant changes that occurred in hospice since 1982, the majority of which took place in the previous 7 years (MedPAC, 2008). The major changes noted were the increased numbers of proprietary hospices that coincided with rapid increases in Medicare expenditures for hospice. The report cited pervasive policy-induced incentives for some hospices to provide care in a manner that maximized reimbursement versus being solely driven by the patient's clinical needs. There are also other important ways that integration has affected hospice programs. In 1983, the average length of stay (LOS) was 70 days (US General Accounting Office, 1979), the optimal LOS from the perspective of the hospice's effectiveness both in terms of care and costs. In 2000, almost two thirds of patients received hospice care for less than 30 days, and one third of these patients were in hospice programs for less than a week before dying (Haupt, 2003). The decline in LOS has been attributed to a variety of factors, including provider practices, patient preferences, public awareness, federal oversight and regulation, and hospice program closure. Between 2000 and 2005, however, the average length of stay increased by 40%, from 48 days to 67 days (CMS, 2007). Additionally, health services research reveals variability in the quality and cost-effectiveness of hospice programs, differences in the types of service provided based on location and ownership type, and disparities in access to services among marginalized populations (McCarthy, Burns, Davis, & Phillips, 2003; Moon & Boucotti, 2002).

Perhaps one of the most enigmatic impacts of the Medicare hospice benefit is that it resulted in the division of personhood into living and dying components. The hospice philosophy of care was predicated on the concepts of holism and integration of mind, body, and spirit. The Medicare hospice benefit required hospices to provide comprehensive care for persons with a terminal diagnosis with 6 or fewer months to live. It did not require hospices to provide care related to coexisting "nonterminal diagnoses," which are covered by traditional Medicare benefits. Ostensibly, this policy was intended to reduce the cost and care burdens of hospice organizations and allowed Medicare recipients more treatment options. Yet it also renders people into their living and dying components, thus requiring them to navigate two different systems of care. In medically complex patients, delineating which disease and/or treatment is causing which symptom is problematic at best, if not impossible. This reductionist division of the body into its nonterminal and terminal parts is confusing to patients and their caregivers and can result in both physical and psychological harm.

ACKNOWLEDGMENTS

The following funders generously supported research and preparation for this chapter: Center for Nursing Historical Inquiry at the University of Virginia; Barbara Bates Center for the Study of the History of Nursing, University of Pennsylvania; National Institute for Nursing Research (F31 NR08301-01) and Advanced Training in Nursing Outcomes Research (T32-NR-007104), Center for Health Outcomes & Policy Research, University of Pennsylvania; American Nurses Foundation; Anne Zimmerman Fellowship (2006); and National Institutes for Nursing Research (1R15NR012298-01), 2010–2013.

NOTE

1. The interview was conducted as part of an ongoing research project. The name of the participant and location of the interview are kept anonymous at the participant's request.

REFERENCES

Amenta, M. O. (2001). History of the Hospice Nurses Association 1986–1996. *Journal of Hospice and Palliative Nursing, 3*(4), 128–136.

Amenta, M. O., & Bohnet, N. L. (1986). *Nursing care of the terminally ill.* New York, NY: Little, Brown.

Backer, B., Hannon, N., & Russell, N. (1982). *Death and dying: Individuals and institutions.* New York, NY: Wiley.

Benjamin, A. E. (1993). An historical perspective on home care policy. *The Millbank Quarterly, 71*(1), 129–166.

Beresford, L., & Connor, S. (1999). History of the National Hospice Organization. In I. Corless & Z. Foster (Eds.), *The hospice heritage: Celebrating our future* (pp. 15–31). Binghamton, NY: Haworth.

Buck, J. (2007a). Netting the hospice butterfly: Politics, policy, and translation of an ideal. *Home Healthcare Nurse, 25*(9), 566–571.

Buck, J. (2007b). Reweaving a tapestry of care: Religion, nursing, and the meaning of hospice, 1945–1978. *Nursing History Review, 15,* 113–145.

Buck, J. (2010). Nursing the borderlands of life: Hospice and the politics of health-care reform. In S. Lewenson & P. D'Antonio (Eds.), *Nursing interventions through time: History as evidence* (pp. 203–220). New York, NY: Springer.

Buhler-Wilkerson, K. (2001). *No place like home: A history of nursing and home care in the United States.* Baltimore, MD: Johns Hopkins University Press.

Centers for Medicare and Medicaid Services (CMS). (2007). *Medicare hospice data, 1998–2005.* Baltimore, MD: Centers for Medicare & Medicaid Services.

Chun, A. (1978). *A special supplement of C/HH News on Hospice.* [Visiting Nurse Association of South Central Connecticut Archives Series I, Box 3, Folder 38]. Barbara Bates Center for the Study of the History of Nursing, School of Nursing, University of Pennsylvania, Philadelphia.

Coser, R. L. (1962). *Life in the ward.* East Lansing: Michigan State University Press.

Daubert, E. A. (1981, August). *A position paper on strategic planning.* [Visiting Nurse Association of South Central Connecticut Archives, Box 7, Folder 103]. Barbara Bates Center for the Study of the History of Nursing, University of Pennsylvania, Philadelphia.

Dobihal, E. (1971). *Letter to Mr. C. Pierce Taylor, Executive Director, Connecticut Hospital Planning Commission.* [Edward Dobihal Papers, Manuscripts and Archives Box 1, Folder 3], Sterling Memorial Library, Yale University, New Haven, CT.

Duff, R. S., & Hollingshead, A. d. B. (1968). *Sickness and society.* New York, NY: Harper & Row.

Feldstein, P. (1996). *The politics of health legislation: An economic perspective.* Chicago, IL: Health Administration Press.

Glaser, B., & Strauss, A. (1965). *Awareness of dying.* Chicago, IL: Aldine.

Haagensen, C. D. (1947). Recent advances in cancer therapy. *Bulletin of the New York Academy of Medicine, 23*(3), 123–135.

Haupt, B. J. (2003). *Characteristics of hospice care discharges and their length of service: United States, 2000.* [DHS Pub. No. 2003–1725]. Retrieved April 2014, from http://www.cdc.gov/nchs/pressroom/03facts/hospicecare.htm.

Hospice, Inc. (1971, March 3). *Steering Committee Minutes.* [Florence and Henry Wald Papers, Series I, Box 1, Folder 9]. Sterling Memorial Library, Yale University, New Haven, CT.

Humphreys, C. (2001). Waiting for the last summons: The establishment of the first hospices in England 1878–1914. *Mortality, 6*(2), 146–166.

Josephs, D. (1971, September 25). The right to die with dignity. *The New York Times,* p. 31.

Kemp, N. D. A. (2002). *Merciful release: The history of the British euthanasia movement.* Manchester, UK: Manchester University Press.

Klagsbrun, S. (1969, June 20). Death in a cancer ward. *Time,* p. 56.

Lack, S., & Buckingham, R. (1978). *First American hospice: Three years of home care.* Branford, MO: Hospice.

Lerner, M. (1970). Where, why, and when people die. In O. G. Brim, H. E. Freeman, S. Levine, & N. A. Scotch (Eds.), *The dying patient* (pp. 5–29). New York, NY: Russell Sage Foundation.

Lynaugh, J., & Reverby, S. (1987). Thoughts on the nature of history. *Nursing Research, 36,* 67, 69.

Marx, M., Blendon, R., & Aiken, L. (1978). *Study of the cost and efficacy of hospice care.* [Linda H. Aikens Papers, Box 1, Folder 39]. Center for the Study of the History of Nursing, University of Pennsylvania, Philadelphia.

McCarthy, E. P., Burns, R. B., Davis, R. B., & Phillips, R. S. (2003). Barriers to hospice care among older patients dying with lung and colorectal cancer. *Journal of Clinical Oncology, 21*(4), 728–735.

Medicare Payment Advisory Commission (MedPAC). (2008). Evaluating Medicare's hospice benefit. In *Report to Congress: Reforming the delivery system* (pp. 203–240). Retrieved April 2014, from http://medpac.gov/documents/Jun08_EntireReport.pdf.

Minutes of the Hospice Nurses Association. (1987, January 12–April 26). [Madalon O'Rawe Amenta papers (unprocessed)]. Barbara Bates Center for the Study of the History of Nursing, University of Pennsylvania School of Nursing, Philadelphia.

Minutes of the organizational meeting of the Hospice Nurses Association. (1986, September 19). [Madalon O'Rawe Amenta papers (unprocessed)]. Barbara Bates Center for the Study of the History of Nursing, University of Pennsylvania School of Nursing, Philadelphia.

Moon, M., & Boucotti, C. (2002). *Medicare and end-of-life care.* Washington, DC: The Urban Institute. Retrieved April 2014, from http://www.urban.org/UploadedPDF/1000442_Medicare.pdf.

Mor, V. (1988). The research design of the National Hospice Study. In V. Mor, D. Greer, & R. Kastenbaum (Eds.) *The hospice experiment* (pp. 28–47). Baltimore, MD: Johns Hopkins University Press.

Mor, V., Greer, D., & Kastenbaum, R. (Eds.). (1988). *The hospice experiment.* Baltimore, MD: Johns Hopkins University Press.

National Hospice & Palliative Care Organization (NHPCO). (2009). *NHPCO facts and figures: Hospice care in America.* Alexandria, VA: National Hospice & Palliative Care Association.

Rauch, F. S. (1967, November 2). *Annual report of the president.* [Archives of the Visiting Nurses Society of Philadelphia, Series I, Box 5, Folder 86]. Barbara Bates Center for the Study of the History of Nursing, University of Pennsylvania, Philadelphia.

Raven, R. (1949). Radical surgery in advanced squamous carcinoma. *Lancet, 253*(6546), 261–263.

St. Christopher's Hospice. (1971, September 22). *Discussion group on religious foundation 6.* [Edward Dobihal Papers, Manuscripts and Archives, Box 1, Folder 3], Sterling Memorial Library, Yale University, New Haven, CT.

Saunders, C. (1959, October 9). Care of the dying 1—The problem of euthanasia. *Nursing Times*, pp. 960–961.

Saunders, C. (1966, April 28). *The moment of truth—some aspects of care of the dying patient.* [Cicely Saunders Papers, Box 57]. Hospice History Project, Trent Palliative Care Centre, Sheffield, UK.

Saunders, C. (1971). The patient's response to treatment: A photographic presentation. In *Catastrophic illness in the seventies: Critical issues and complex decisions* (pp. 33–46). New York, NY: Cancer Care.

Social Security Administration. (2003). *History of SSA during the Johnson Administration 1963–1968.* Retrieved April 2014, from http://www.ssa.gov/history/ssa/lbj-leg1.html.

Technical Committee on Medical Care, Interdepartmental Committee to Coordinate Health and Welfare Activities. (1938). *The Need for a National Health Program.* Retrieved April 2014, from http://www.ssa.gov/history/reports/Interdepartmental.html.

Transcript of President's State of the Union message to nation. (1982, January 27). *The New York Times.* Retrieved from http://www.nytimes.com/1982/01/27/us/transcript-of-president-s-state-of-the-union-message-to-nation.html?scp=9&pagewanted=all.

TRICARE. (2008). Hospice reimbursement—general overview. In *Tricare Reimbursement Manual 6010.58-M.* Retrieved April 2014, from http://manuals.tricare.osd.mil/DisplayManual.aspx?SeriesId=T3TRM.

United States General Accounting Office. (1979). *Report to the Congress of the United States: Hospice care—a growing concept in the United States (HRD 79-50).* Washington, DC: Author.

Wald, F. (1986). In search of the spiritual component of hospice care. In F. Wald (Ed.), *In quest of the spiritual component of care for the terminally ill: Proceedings of a colloquium* (pp. 24–37). New Haven, CT: Yale University Press.

Walsh, J. (1929). *The history of nursing.* New York: P.J. Kennedy.

Webb, M. (1997). *The good death: The new American search to reshape the end of life.* New York, NY: Bantam Books.

Weikart, R. (2004, January/February). Killing them kindly: Lessons from the euthanasia movement. *Books and Culture: A Christian Review.* Retrieved from http://www.booksandculture.com/articles/2004/janfeb/22.30.html.

CHAPTER 2

Hospice Care As a Moral Practice

Exploring the Philosophy and Ethics of Hospice Care

TIMOTHY W. KIRK

Karen Brown is a liaison social worker with Good Care Hospice and Home Care in New York City. She loves her job, is proud to represent her hospice, and likes being onsite at New York Prestigious Hospital, a major academic medical center in Manhattan. Increasingly, however, several members of the oncology service—an important and reliable source of referrals for her—have pulled her aside before she visits with families and made a troubling request: "Please do not use the word 'hospice' when talking with the patient and family." These requests usually come with the added information that some member of the family—sometimes the patient—has not acknowledged that the patient is terminally ill. The referring physician believes the patient would benefit from hospice care but fears that talking about it explicitly would prevent the family from electing to receive such care.

Karen is not comfortable with these requests. She believes strongly that honesty is a core ethical value of hospice care, and that requests to not use the word "hospice" violate that value. Some of her colleagues say she is overreacting; they believe that it is quite possible to accurately describe all of the care and services that comprise hospice care without using the word "hospice," thereby being completely honest and keeping important referral sources happy by honoring their requests. Karen and her colleagues agree that honesty is important in hospice care. They disagree, however, about whether Karen can be honest without using the word "hospice." In other words, in this situation they disagree about what it means to be "honest."

How can Karen and her colleagues gain clarity about whether honoring such a request constitutes being dishonest? Moreover, how do they know that honesty is a core ethical value of hospice care? Indeed, what does it mean to say that honesty is a core ethical value in hospice care? Where do such values come from, and how do we know what they are? One answer resides in the close connection between hospice ethics and hospice philosophy, a connection explored in this chapter.

INTRODUCTION

This chapter explains the interrelationship between a clearly formulated philosophy of hospice care and the possibility of ethical reflection and analysis in hospice care, suggesting that the latter is more clear, robust, and helpful when it draws upon the former. In so doing, it proposes that the reader consider hospice care to be a special kind of *practice*. I argue that hospice care is a moral practice with well-defined goals and values internal to itself. Hospice caregiving is also situated in a larger society, and therefore its internal values interact with a broad set of social values; the practice of hospice care interacts with many other social practices, some that support hospice and some that are in tension with it. This situation of internal ethical coherence within a context of social and cultural plurality provides an important orientation and framework for ethical decision making in, and about, hospice care.

The remainder of this chapter is arranged in five sections. First, I offer a discussion of a particular way to think about ethics. Second, I explain how such an approach to ethics relies on its connection to philosophy via the concept of a *moral practice*. Third, I offer an explanation of four core concepts that, I argue, constitute the "heart" of the hospice philosophy of care. Fourth, I argue that the way these four core concepts are operationalized into hospice care constitutes a profound paradigm shift from a focus on underlying causes of medical conditions to the lived experience of patients and families. Finally, I conclude with an invitation to consider hospice care as a practice in which the interplay of its internal ethical values and the hospice philosophy of care creates a living lens through which to understand the distinctiveness and importance of hospice ethics. This perspective also provides a lens through which to read the diverse analyses and arguments contained in the other chapters of this book.

As an activity, what ethics does is deceptively simple: It helps us think about right and wrong. I say "deceptively" simple because *how* ethics does this is both complex and the subject of heated debate. One way to think about ethics as an enterprise is to consider it a process that serves three important functions:

1. *Values identification.* Ethics helps us identify and justify which values are most important to us and why. Values are simply experiential objects— character traits, states of affairs, qualities of interactions, and so on— that it is reasonable to believe are desirable or preferable over others.
2. *Values implementation.* Ethics helps us use the values identified in (1) as guides to set goals, establish norms, develop rules and practices, and think about the kinds of persons we want to be in our personal and professional lives.
3. *Ethical evaluation.* Finally, ethics helps us evaluate goals, rules, processes, persons, and phenomena like intentions, actions, decisions, and outcomes—and the structures and practices that influence these phenomena. The criteria used in ethical evaluation are the values themselves; we want to know the extent to which a particular decision, practice, or goal promotes and is consistent with our most important values. Loosely speaking, one that does is often called "right." One that is inconsistent with, or violates, our most important values is often called "wrong."

Returning to the earlier example of Karen, the value that Karen is most explicitly concerned with is honesty. She values honesty in her practice, and she strives to make choices in her interactions with colleagues and patients that favor honesty over dishonesty. Karen's choice of honesty as a moral value means that she will exhibit a preference for interactions that are honest over interactions that are dishonest. Given her referral source's request to not use the word "hospice," Karen is prospectively exploring how she will respond to that request by identifying and evaluating the options before her, attempting to determine which response best reflects both her definition of honesty as a moral value and the role she wants that value to play in her professional life. By engaging in this kind of ethical reflection and decision making, Karen is acting as an *agent*: one who has the power to identify and implement values in her practice and evaluate her actions according to those values.

Not all values, however, are ethical values. Investors in economic markets, for example, strive to realize the values of productivity and efficiency in the companies that participate in those markets. Companies who are relatively less productive and efficient than their competitors will lose favor with investors because they fail to fulfill these important economic values. While this might put them at an economic disadvantage, it would be a stretch to say that inefficiency is an ethical value or that a company's inefficiency is, in itself, *ethically wrong*. Indeed, one of the defining elements of an *ethical* value that distinguishes it from, say, a market value, is that an ethical value is not merely about instrumental or practical success. Rather, an ethical value enables me to make judgments about, and discern the meaning of, *right and wrong*.

"Right" and "wrong" are terms used to communicate a particular kind of value: normative value. Normative value carries with it a certain force—in academic ethics parlance, "normative force"—that suggests that things *should* be a certain way. If honesty is an ethical value, it means that evaluating a certain action and concluding that it is *dis*honest carries with it at least two meanings. First, it means the action is not consistent with the definition, qualities, and stated goals of honesty as a concept. This can be thought of as the "descriptive" meaning of the evaluation. Second, it means that because the action was not consistent with honesty it was *wrong*—that is, it should have been otherwise (namely, it should have been consistent with honesty). This is the normative meaning of the evaluation. If honesty is functioning as an ethical value, actions inconsistent with honesty are *both* dishonest *and* wrong.

The normative force that accompanies ethical values creates a phenomenon of *obligation* related to those values. This means that a state of affairs inconsistent with the ethical values of a person or profession is not a neutral state of affairs, but rather one which obligates some agent (or group of agents) to change the state of affairs such that it is brought into alignment with those values. Presuming it is possible to identify one or more agents who have causal influence over the current state of affairs, and have the power to effect change, those agents are then (at least, partially) ethically *culpable* for whether the state of affairs is consistent with, or violates, the ethical values in question. That is, they can be blamed or praised for the extent to which what is currently being experienced is consistent with, or violates, relevant ethical values.

Yeo (2010) offers a helpful supplement to this way of looking at the distinction between ethical values and other kinds of values. He writes that ethical values are those values that, in addition to being reasonably linked to judgments about right and wrong, are so important that they can be considered central to the identity of an agent or an activity. As such, actions, intentions, or other kinds of experiences that are either inconsistent with, or in opposition to, ethical values create harm (or the potential for harm) not only to the particular object valued but to the people or processes involved.

Let's return to the example of Karen Brown, the hospice liaison who values honesty. If being involved in exchanges that are dishonest is experienced by Karen and others as merely an inconvenience, but everyone still feels that who they are as persons and the ability to give and receive her services as a hospice liaison are able to thrive and flourish, then honesty may not be an *ethical* value central to Karen's practice as a liaison hospice social worker.

If, however, she considers honesty to be fundamental to who she is as a person, such that repeated involvement in dishonest exchanges would *change* who she is in a way she believes to be harmful, or if honesty is a necessary condition to give and receive liaison services such that frequent dishonest exchanges would change what it means to give and receive such services in a way that harms her practice and the larger hospice care efforts of which it is a part, honesty could be considered an ethical value.

To summarize, ethics provides a systematic framework in which to (a) identify and justify important ethical values; (b) integrate those values into goals, processes, and practices; and (c) evaluate intentions, actions, processes, and people by using a set of values that carry normative force and are central to the identity of persons and their practices. The results of such evaluations tell us whether certain states of affairs— and/or the actions, agents, or conditions that produced them—are consistent with the ethical values. The results also tell us whether such states of affairs are "right" or "wrong." Agents who have causal influence over, and the ability to change, such states of affairs can be ethically culpable for actions or inactions that affect if and how valued states of affairs are present or absent. Such culpability arises from their obligation to acknowledge and use their power in a manner that honors and promotes the relevant ethical values.

Thus far, this section of the chapter has explained what might be called the "functional domains" in which ethics operates; it has painted a picture of ethics that tries to capture the role that ethics can play in the lives of individuals, organizations, and communities. What it has not explained, however, is how someone like Karen Browning can know that honesty is a core ethical value of hospice care, or how Karen and her colleagues can gain clarity on whether using the word "hospice" with patients and families is necessary to practice honestly. For such understanding, the next sections of the chapter address how and why hospice ethics is closely intertwined with the hospice philosophy of care.

ON THE RELATIONSHIP BETWEEN ETHICS AND PHILOSOPHY: HOSPICE AS A MORAL PRACTICE

For Karen Browning to know that honesty is a core ethical value of hospice care (and for that knowledge to be accurate), Karen must know that honesty is central to what it means to give and receive hospice care. If it is, then Karen must understand that, absent honesty, care given by professionals—even hospice professionals—is not the best hospice care possible. For Karen to have such knowledge and understanding, she must be drawing on some belief about what hospice care *is*. That is, she must have a belief—whether explicit or implicit—concerning which defining goals, actions, intentions, and ideas together constitute the defining elements of hospice care. For anyone—including Karen herself—to assess whether Karen is correct that honesty is a core ethical value of hospice care, Karen's belief about the nature of hospice care needs to be made explicit. Karen can sufficiently justify her claim that honesty is integral to hospice care only if she can explain *how* and *why* honesty is so central to what it means to give and receive hospice care.

One way for Karen to explain the philosophy of hospice in a way that illuminates whether, and why, honesty is a necessary part of hospice is to think of hospice care as a *moral practice*. It is important now to explore the ways in which hospice care can be considered a moral practice, and how doing so can inform the relationship between philosophy and ethics in hospice care.

In moral philosophy, "practice" is a technical term. Macintyre defines it as follows:

> By a 'practice' I am going to mean any coherent and complex form of socially established cooperative human activity through which human goods internal to that form of activity are realized in the course of trying to achieve those standards of excellence which are appropriate to, and partially definitive of, that form of activity, with the result that human powers to achieve excellence, and human conceptions of the ends and goods involved, are systematically extended. (MacIntyre, 1981, p. 30)

In simpler language, a "moral practice" is an activity in which people work together using specific skills and methods toward a shared goal. Further, the goal itself is considered good—both for those who achieve it and for society at large. And the habits and character traits one develops in working to achieve the goal are also considered good—both for the practice and for society at large.

For example, we often speak of nursing as a "practice." And, while we may not have Macintyre's formal sense of "practice" in mind when we do so, nursing does fit the formal definition of "practice" quoted earlier. It is a cooperative endeavor that requires the development of specialized skills *and* the development of certain character traits to engage patients therapeutically and deliver quality care. It has a set of "internal goods"—abilities, values, and goals—required to achieve and measure "good" nursing care. And that set of internal goods is consistent with, and contributes to, a set of "external goods" in society at large. That is, the habits and traits one develops in becoming a good nurse are consistent with being a good person in general, and the goals of nursing—restoration of health, engaging patients in self-care, teaching preventative practices that promote wellness, and so on—promote the larger goals of a thriving society (Sellman, 2000, 2011). For one to know which actions, values, or character traits are parts of what constitutes "good" nursing, one must have a solid understanding of the defining elements of nursing as a practice.

Hospice care, like nursing, can also be seen as a "practice" in the formal sense of the term.[1] Hospice has internal goods that are consistent with—and contribute to—larger social goods. It requires the development of specialized skills and the nurturance of certain character traits to effectively partner with patients and families to create the conditions in which good end-of-life care can be given and received. And, when successful, hospice helps those patients and families achieve a goal—a good death—that promotes both the integrity of individuals and the flourishing of society. For one to know which actions, values, or character traits are parts of what constitutes "good" hospice care, one must have a solid understanding of the defining elements of hospice care as a practice. Understanding the basic philosophical structure underlying hospice care is a good way to uncover those elements.

The defining nature of practices and professions—the defining elements, for example, of nursing without which nursing would no longer be nursing—is something that philosophy is especially well equipped to address. Indeed, in the case of nursing, there is an entire subdiscipline of philosophy (the philosophy of nursing) dedicated to exploring such questions. While there is no similar subdiscipline of philosophy devoted to exploring the philosophy of hospice, the hospice movement—perhaps because of its very origins as a "movement"—has been from its start explicitly philosophical.

The modern hospice movement has from its beginning asserted an important relationship between what it does and the enterprise of philosophy. In an essay titled "The Philosophy of Terminal Care," Cicely Saunders, widely considered to be the founder of the modern hospice movement, discusses the way in which philosophical questions and commitments lie at the heart of the meaning and structure of hospice care. She writes:

> The Shorter Oxford Dictionary includes as definitions of philosophy—[1] that department of knowledge or of study which deals with ultimate reality, and also, [2] the study of the general principles of some particular knowledge, experience, or activity. Both definitions have been used to cover the substance of this book in the belief that, as in any field of care, we will only respond fully to the second if we give heed to the first. Here we are concerned with the nature of man, with living and dying, and with the whole man—body, mind, and spirit—part of some family unit, with physical, practical needs for us to tackle with maximum competence. (1978, p. 193)

For Saunders, hospice philosophy was both practical and theoretical philosophy. That is, it reflected both a certain philosophy of care—the "general principles of some particular knowledge, experience, or activity"—but also a more fundamental philosophy of the nature and meaning of human existence, such as claims about the nature of "ultimate reality." Consistent with the formal idea of a "practice" explained earlier, Saunders believed that the concrete pieces of good hospice care—pieces that constituted the hospice philosophy—were embedded in a larger vision of the good life in general. The core concepts of that philosophy are explained in the next section of the chapter.

THE HOSPICE PHILOSOPHY OF CARE: FOUR CENTRAL CONCEPTS

As noted in Chapter 1, the shape and content of hospice care in the United States is the product of many (and sometimes conflicting) social, economic, political, and regulatory forces. Understanding those forces and their influence on the current state of hospice care is important. There are also, however, some hallmark philosophical commitments that powerfully shaped the evolution of US hospice care in the 1970s and 1980s. Many of these commitments continue to inform the practice of hospice care in 2014, both explicitly and implicitly. This section of the chapter will explain four of those commitments—three arising out of Saunders's original philosophy and a fourth that, while important for Saunders's work, has become modified and paramount in the distinctly American version of hospice care delivered in the United States—and discuss how the structure and practice of hospice care attempts to operationalize them into the experience of dying for patients and families.

Saunders herself recognized the ways in which her philosophy of terminal care bore the unmistakable imprint of her training as a nurse, social worker, and physician and her many years of studying and caring for dying persons. In describing the origin of her philosophy, she writes:

> The following list of the essential components of terminal care is the fruit of years of working in different units and of endless discussions with others working and interested in this field (Kastenbaum, 1976; Wald, 1976). Above all, it is the outcome of the good fortune which gave me the opportunity of listening to patients and their families during the 30 years since that first patient told me that he wanted 'What is in your mind and in your heart.'" (Saunders, 1978, p. 195)

In what is perhaps her clearest and most direct writing on "the hospice concept," Saunders (1979, pp. 641–651) outlined 13 "General Principles of Hospice Care":

1. Management by an experienced clinical team
2. Understanding control of the common symptoms of terminal disease, especially pain in all its aspects
3. Skilled and experienced team nursing
4. A full interdisciplinary staff
5. A home care program
6. Recognition of the patient and family as the unit of care
7. A mixed group of patients
8. Bereavement follow-up
9. Methodical recording and analysis
10. Teaching in all aspects of terminal care
11. Imaginative use of the architecture available
12. An efficient administration
13. The cost of commitment and the search for meaning

These 13 elements, I argue, can be derived from four core philosophical concepts that lie at the heart of Saunders's hospice philosophy: (1) dying as an experience pregnant with meaning; (2) family-centered care; (3) the nature and relief of suffering; and (4) the integrity of persons as a condition of creating and experiencing meaning in life and exercising moral agency.

Dying As an Experience

Hospice care is focused on the *experience of dying*. There are several important nuances surrounding the way in which the "experience of dying" is conceptualized. The first is that dying is not an event but a process. That is, dying is not something that occurs at the moment one satisfies the criteria for cardiopulmonary or brain death. Rather, dying is the process one goes through in the months and weeks preceding that moment.

Second, this conceptualization of dying implies that dying is not simply a biological event experienced by physiological organisms. Rather, the invocation of dying as an "experience" reflects a commitment to the idea that when persons die the process involves all of the different elements of their personhood—their emotional lives, their spiritual lives, their relational lives, their professional lives, and many others—and not just their bodies. So, while the death of the body occasions the end of these different pieces of personhood in their current forms (they are, after all, embodied), to consider death as *merely* a bodily process fails to capture the full meaning of the process for all involved.

Third, it reflects the idea that the experience of dying itself can be meaningful—both for the one dying and for that person's loved ones. The focus in hospice care on dying in one's home—rather than the hospital, for example—is rooted in this commitment to the experience of dying as a valuable one: being surrounded by the conditions in which one has built and discovered meaning throughout life is thought to maximally enable persons to create and find meaning in the last weeks to months of life as well. The conceptualization understands dying as a process that is experienced by persons (not just bodies) that is still pregnant with meaningful possibilities. This conceptualization also informs the second philosophical commitment of hospice care: family-centered care.

Family-Centered Care

Because hospice care has conceptualized the dying process as explained earlier, a core goal of care is to support the patient in a manner that allows the experience of dying to be as meaningful as possible. And, because our identities as persons have emerged and evolved in the context of intimate relationships with families and loved ones, those intimate relationships can be structures through which we have learned to create and discover meaning throughout our lives. It then makes sense conceptually that hospice care would seek to incorporate relationships with families and loved ones in the care of dying persons. Indeed, rather than disrupt the relational structures through which we have given and received care across our lives—a disruption that the founders of hospice thought was a significant drawback of hospital-based care—hospice seeks to support patients through those very structures. Family-centered care, in the hospice model, involves conceiving of the family as the direct recipient of support and services, with the goal of allowing the family to then care for the dying person through its already-established structures of familial intimacy and support. The logic is rather straightforward. Just as allowing patients to remain in their homes is thought to give persons the benefit of leaning on their familiar surroundings while engaging the dying process (rather than having to learn the new patterns, structures, and spaces of the hospital environment *in addition* to engaging the dying process), so, too, allowing care to be delivered through the already-existing family structure is thought to give persons the benefit of receiving care and support through the patterns of interaction and intimate obligation that have (hopefully) already been established through trial and error and agreement across the life span of the family.

Acknowledgment of the important influence of relationships in the formation and expression of identity also recognizes that the impact of intimate relationships is often reciprocal; that is, just as the suffering of dying persons can be significantly impacted by the involvement of their family members as caregivers, so, too, the dying of persons can significantly impact the lives of those who love them. Caring for dying persons in a manner that supports as many elements of their personhood as possible requires supporting and including their loved ones, because relationships with those loved ones constitute a profound and ongoing influence in the identity of dying persons. Therefore, caring for the family is not

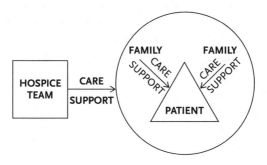

Figure 2.1
The hospice model of family-centered care.

disconnected from caring for the patient. Indeed, as illustrated in Figure 2.1, it is part of the same process.

The Nature and Relief of Suffering

The third commitment, though perhaps for many hospice clinicians the first in order of priority, is that hospice care has one primary goal which informs all of the others: the relief of suffering. Similar to the way in which the "experience of dying" is an expansive and holistic concept, the phenomenon of suffering is equally expansive and holistic. In hospice care, suffering can occur in relation to any aspect of the personhood of the patient who is dying (and, following from the earlier explanation of family-centered care, can also occur via the experience of the patient's loved ones). Saunders developed this idea in her concept of "total pain."

For Saunders, total pain was not simply a bodily phenomenon. Rather, it had the potential to insinuate itself into multiple aspects of personhood, becoming a noxious inhibitor of one's ability to engage the world in many ways—emotionally, spiritually, psychologically, relationally, and intellectually as well as physically. In short, it could arise from—or find its way into—the totality of one's existence (Clark, 2000). To *treat* such pain in a biomedical model would require identifying and eliminating its cause. Given that this is often not possible in patients with advanced disease (especially the cancer patients whom Saunders had in mind for hospice), the goal shifted from treating disease to addressing symptoms.

To address such total pain effectively meant finding ways to support and intervene in patients' lives that covered up the suffering and kept it below the level of phenomena experienced by the patient. For Saunders, the kind of care required to address total pain had to engage patients at the level of experiencing persons, not metabolizing bodies. And it had to do this because it was precisely at the level of experience—where you and I engage with the world, where we give the things, people, and places we experience meaning, and where we develop feelings about those meanings—that total pain manifested itself during the experience of dying. If (recall from earlier) dying is not simply a biological process in organisms but instead is a meaningful process in persons (hence the difference between dying per se and the *experience* of dying), then care of persons who are going through the experience of dying needs to engage them precisely via the openings through which they are experiencing their own dying.

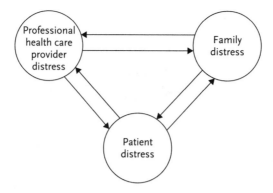

Figure 2.2
The interrelationship between the distress of the patient, family, and health care providers.
(Reprinted from Cherny, 2005, p. 7, by permission of Oxford University Press.)

The second and third commitments interact in important ways, insofar as suffering is not always an entirely individual phenomenon. That is, suffering can be experienced individually, but it can also be experienced as a *shared* phenomenon. Similar relational themes emerge in a robust conceptual model of suffering by Cherny, Coyle, and Foley (1994), and again by Cherny (2005), who notes that the suffering of loved ones can exacerbate one's own suffering and, inversely, the relief of a loved one's suffering may help ameliorate suffering of one's own (see Fig. 2.2).

Restoring and Supporting Moral Agency

The fourth philosophical commitment informing hospice care is delivering care that maximally supports patients such that they can continue to live with the integrity and sense of self required to find and create meaning until the moment of death. For Saunders, this could be conceptualized as a commitment to moral agency: supporting the patient such that she can explore and express who she is, continuing to live in a manner that honors what she finds most valuable and meaningful in life up until the moment of her death. Supporting and restoring the agency of persons did play a significant role in Saunders's writings about the hospice concept. (Indeed, she was very distressed at how advanced cancer patients were often exiled from the decision-making process in hospital-based oncology care.)

However, the way in which this aspect of the hospice philosophy has been translated into a liberal notion of patient autonomy focused on choice and control (and has been given such a central place in the rhetoric and practice of contemporary hospice care) is a more recent, and distinctly American, development. As shown later in this chapter, the Americanized version of this fourth component of the philosophy of hospice care can create some interesting tensions with the three philosophical commitments outlined earlier.

Saunders speaks directly to supporting moral agency and honoring patient preferences in her writing about the hospice concept, noting the following:

> Continuity of care for people suffering from persistent cancer aims to ensure that throughout the whole course of the disease they receive treatment appropriate to each stage *and that, as far as possible, this is carried out in the place that accords best with their own way of life and its commitments.*
>
> We owe our patients the attempt to decide when our management has finally turned into care for their dying, even though this may be a difficult moment to identify. We define it as occurring when all active treatments only hold out diminishing returns coupled with increasing morbidity, when the incidence of side effects or the management required by the treatment itself serve only to isolate the patient from those around him and *hinder him from completing life in his way.* (Saunders, 1979, p. 636, my emphasis)

Saunders believed it was quite possible for medical treatment to impede and violate a patient's sense of self, thereby compromising her moral agency. As such, one of the prime motivations in her development of hospice as a concept and practice was to offer patients a care alternative at the end of life that did not require sacrificing the integrity of who the patient was as a person. Consistent with the hospice concepts of suffering, family-centered care, and dying as a meaningful experience explained earlier, a core component of the hospice philosophy is to care in a way such that support of the patient and family empowers the patient to recover/rebuild/maintain the wholeness and integrity of self through which to find and create meaning across the entire dying experience. "At no time," writes Saunders, "in the total care of a cancer patient is the awareness of him as a person of greater importance" (Saunders, 1979, p. 636). Indeed, for Saunders, death is the final act in the life of an agent, and the experience of dying is the final opportunity for that agent to create and discover meaning. As such, preserving and respecting agency was an important requisite for actualizing the first piece of hospice philosophy: focusing on the *experience* of dying.

It would not be an overstatement to say that Saunders conceived of hospice care as "agency-conserving" care at the end of life, predating the current "patient-centered" care movement in medicine by several decades. And, when one considers the kinds of complementary care and services offered in many hospices—music therapy, life review, massage therapy, and many others—they can all be seen as ways to help patients restore a sense of self by reintegrating pieces of their lives (and their bodies) that have been disintegrated by their terminal illness and its previous treatments.

In US hospice care, however, this focus on patient integrity and moral agency has an added valence of liberal autonomy, which is focused on the right of patients to choose (or to refuse) certain elements of their care, how they are delivered, and in what circumstances. One sees this emphasis on choice, as well as the tension with some of the other concepts noted earlier, in the following definition of "hospice" recently offered by the National Hospice and Palliative Care Organization:

> Considered to be the model for quality, compassionate care for people facing a life-limiting illness or injury, hospice care involves a team-oriented approach to expert medical care, pain management, and emotional and spiritual support expressly tailored to the patient's needs and wishes. Support is provided to the patient's loved ones as well. At the center of hospice and palliative care is the belief that each of us has the right to die pain-free and with dignity, and that our families will receive the necessary support to allow us to do so. (NHPCO, n.d.)

Note the idea in this statement that hospice care is "expressly tailored to the patient's needs and wishes." This resonates well in a culture that has taken on the mantle of patient rights and autonomy as perhaps the most popularized product of health care ethics. Indeed, hospice is often presented to patients, families, and the public as way to put patients "back in control" of their care at the end of life.

Mesler (1994) points out that, while autonomy and patient control are signature components of the rhetoric of American hospice care, his observational research of several hospices in the 1990s revealed a tension between this rhetoric of choice and control, and the limits on care options that arose from the structure and processes of hospice care as actually given. For example, patients who make considered and thoughtful decisions to continue to live at home when hospice staff deem it unsafe to do so can face significant pressure from the team to move into in a residential care facility, sometimes with the implicit message that doing so is a condition of receiving continued care. Patients who choose to suffer even when safe and effective interventions to assuage their suffering are available seem to simultaneously (a) invoke the core hospice concept of supporting patient agency and (b) challenge the core hospice concept of relieving suffering.

And, of course, "electing" hospice care requires—if one's care is being paid for by Medicare or another insurance provider—"giving up" reimbursement for curative treatments related to one's terminal illness. Indeed, in the United States, the price of gaining a care modality presumably centered on patient control requires giving up control over one's treatment; nonpalliative interventions will no longer be covered, giving patients an "either/or" set of choices, which artificially renders reimbursement for some care options mutually exclusive to reimbursement for others. Despite the implication of voluntariness embedded in terms like "election," it borders on chicanery to speak of autonomy and control when such autonomy and control are conditioned upon choosing from among only a small subset of the care and treatment options available.

Indeed, this tension is embedded in the NHPCO statement itself which, two sentences following the claim about honoring patients' wishes, emphasizes that all patients have "the right to die pain-free and with dignity." This works well in the case of patients for whom "dying with dignity" means dying "pain free." For patients who don't have such an association, however, and who might either wish to die in pain or without dignity, or— perhaps most interestingly—both in pain *and* with dignity, the hospice philosophy develops some cracks. Jennings (1997) argues that the individualism embedded in a rhetoric of control and choice is not consistent with the primacy of community and relational identity at the heart of the hospice philosophy. Hence, there is a tension—conceptually and practically—between the language of control and choice that has become one of the hallmarks of discussion and marketing in US hospice care and some of the other philosophical cornerstones of hospice care explained earlier.

I would argue that the potential problems here are not with the hospice philosophy itself. Or, perhaps, not with the hospice philosophy as conceived by Saunders and further refined in the 1970s and 1980s by Wald and other early US hospice pioneers. Rather, the problems arise when one takes the component of the hospice philosophy that emphasizes caring for patients and families in a way that restores and supports their integrity and moral agency such that they can experience meaning during the dying process—an emphasis perfectly consistent with the other three components of the hospice philosophy described earlier—and transforms/reduces that component to a much simpler and far more individualistic notion of liberal autonomy that then gets simply translated as giving patients "control" and respecting their "choices."

While Saunders's commitment to restoring and respecting patients' integrity as moral agents is not inconsistent with an emphasis on patient control and choice, the two are not equivalent. However, as the material referenced earlier from NHPCO, Mesler, and Jennings, and much of the current lay literature on hospice make quite clear, the "Americanized" version of this piece of the hospice philosophy has been transmuted into a notion of liberal autonomy. And this transmutation can be the source of tension and conflict—both in the delivery of hospice care and within the philosophy that explains and defines what constitutes hospice as a concept.

HOSPICE CARE AS A PARADIGM SHIFT

The paradigm shift that resulted in hospice care occurred along several axes simultaneously, but it can be captured in the shift from the "cure of disease" paradigm to the "care of ill persons" paradigm. Perhaps the most important feature of this paradigm shift is the change in the target of intervention— from an underlying cause of disease to the lived experience of illness.

All health care occurs at the level of personal experience insofar as it involves real human beings interacting with one another in a way that attempts to improve the life of the patient. What is significant about hospice care, however, is that the symptoms and suffering the care seeks to address, and the interventions used to address them, are all conceptually designed and delivered through the lens of experience. This is a departure from the dominant allopathic medical model in the United States.

In US allopathic medicine, symptoms and functional impairments are treated as signs—signs that indicate the presence of an underlying cause (an infectious process; a chemical imbalance; an injury to bone, nerve, or connective tissue, etc.). In such a paradigm, the target of intervention is the underlying cause of disease or impairment. Once that cause is eliminated or that injury repaired, the symptoms are expected to resolve because they were simply signs of the true cause of disease/impairment. Symptoms are important, and they gain their legitimacy and meaning because of their relationship to an underlying biomedical cause.

From initial history taking, through the diagnostic examination, and into the formation of a treatment plan, the goal is to come up with a "medical diagnosis" that identifies the underlying cause of the symptoms so that one can then identify a "treatment" to address the cause. In contradistinction to the hospice model, this approach is sometimes (and, on occasion, derisively) called the "curative" model, insofar as it seeks to cure the underlying cause of symptoms and impairments. Absent a diagnosis, contemporary allopathic medicine is often unable to proceed (or, at least, to proceed coherently). It is unable to proceed because what it is designed to treat is underlying causes. If one is not identified, there is no target for treatment.

This can lead to patients experiencing prolonged journeys in search of a cause, characterized by increasingly invasive diagnostic tests and procedures. Or it can lead to unfocused, scattershot treatment plans targeting "presumed" or "likely" causes. The focus, however, remains on the cause, and not the symptom.

If the underlying cause cannot be successfully treated (for example, a very late stage IV pancreatic malignancy that has broadly metastasized), or if a patient—for whatever reason—does not wish to treat the underlying cause, then the contemporary allopathic medical model has little to offer. It has little to offer not because providers don't care about their patients. It has little to offer because its defining explanatory paradigm—the use of the scientific method, a causal theory of disease, and interventional treatments designed to eliminate causes or repair injuries—is no longer relevant to the patient's situation.

Saunders's vision of hospice, as explained in her writing and as evident in her design of St. Christopher's Hospice in London, was that it could step into the care gap created by the disconnect between a curative medical model and patients who were suffering but could not be (or did not want to be) cured. As it was attempting to do something different than medicine was doing, it reflected not simply a different method of care. It was, in fact, a completely different *philosophy* of care—a different explanatory model, a different definition of what it meant to "intervene" or "treat," and different kinds of outcomes that would help define what it meant to give "good" or "successful" care (see Fig. 2.3).

This paradigm shift is nicely captured in something as simple as Saunders's redefinition of "vital signs." Explaining this notion, she writes:

Vital signs in a ward specializing in the control of terminal pain include the hand steady enough to draw, the mind alert enough to write poems and to play cards,

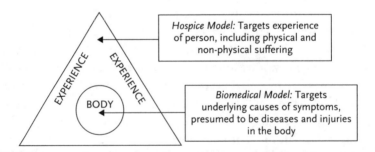

Figure 2.3
Clinical engagement with persons: the hospice model versus the biomedical model.

and above all the spirit to enjoy the family visits and spend the last weekends at home. (1979, p. 637)

Passages like this indicate that her vision of hospice care was not simply a change in emphasis. Rather, she was redefining basic medical concepts like "vitality" and its measurements; shifting their meaning to the realm of lived experience. One was not simply documenting, for example, whether a patient was awake, alert, and oriented *per se*. Rather, one was assessing whether a person was alert and aware enough to engage in the world around her *in a manner that was meaningful to her*. As such, it was not a measure of neurobiological function but an assessment of one's ability to express oneself as a moral agent.

Seeing the hospice philosophy as a paradigm shift—a new and different explanatory structure through which to understand what it means to give and receive care at the end of life—and not just as a supplement to, or change in emphasis from, the biomedical model of disease treatment, requires us to acknowledge that there are deep philosophical commitments informing hospice care as a practice. Four of those commitments have been explained earlier. Any attempt to clearly formulate, thoroughly explain, or robustly justify ethical claims in and about hospice care, then, will have to draw upon and be consistent with these four core components of the philosophy of hospice care.

HOSPICE PRACTICE: HOSPICE ETHICS IN DIALOGUE WITH HOSPICE PHILOSOPHY

The core philosophical commitments of hospice create the space in which normative value takes shape and concrete ethical values can become clear and well defined. Actions, intentions, decisions, character traits, and policies/procedures that embrace and promote conditions in which the core components of the philosophy can be actualized are those that should be promoted as ethically sound. For it is under these conditions that good hospice practice can flourish. Likewise, actions, intentions, decisions, character traits, and policies/procedures that embrace and promote conditions which inhibit the actualization of one or more core components of the hospice philosophy should be considered "unethical." For in such conditions good hospice practice fails to flourish.

Persons or groups of persons with the power and ability to affect conditions in which hospice care is given and received then become ethically culpable for the extent to which such conditions promote and reflect actions, intentions, decisions, character traits, and policies/procedures consistent with the hospice philosophy—they can be praised and blamed accordingly.

The relative importance of different ethical values in hospice is a reflection of (a) the extent to which they can be demonstrated to promote or inhibit good hospice practice and (b) the degree to which it makes sense to hold persons and organizations ethically culpable for meeting or failing to meet obligations structured by those values. For example, failure to adequately relieve the suffering of a hospice patient who has declared such relief to be a primary goal of her end-of-life care violates an ethical value at the core of the hospice philosophy: the relief of suffering. The extent to which a hospice organization or its care team is ethically culpable for this failure is directly tied to its ability to affect the conditions that resulted in the unrelieved suffering. The intentional withholding of opioid medications by a hospice nurse, the pharmacy courier not delivering medication on time, fear of a family member to administer the medication, or unnoticed theft of the medication by a third party are all circumstances that suggest different degrees and loci of ethical culpability. These different circumstances do not change the fact that unwanted, unnecessary suffering violates a basic ethical value of hospice care. What they do determine is the answer to two key questions: What person or group of persons is responsible for the violation? And what steps need to be taken to remedy the failure and bring the circumstances back in line with the values that promote and sustain good hospice practice? Those values, in turn, arise from—and help to shape—the core philosophical concepts that define the goals and nature of hospice care as a moral practice.

CONCLUSION

To what extent, then, should we accept Karen Browning's claim that honesty is a core ethical value of hospice care? The answer depends upon the extent to which the following propositions, drawn from the hospice philosophy of care, are true. First, honest interactions with patients and colleagues enable the creation of conditions in which the process of dying can be a meaningful experience for the patient and family. Second, honesty facilitates family-centered care. Third, honesty promotes the relief of suffering. And fourth, honesty supports the moral agency of hospice patients. If these propositions are true, Karen's claim that honesty is a core value of hospice care is well supported.

Whether using the word "hospice" is the right thing to do, then, hinges not so much on figuring out whether one can do so and still be "honest."

Rather, gaining clarity on the right thing to do in Karen's situation depends on the extent to which honoring the oncology physicians' request promotes or inhibits the ability of her patients, families, and team to give and receive care that embraces the core philosophical commitments of hospice. If hospice is just a word and its care can be given and received in a manner that constitutes good hospice care without using that word, Karen's colleagues may be right. If, however, not using the word "hospice" also hides the truth—from the patient or her family—that the patient is dying, it is hard to imagine how the patient and family can express their moral agency and fully explore the meaning of the dying experience absent knowledge that death is imminent.

In the following chapters of *Hospice Ethics*, one way for the reader to think about the ethical significance of the topics addressed and the strength of the claims made by chapter authors is to evaluate the extent to which the topics and claims can be connected to, or derived from, the philosophy of hospice care. Similarly, identifying which values are important in hospice care—and understanding what those values mean and how best to apply them to the topics addressed in the chapters—can be a function of the extent to which those values promote the conditions necessary for hospice care to flourish as a moral practice. In so doing, the reader is invited to consider the philosophy explained herein, and to do so in concert with reflection on the reader's own philosophy of hospice care. Attunement to both philosophies will be valuable resources in the larger enterprise of hospice ethics.

NOTE

1. Thanks to Bruce Jennings for assistance in developing this point.

REFERENCES

Cherny, N. (2005). The challenge of palliative medicine. In D. Doyle, G. Hanks, N. Cherny, & K. Calman (Eds.), *The Oxford textbook of palliative medicine* (3rd ed., pp. 8–13). New York, NY: Oxford University Press.

Cherny, N. I., Coyle, N., & Foley, K. M. (1994). Suffering in the advanced cancer patient: A definition and taxonomy. *Journal of Palliative Care, 10*(2), 57–70.

Clark, D. (2000). Total pain: The work of Cicely Saunders and the hospice movement. *APS Pain Bulletin, 10*(4), 13–15.

Jennings, B. (1997). Individual rights and the human good in hospice. *Hospice Journal, 12*(2), 1–7.

MacIntyre, A. (1981). The nature of the virtues. *Hastings Center Report, 11*(2), 27–34.

Mesler, M. A. (1994-1995). The philosophy and practice of patient control in hospice: The dynamics of autonomy versus paternalism. *Omega: Journal of Death and Dying, 30*(3), 173–189.

National Hospice & Palliative Care Organization (NHPCO). (n.d.). *Hospice care*. Retrieved April 2014, from http://www.nhpco.org/i4a/pages/index.cfm?pageid=4648.

Saunders, C. (1978). The philosophy of terminal care. In C. Saunders (Ed.) *The management of terminal disease* (pp. 193–202). London, UK: Edward Arnold.

Saunders, C. (1979). The nature and management of terminal pain and the hospice concept. In J. J. Bonica & V. Ventafridda (Eds.), *Advances in pain research and therapy* (Vol. 2, pp. 635–651). New York, NY: Raven Press.

Sellman, D. (2000). Alasdair Macintyre and the professional practice of nursing. *Nursing Philosophy, 1*(1), 26–33.

Sellman, D. (2011). Professional values and nursing. *Medicine, Health Care, and Philosophy, 14*(2), 203–208.

Yeo, M. (2010). A primer in ethical theory. In M. Yeo, A. Moorhouse, P. Kahn, & P. Rodney, *Cases and concepts in nursing ethics* (3rd ed., pp. 37–72). Peterborough, ON: Broadview Press.

The Interdisciplinary Team: Ethical Opportunities and Challenges

CHAPTER 3

The Pharmacist As an Integral Member of the Hospice Interdisciplinary Team

R. TIMOTHY TOBIN

Pharmacists are specializing in palliative care in increasing numbers. Pharmacists have long been involved in monitoring drug therapy in terminally ill patients. Until recently, however, this was often limited to screening for drug interactions, redundant therapies, contraindications, and appropriate doses. Today palliative care is a specialty in medicine, nursing, and pharmacy. Some of the changes have evolved from new knowledge and experience in treating end-of-life symptoms, and some have been mandated by more stringent conditions of participation (CoPs) in Medicare-approved hospices and more refined guidelines and goals established by accrediting agencies, such as the Joint Commission and the Community Health Accreditation Program (CHAP).

Medicare CoPs require that a pharmacist or similarly qualified member of the palliative care team be available to consult with the interdisciplinary team (Centers for Medicare and Medicaid Services, 2013). Smaller hospices utilize pharmacy service providers that specialize in palliative care and provide medications and consultations from clinical pharmacists. Some pharmacy schools are including specialized training in palliative care, including postgraduate pharmacist residencies. Pharmacists with experience in palliative care are working with educators and professional societies to establish core competencies and credentialing for pharmacists who specialize in this field.

Along with the increased intensity and visibility of the role of the palliative care pharmacist come ethical challenges and responsibilities that are often unarticulated in the hospice and palliative care literature. This chapter explains and explores the role of the palliative care pharmacist by focusing on the following six areas of practice that raise interesting and complex ethical questions:

1. Responsibilities of the hospice pharmacist on the interdisciplinary team (IDT)
2. Ensuring expertise and competence in palliative care pharmacology for hospice pharmacists
3. Balancing the needs and wants of the patient with stewardship of resources (use of expensive or rare medications and consideration of whether a less expensive or more available alternative is acceptable), or dealing with a patient or caregiver's desire for a treatment that may be inappropriate or even futile
4. Establishing a drug formulary or list of medications that are appropriate to use for palliation of symptoms related to the patient's hospice diagnosis (this may include consideration of costs, benefits vs. risks, whether the drug is disease modifying, and whether it is truly related to the hospice diagnosis and therefore covered under the hospice benefit)
5. The use of a "collaborative prescribing protocol" that allows pharmacists to initiate, modify, and discontinue medications under a protocol approved by most states and supervised by the hospice medical director
6. Pharmacists as members of the hospice ethics committee

RESPONSIBILITIES OF THE HOSPICE PHARMACIST ON THE INTERDISCIPLINARY TEAM

This section summarizes some of the responsibilities of the palliative care pharmacist in my hospice agency. Pharmacists who work for other agencies, hospice providers, or inpatient hospice facilities may perform these and other duties, such as mixing, compounding, or administering pharmaceuticals, and managing infusion devices. My contributions to the IDT include the following:

- Attend team meetings and review all new admissions and patients due for recertification (as outlined under "Roles and Duties of the Hospice Pharmacist" in the next section)

Box 3.1: DRUGS COMMONLY IMPLICATED IN TRIGGERING HOSPICE PHARMACIST SCRUTINY OR INTERVENTION

- Drugs with caution warning in elderly via Beers Criteria (Beers, 1997), drugs associated with increased fall risk
- Methadone combined with other drugs known to increase risk of cardiac arrhythmia or known to interact with it
- Warfarin or other blood thinners
- Any drug with high potential for drug interactions (cytochrome P-450 inhibitors or inducers)
- More than one benzodiazepine (lorazepam, alprazolam, clonazepam, etc.)
- Therapeutic duplication such as lisinopril + losarten, or omeprazole + ranitidine, or multiple long-acting opioids
- Nonpalliative drugs such as statins, fibrins, cholinesterase inhibitors, bisphosphonates, antiplatelet drugs
- Disease-modifying drugs (may or may not be appropriate to continue)
- Missing drugs (furosemide without potassium, opioids without bowel care, etc.)
- Steroids or nonsteroidal anti-inflammatory drugs (NSAIDs), such as ibuprofen, ordered without gastrointestinal (GI) protective medications such as omeprazole
- Steroids in diabetic patients or patients with history of GI bleed
- Inappropriate doses of immediate-release opioid for breakthrough pain
- Fentanyl patches in cachectic patients
- Visceral or bone pain not currently being treated with a steroid or an NSAID
- Adjuvant pain medications missing (unless contraindicated)
- Neuropathic pain without a tricyclic, anticonvulsant, or steroid (unless contraindicated)
- Broad spectrum antibiotics, especially long term
- Atypical antipsychotics in dementia patients
- Use of total parenteral nutrition (TPN) or tube feedings
- Unnecessary drugs or supplements
- Orphan drugs (drugs developed specifically to treat a rare condition affecting fewer than 200,000 Americans)
- Expensive drugs that may have a role in specific cases, and drugs that may have value in early stages of disease but are not effective in end-stage disease where the goal of the plan of care is comfort

- Write a case conference note on each new patient's electronic medical record (EMR) including a review of the patient's medications, any comorbidities that could affect drug therapy (such as diabetes, Parkinson's disease, dementia, chronic pain, chronic obstructive pulmonary disease, liver or kidney disease, etc.), and document any recommendations to initiate, modify, or discontinue any drug therapy (medications listed in Box 3.1 are reviewed with increased scrutiny and are likely to trigger an intervention)
- Follow up with nurse case manager and/or patient's hospice physician for any urgent recommendations
- Review patient's history and physical when appropriate (the pharmacist should be familiar with the EMR and know where to find history and physical, previous drug histories, demographics such as patients' height and weight, labs such as electrolytes, drug levels, kidney and liver function, albumin, etc.)
- Review previous recommendations at time of patient's recertification, following up on those that have not been implemented
- Review formulary compliance monthly
- Enter prescription and medication orders, including refills per algorithm protocol or on behalf of the medical director
- Monitor prescription usage to check for compliance, noncompliance, or diversion
- Provide teaching, in-service education, and drug information to staff, facilities, pharmacies, nurses, patients, and families
- Participate in ethics committee meetings and ethics consultations

ENSURING EXPERTISE AND COMPETENCE

Palliative care pharmacists must possess the capacities and competence to satisfy and evaluate several core role responsibilities. Responsibilities discussed in detail in this section include the following:

- Operate with collaborative prescribing agreements, where the interdisciplinary team works together to manage symptoms, such as using an "assessment and treatment algorithm protocol" that allows the pharmacist prescriptive authority to initiate, change, or discontinue drug therapy
- Perform an initial assessment within 48 hours of admission and a comprehensive assessment to include a review of all of the patient's prescription and over-the-counter medications, herbal remedies, and other

alternative treatments that could affect medication therapy. This review should include identification of the following:

- Effectiveness of drug therapy
- Drug side effects
- Actual or potential drug interactions
- Duplicate drug therapy
- Unnecessary or potentially harmful drugs
- Drug therapy concurrently associated with laboratory monitoring
- Establish and maintain a drug formulary
- Determine which medications of a patient's regimen are related to the terminal diagnosis and are appropriate for payment by hospice
- Assess the need to continue with nonpalliative or nonessential medications
- Convert safely to appropriate alternate opioids when opioid toxicities occur
- Provide expertise in identifying types of pain (somatic, neuropathic, visceral, bone metastases) and the most effective drug treatment for each type of pain
- Minimize side effects from multiple drugs
- Develop a policy for the disposal of controlled drugs maintained in the patient's home when those drugs have been discontinued or are remaining at the time of death (a Medicare requirement)
- Exploit favorable side effects, such as knowing when to choose a less sedating versus more sedating drug of the same class, or choosing a drug known to cause dry mouth when the patient is experiencing excessive secretions
- Recommend drugs and doses when performing "aggressive management of unrelenting symptoms," also known as "palliative sedation"
- Communicate concise, relevant information to the patient, family, and caregivers on behalf of the IDT in cases where a difficult decision about a medical or ethical dilemma involving medications could influence a patient's well-being
- Participate as members of multidisciplinary ethics committees

Many larger hospices employ their own pharmacists, and others contract with compounding pharmacies, community pharmacies, and specialized providers such as Hospice Pharmacia, Outcome Resources, HospiScript, and others. The companies that specialize in providing services to hospices have clinical pharmacists on staff and are often available for consultation 24 hours per day. They may use mail order for routine medications or contract with local community pharmacies for urgent medication needs. Some hospices that employ their own pharmacists may not provide 24-hour coverage, but they may have other resources such as an affiliation with a hospital that has 24-hour pharmacy services.

Recognizing Opioid Toxicities

Opioids are one of the most common classes of drugs in hospice patients for controlling pain and shortness of breath. Of all of the opioids, morphine remains the gold standard because of its low cost and known pharmacologic properties, and pain can be controlled in the vast majority of hospice patients by utilizing the oral or rectal route of administration (Dahl, 1996). Although true allergies such as anaphylaxis to morphine or other opioids are rare, many patients who initially receive them will experience common side effects such as nausea, vomiting, urinary retention, central nervous system changes ranging from euphoria to dysphoria and hallucinations, constipation, and itching. All opioids can cause a release of histamine that can result in itching and even a rash, but this is not considered an allergy. Patients who claim an "allergy" to morphine or other opioids may tolerate a rechallenge with the drug, especially if they are counseled on the expected side effects and how to manage them. Some patients will tolerate a particular opioid better than another. The selection of a particular opioid should be guided by the clinician's experience and patient preference. There may be cases where a particular opioid has a "stigma" with a patient or caregiver that can range from an association with drug addiction, the experience of a friend or relative, or some irrational fear. Sometimes careful education can overcome this, and other times it may be easier to select an alternate drug that the patient or caregiver does not associate with this stigma.

Respiratory depression can occur with overdose but is rare when doses are titrated carefully, even in patients with respiratory disease. Pain is a powerful respiratory stimulant that counteracts opioid-induced respiratory depression, and as long as the patient's pain is not controlled, respiratory depression from an opioid is rare (Bonica, 1990). Some less common toxicities of opioids are myoclonus and seizures. These are more likely to occur with very large doses of morphine or hydromorphone, or in patients with renal impairment. A likely explanation is that a metabolite of the opioid accumulates to levels that cause toxicity. Ordinarily the kidneys rapidly excrete these metabolites, but in cases of renal impairment or when very large doses of opioids are required, accumulation to toxic levels can occur. In cases where myoclonus is mild (jerking occurs occasionally over an hour) and it is not distressing to the patient, it does not need to be treated. Sometimes myoclonus can be more distressing to family members who observe it than to the patient. But when it is occurring several times per minute or becomes painful or interferes with sleep, it needs to be treated (Mercande, 1998). Drugs such as lorazepam or clonazepam can lessen symptoms. Other times opioid rotations are required. This is where a patient is converted from the offending opioid to a different opioid, such as from morphine to fentanyl or hydromorphone (Mercande, 1998).

Opioid Conversions and Opioid Rotations

There are subtle differences in how a particular patient might respond to different opioids. Sometimes a patient might experience a side effect such as itching or nausea from a particular opioid but not from another related opioid. Sometimes intolerances develop to a particular opioid when the dose is escalated. When the currently used opioid is not well tolerated, rotating to a different opioid can often restore symptom management. When performing opioid rotations, opioid equivalency tables are used (McPherson, 2009; NHHPCO, 2009). But with opioid doses exceeding 60 mg of oral morphine equivalent per 24 hours, the calculated equivalent dose should be further reduced by 30% to 50% to account for the difference in cross tolerance between the opioids at these higher doses (Arnold & Weissman, 2005). A patient who experiences intolerable myoclonus with morphine might be successfully converted to hydromorphone using this method, since the hydromorphone would be effective at a 30% lower dose than the tables indicate due to differences in cross tolerance. Offending metabolites would be less likely to accumulate with the 30% lower dose. Some clinicians prefer rotating to fentanyl or methadone when myoclonus occurs because these opioids do not produce toxic metabolites that are thought to cause some opioid toxicities (Teutebert, 2005). Fentanyl should be considered because its cost has decreased since it became available generically to about that of equianalgesic doses of morphine, and it is much less expensive than equianalgesic doses of hydromorphone. Methadone conversions are much trickier due to complex pharmacokinetics and numerous drug interactions, and they are best performed by experienced clinicians (McPherson, 2009).

There are other reasons for needing to do opioid conversions besides opioid rotation. They include the need to switch between an oral and a parenteral/epidural/intrathecal/topical or rectal opioid. Some opioids are not available in all dosage forms. The clinician should always consult with a colleague or an experienced palliative care practitioner whenever performing these conversions (McPherson, 2009).

Tolerance, Addiction, Physical Dependence, and Pseudo-Addiction: Understanding the Differences

Tolerance, addiction, physical dependence, and pseudo-addiction are all possible consequences of the use of opioids, and it is exceedingly important that clinicians, patients, and caregivers understand the definitions of these terms and the differences between them (Weissman, 2006).

Tolerance is a consequence of the chronic administration of a drug where the patient requires escalating doses to achieve the same effect. It can occur with chronic dosing of opioids (and many other drugs). Tolerance is common with opioids, and the dose should be increased when the patient's pain is no longer controlled. Tolerance can also develop to the opioid side effects such as nausea and sedation (but not constipation), which is why these side effects become less troublesome with continued use.

Physical dependence occurs over time when a patient becomes tolerant to the effects of a drug and may experience a "withdrawal effect" that can be associated with unpleasant symptoms such as cravings, nausea, cramping, sweating, chills, diarrhea, anxiety, and muscle pain if the drug is suddenly stopped. Withdrawal symptoms can be avoided by tapering the dose of the drug. Physical dependence should not be confused with addiction.

Addiction is a neurobehavioral syndrome with genetic and environmental influences that results in psychological dependence on the use of the substances for their psychic effects. It is characterized by compulsive use despite harm.

Pseudo-addiction is a drug-seeking behavior that in some ways simulates that seen in addiction (hoarding medication, using multiple prescribers and pharmacies), but the cause is from inadequately treated pain. Unlike true psychological addiction, those behaviors tend to stop when pain is adequately treated.

Types of Pain and Specific Treatments

Somatic pain is a nociceptive pain (a pain perceived through specialized nerve cells that detect tissue damage from heat, crushing or tearing, or chemical disruption) that arises from nerve endings in skin, muscle, and bone throughout the body other than the viscera. The opioids are very effective for this type of pain. They can be used with adjuvant analgesics such as acetaminophen that work synergistically with the opioids and may have an opioid sparing effect (i.e., provide symptom relief with lower doses of opioid, resulting in less sedation and other opioid toxicities).

Neuropathic pain is pain caused by nerve damage. It can often be a component of chronic pain, and it is often described as "burning, stabbing, tingling, electric shock, or pins and needles." Neuropathic pain can remain after an injury has apparently healed. Chronic pain can sometimes stimulate new nerve pathways that are not associated with injury. Postherpetic neuralgia is a type of neuropathic pain sometimes described as "stabbing" or "electric shock" that sometimes occurs after shingles. Neuropathic pain can sometimes be resistant to all but large doses of opioids, with the possible exception of methadone. Methadone is the only opioid that antagonizes a receptor known to be involved in perceiving neuropathic pain (NMDA receptor antagonist), giving it a dual mechanism of action. Other adjuvants that are effective for treating neuropathic pain include several anticonvulsants and the tricyclic antidepressants. Steroids can also be useful adjuvants for neuropathic pain.

Visceral pain is a nociceptive pain that originates in the gut. The viscera are innervated differently—from muscle, bone, and skin. Visceral pain is often described as dull, aching, or cramping and may be difficult to localize. Patients will often use their whole hand to circumscribe an area of the gut where pain radiates. Visceral pain can radiate to areas unrelated to the injury, which is called "referred pain." Steroids such as dexamethasone or prednisone are often helpful in relieving visceral pain, and they can often have an opioid sparing effect (Christo & Magloomdoost, 2008).

Bone metastases are areas where tumor invades bone and can cause severe bone pain. This is a type of somatic pain, but bone metastases often respond to steroids, nonsteroidal anti-inflammatory drugs (NSAIDS), or other adjuvants better than to opioids alone. Opioids are still useful, but these adjuvants may have an opioid sparing effect and allow good pain control with lower doses of opioids and thus fewer opioid toxicities (Christo & Magloomdoost, 2008).

Adjuvant Pain Medications

The ideal but goal in pain management would be to reduce pain to 0 or 1 on a scale of 0–10, or to a level of pain identified as ideal by the patient. The ideal goal will vary between patients and should balance the side effects of the drugs with the patient's desire to remain alert and functioning. These goals will change as the patient's condition progresses. Opioids used alone to control pain may decrease the pain score satisfactorily but leave the patient feeling unacceptably sedated, with reduced function or unacceptable side effects. Other pain medications, even those considered "mild

analgesics" such as aspirin, ibuprofen, or acetaminophen often work synergistically with the opioids and have an opioid sparing effect. There are
other classes of medications that treat specific types of pain (such as neuropathic, visceral, or bone metastases pain) better than the opioids alone.
These include the tricyclic drugs such as nortriptyline and desipramine, the
anticonvulsant drugs gabapentin and carbamazepine, and the steroids or
NSAID drugs such as dexamethasone or naproxen. These should always be
used in conjunction with the opioids unless contraindicated. A palliative
care pharmacist may be the best resource for choosing appropriate and
cost-effective adjuvant medications.

BALANCING THE NEEDS AND WANTS OF THE PATIENT

Polypharmacy

It is not unusual for a patient to be admitted to hospice on five, ten, or
even twenty or more medications. Some of these medications may be prophylactic, such as to prevent cardiovascular disease or osteoporosis. Some
may offer long-term benefit but little short-term benefit. Some are useful
in early stages of a disease but offer little benefit in advanced disease, and
withdrawing them when they are no longer beneficial should be considered. Some patients may also take multiple nutritional or herbal supplements that could potentially interact with other medications. If the patient
perceives that a treatment is helping, or is possibly experiencing a positive
placebo effect, and there are no contraindications, there may be justification in continuing. Sometimes patients are pressured by loved ones to try
alternative therapies. If the IDT has concerns that these therapies may
potentially interfere with the hospice plan of care, the team should try to
educate the patient and family that these therapies are unlikely to provide
benefit but could interfere with more effective therapies.

Some patients may desire to remain on a medication that is no longer
clinically indicated, but the medication may provide a sense of security or
even have sentimental value. ("My mother took Geritol every day and she
lived to be 94.") Patient autonomy is important here, but education can
help patients understand when a treatment is no longer beneficial or even
harmful. Following are some examples of commonly prescribed media-
tions that a hospice patient might be using when beginning service that
should trigger a discussion between the IDT and the patient or caregivers
about whether the therapeutic goals still fit the hospice plan of care and
are still beneficial.

- *Statins*: Medications such as the "statins" (atorvastatin [Lipitor], rasu-vastatin [Crestor], simvastatin [Zocor], etc.) have been proven to lower the risk of future cardiovascular disease, but for a hospice patient with a prognosis of less than 6 months, statins offer very little risk reduction or effect on longevity. Conversely, they may contribute to myopathies and interact with other medications. They are not palliative medications, and they may be expensive. Hospice clinicians often advise new patients that statins may be stopped with little risk. Many patients heed this advice, but others resist stopping these medications for varying reasons. Sometimes it is because their doctor told them that they would have to take these drugs "for the rest of their lives" or from the influence of direct to consumer advertising. It is certainly within the patient's prerogative to continue these medications, but the hospice clinician has an obligation to teach and counsel so that the patient can make an informed decision.
- *Bisphosphonates*: In intravenous (IV) form (pamidronate [Aredia], zole-dronic acid, others), these can sometimes have a role in palliating severe bone pain caused by metastases, but they are more frequently prescribed orally (as alendronate [Fosomax], risedronate [Actonel], others) to reduce bone density loss in patients with osteoporosis. As with the statins, bisphosphonates prescribed for osteoporosis offer minimal benefits for hospice patients, and they commonly cause side effects.
- *Cholinesterase inhibitors*: These include donepezil, rivastigmine, and others. These drugs offer modest benefit to some patients with early stages of dementia, but when a patient's symptoms advance to the point that the patient meets Medicare criteria for hospice (functional assessment staging [FAST] scores >7C), these medications offer little benefit. They can, however, increase the risk of falls or the need for cardiac pacing due to the cholinergic effects on the heart (Birks, 2006; Gill et al., 2009). There is some evidence that abruptly stopping these medications can cause agitation, so they should be tapered over several days rather than abruptly withdrawn (Overshot & Burns, 2005).
- *Platelet inhibitors*: These include aspirin, clopidogrel (Plavix), prasugrel (Effient), and others. They are often prescribed for prophylaxis of thromboembolic events and therefore are prophylactic rather than palliative. The patient's physician should consult with the patient and the IDT as to whether the benefits of continuing antiplatelet therapy outweigh the risks of bleeding or hemorrhagic stroke.
- *Warfarin*: Patients who have experienced a blood clot due to cancer or cancer treatment should be maintained on anticoagulants as long as they are able to take them and the risk of a clot exceeds the risk of a

potential bleed. Those patients who require anticoagulation that is resistant to warfarin may need to be maintained on injectable anticoagulants such as daltaparin (Fragmin) or enoxaparin (Lovenox). But as a patient's condition deteriorates, the risks of continuing anticoagulation therapy may eventually outweigh the benefits. Decreasing albumin levels, low platelets, a gastrointestinal bleed, or treatment with steroids can all complicate anticoagulation therapy or make it impossible to maintain a patient's international normalized ratio (INR) in the therapeutic range. In these cases, the IDT should consider terminating anticoagulation therapy and concentrating on comfort care. There are cases where hospice patients are taking warfarin for conditions with a low risk of embolism, such as atrial fibrillation or a long resolved deep venous thrombosis (DVT). If these patients are still ambulatory, receiving adequate nutrition, and their INR is stable, they or their doctor may wish to continue with warfarin.

- *Insulin, oral antidiabetic drugs, and blood sugar testing*: A goal of treating diabetes is to prevent the long-term complications of kidney and cardiovascular disease, neuropathies, and blindness. When a patient begins hospice, the risk from those complications diminishes with their decreased life expectancy. The risks of trying to maintain a patient's blood sugar in a tight range when the patient has a poor appetite and is not eating and losing weight may exceed the benefit. For example, in some hospice patients aggressive dietary management can increase the risk of hypoglycemia at a time when the risk of harm from mild hyperglycemia is decreased. Patients with labile diabetes should still maintain their blood sugars at levels that will avoid catastrophic complications such as diabetic ketoacidosis, but as long as their blood sugars are stable, even if moderately elevated, they may not need to be as aggressively managed. Painful and intrusive finger stick testing should also be minimized when appropriate.

- *Antibiotics*: Patients often express their wishes regarding the desire to receive antibiotics in their advanced directives or their physician orders for life-sustaining treatment (POLST). There are many circumstances where the use of an antibiotic in a hospice patient is a comfort measure and certainly appropriate. Urinary tract infections and pneumonia are common in hospice patients and can cause severe pain and even delirium. If symptomatic, they should be treated with a course of antibiotics. But in cases where an infection recurs despite aggressive antibiotic treatment, and the patient is likely to ultimately die from this process, it may be unethical to prolong the patient's suffering with continued aggressive courses of antibiotics. Sometimes there is not a clear line as to when aggressive treatments become futile. The IDT should discuss these cases before they get to that point.

- *"Futile" drug therapy*: The concept of futility is beyond the scope of this chapter, mostly due to the difficulty in defining it (Rubin, 2007). But if there is disagreement between the patient, caregiver, and clinicians as to whether a particular drug or treatment may be beneficial, harmful, or futile, the entire hospice IDT and even the ethics committee should become involved. The hospice pharmacist can provide valuable input regarding the pros and cons of using a particular medication for a possibly futile endeavor, and advise whether there might be an alternative medication with greater benefit, smaller risk, or lesser impact on resources.

ESTABLISHING A DRUG FORMULARY

Hospice covers the cost of only those drugs that are useful for symptom management related to the patient's terminal diagnosis. According to Medicare regulations, the cost of medications not related to relieving symptoms of the terminal diagnosis are the responsibility of the patient. This means that different hospice diagnoses will cover different drugs, and that some drugs that are appropriate to cover for end-stage cardiac disease may not be appropriate to cover for pancreatic cancer.

Medicare does not maintain a formulary of drugs that are covered by hospice; it simply states that medications used for palliation of symptoms related to the terminal diagnosis will be covered. The "formulary" of covered drugs is presently left up to the individual hospice providers who must consider the ethical principals of justice, autonomy, and beneficence to decide whether a certain drug should be covered for a particular symptom, keeping in mind the capitated payment that the agency receives. Some medications such as opioids are clearly palliative, but there are other medications that could be considered palliative in certain circumstances but also may be disease modifying to the point where they could affect the patient's eligibility to remain on hospice. An example is chemotherapy, which can clearly be palliative when it successfully shrinks a tumor that is causing pain. However, that same chemotherapy may also extend the patient's prognosis past the 6-month time period that allows a patient to be on hospice. For this reason, chemotherapy is generally not considered valid drug therapy to cover under the hospice benefit. (There may be exceptions where a medical director will determine that a chemotherapy treatment is truly palliative and not necessarily life extending.) Patients who are on hospice may elect to discharge from hospice in order to try a promising chemotherapy regimen, with the intent of returning to hospice care if and when the treatment is no longer effective.

Some hospices have their own pharmacy or network of pharmacies that may offer custom compounding, delivery, mail order, and specialized medication management. It is easy for these hospices to design their own formularies through collaboration of their medical directors, pharmacists, and IDT members. But for smaller hospices or hospices that serve a large geographical area, the problem is more complex.

Box 3.2: STEWARDSHIP, JUSTICE, RESPECT FOR AUTONOMY, AND NONMALEFICENCE: ONE HOSPICE'S EXPERIENCE WITH RESTRUCTURING ITS PHARMACY SERVICE

BACKGROUND

In the case of Providence Hospice of Snohomish County in Washington State, I currently practice as the sole palliative care pharmacist for the agency. Our hospice is the largest Medicare certified hospice provider in a county of over 650,000 people covering over 2,000 square miles. We are affiliated with a regional nonprofit medical center that also owns four community pharmacies in our county. There are additionally over 125 private and chain community pharmacies in our service area.

PROBLEM

In 2004, our agency was operating under outdated contracts with each of the individual community pharmacies in our county with prescription pricing based on drugs' published average wholesale price (AWP). Pharmaceutical AWPs can be orders of magnitude higher than the drugs' actual acquisition price, and we had little control over the use of brands versus generics, or formulary restrictions. Our pharmacy costs were over $12 per patient per day, which was 30% higher than other hospices in our peer group. Because of the large geographical area we serve, it was impossible to provide pharmaceutical services to all of the patients in our county with just the four community pharmacies affiliated with our ministry. Additionally, we did not want to interfere with our patients' established patient–pharmacist relationships.

There are several excellent pharmacy hospice providers who employ their own palliative care pharmacists and who offer services nationally. We felt that because of the success of our collaborative prescribing

(continued)

protocol, our large geographical service area, and the importance of maintaining our patients' relationships with their own community pharmacists (some of which had cultivated trust over decades), we could be successful in teaming with a pharmacy benefit manager (PBM) and our own network of community pharmacies to provide medications for our patients without contracting with one of the national services.

We interviewed a number of PBM companies to see whether any of them could help us manage our drug costs. These are the same companies that manage drug plans and formularies for employers who provide prescription benefits to their employees. Many PBMs were unwilling or unable to work with us due to our requirement for a custom drug formulary for each hospice diagnosis.

We finally selected a PBM that was able to manage our formulary requirements and also maintain a friendly working relationship with our community pharmacies.

RESULT

We went live on the Monday after the July 4th holiday in 2004. There were a few snafus and lots of phone calls on the first few days, but we learned from our mistakes and the process was going smoothly after a few days.

After the first month, our drug costs were $50,000 less than our previous monthly average. This exceeded our expectations and we hoped that it was not a fluke, but the next several months continued to be $30,000 to $35,000 below average. In addition, the PBM provided us with a digital statement listing all prescriptions billed to hospice for the month. Previously we received more than 100 different statements from individual pharmacies each month, which contributed to significant administrative costs. Since then, our average drug cost per patient day has continued to decrease from over $12.00 per day to the current average of $6.20 per patient day, almost a 50% reduction. We developed a spreadsheet that sorts the prescriptions by patient, prescriber, pharmacy, drug name, number of prescriptions per drug, and drug cost. This allows us to easily monitor drug usage, to look for duplicate therapies, drug interactions, inappropriate antibiotic usage, and inappropriate usage of expensive medications when an alternative that may be at least as effective has not been tried. The PBM charges our agency a fee for each covered prescription that averages less than 2% of our total drug expenditure per month, or about $880.

NUTS AND BOLTS

Patients of our agency are given a prescription benefit card when they are admitted to our hospice, which they can use the card at their usual pharmacy.

(continued)

The admitting hospice nurse takes detailed drug histories at the time of admit and enters them into the electronic chart. This includes comorbidities, allergies, all current prescription, and over-the-counter (OTC) medications as well as herbal, homeopathic, and nontraditional treatments. The nurse notes whether each medication is paid for by the patient (not palliative or not related to hospice diagnosis) or covered by hospice and discusses this with the patient or caregiver. If the nurse is not sure, he or she consults with the pharmacist or medical director before assigning coverage. The electronic chart software checks for drug interactions and duplications, and the palliative care pharmacist thoroughly reviews each medication profile soon after admission and at least every 14 days thereafter.

The pharmacist may have recommendations for medication intervention at this point. The pharmacist also works closely with the interdisciplinary team to discuss the rationale for continuing a particular drug therapy that no longer has palliative value, is burdensome, or no longer has a favorable risk to benefit ratio.

In redesigning our delivery of pharmacy services, we sought to honor four basic ethical values that are consistent with our hospice's mission statement: stewardship, justice, respective for autonomy, and nonmaleficence. We honored stewardship by dramatically lowering our median per-patient pharmacy costs, thereby freeing up funds to devote to other forms of patient care while still ensuring that symptoms that respond to medical intervention were adequately addressed. We honored justice by establishing an evidence-based formulary that balanced concern for clinical efficacy with concern for cost, such that our pharmacy resources were allocated based on what was needed to effectively treat patient symptoms using lower cost drug equivalencies when possible. This mitigated the phenomenon of some patients getting far more expensive drugs than others simply based on what their prehospice medical team happened to prescribe. We respected our patients' autonomy by working with our pharmacy benefit manager to create a system that allowed patients to maintain their relationships with the community pharmacists they have known and trusted for many years. And we honored nonmaleficence by creating a system that more rigorously checked for and identified unnecessary and dangerous medications or medication combinations, thereby lowering the risk of harm to patients.

Determining Which Medications Are Covered by Hospice

It is the responsibility of the medical director to certify a "hospice diagnosis" with a prognosis of no more than 6 months at the time of admissions.

In the recent past, the majority of patients admitted to hospice had cancer diagnoses. Currently in our hospice, cancer diagnoses still make up slightly over half of the diagnoses at time of admission, while end-stage heart disease, pulmonary disease, neurological disorders, dementia, and organ failure such as kidney and liver make up much of the difference. The number of patients with multiple comorbidities who are clearly approaching end of life, but with ill-defined primary diagnoses, is also increasing. These patients are often admitted with a hospice diagnosis of debility, or "adult failure to thrive." This can create a quandary for the hospice pharmacist and medical director for determining exactly whether a particular medication is providing comfort and symptom relief for a patient with multiple comorbidities. Medications for pain, fever, bowel care, nausea, and shortness of breath would all be covered. But what about a patient who may be suffering from Parkinson's disease, diabetes with renal impairment, dementia, congestive heart failure, decubitus ulcers, and osteoarthritis and is on a regimen of 20 different drugs at admission?

In cases such as this, the team should confirm that the patient meets the criteria for admission to hospice and the team should review which medications are truly beneficial and helpful in controlling the patient's symptoms without potential for harm, and those medications should be covered. Supplements, nonpalliative drugs, and drugs that are burdensome or have potential side effects with little benefit should be stopped. Of course, the patient's autonomy must be considered, as for example when a patient may desire to continue a particular supplement that does not have a documented beneficial clinical effect but may have a powerful placebo effect that is beneficial to the patient.

THE USE OF A "COLLABORATIVE PRESCRIBING PROTOCOL"

Washington State was one of the first in the nation to allow pharmacists prescriptive authority through collaborative prescribing protocols. Now, almost all states recognize protocols that allow pharmacists to initiate, modify, or discontinue drug therapy in varying degrees. This includes therapeutic drug substitution protocols; administering vaccinations; ordering laboratory monitoring tests; following prescription refill protocols; managing medications for diabetes, hypertension, hyperlipidemia; and others. The Washington State Board of Pharmacy was also the first to approve a symptom management algorithm protocol for palliative care in 1993 that gives pharmacists authority to prescribe for hospice patients according to "assessment and treatment algorithms" developed by their hospice team

(Wrede-Seaman, 1999). These algorithms were published in 1999 and have served as a model for many other collaborative prescribing protocols (Wrede-Seaman, 2009). Updated volumes, including algorithms developed for pediatric patients, have been published since (Wrede-Seaman, 2005). Pharmacists must have a physician sponsor for their protocol (usually the hospice medical director) and must submit their protocol to their state board of pharmacy for approval. Pharmacists operating under the protocol are required to demonstrate knowledge and proficiency in palliative care.

The team has access to the patient's previous and current history and physical, lab results, consults, and other medical records. The hospice nurses use this information and the assessment tools from the algorithm protocol to evaluate the patient. In assessing pain, a nurse will assess the type of pain, onset, intensity, duration, location, description, and what exacerbates or alleviates the pain. Patients usually rate their pain on a scale of 0–10, but in cases when a patient is nonverbal or moribund, the nurse will use nonverbal clues to assess pain, such as moaning, grimacing, blood pressure, heart rate, and respirations. If a patient's symptoms are not well managed, the nurse consults with other members of the team, including the medical director, other nurses, social workers, aids, chaplains, and pharmacists. If a medication intervention is required due to unmanaged symptoms or medication side effects, the nurse, pharmacist, and other team members formulate a plan. The pharmacist then writes orders for medication changes, and the team agrees on follow-up assessment plans. The pharmacist initiates the medication changes immediately and transmits the new prescription to the pharmacy. This process expedites the process of medication intervention from a typical 24- to 48-hour process to an immediate process.

A physician order is required to initiate the protocol for a particular patient. Most protocols require that the team notify the physician of interventions made under the protocol within a reasonable time frame. Most interventions occur when the patient contacts hospice about unmanaged symptoms or when a hospice nurse discovers unmanaged symptoms during a routine assessment.

Symptoms Addressed in Our Protocol

The initial algorithms were developed for hospice patients during a time that the vast majority of hospice admissions were related to a cancer diagnosis. Since then, more patients are being admitted to hospice with noncancer diagnoses, including cardiac disease, respiratory failure, renal or hepatic failure, infections such as AIDS, neurological disorders such as Parkinson's disease and dementia, and others. The protocol is periodically modified and expanded to meet changing needs. Some of the symptoms that are managed in our protocol include pain, nausea and vomiting, anxiety, constipation, itching, dry mouth, insomnia, and others. Our protocol allows the hospice pharmacist to authorize routine refills (including controlled substances) when appropriate. All medications prescribed under the protocol by the hospice pharmacist include a notation of whether the medications are to be billed to hospice or to the patient. If the medication in question is one that is sometimes covered depending on the diagnosis, only the hospice pharmacist or hospice nursing supervisor may authorize the pharmacy benefit manager to approve coverage of that mediation.

PHARMACISTS AS MEMBERS OF THE ETHICS COMMITTEE

Most ethics committees affiliated with health care organizations are multidisciplinary. Many of the ethics consultations that have been reviewed since I have been on the ethics committee have in some way involved drug therapy. Specific examples include allocation of vaccine during a pandemic, determining competency of a substance-abusing patient seeking discharge against medical advice, determining whether a pharmaceutical company–sponsored drug trial was ethical or in conflict with our mission, and deciding whether a pharmacist has a right to refuse to fill a medication order due to personal moral values. I was invited to become a member of our hospice's affiliated medical center ethics committee due to the high percentage of ethics consults that involved end-of-life care (about 50% in our ministry), my involvement in hospice, and my experience with palliative sedation therapy (PST), which provides aggressive symptom management of unrelenting symptoms.

Palliative sedation therapy has been reviewed by ethical experts and even the US Supreme Court (*Cruzan v. Director, Missouri Department of Health*, 1990). It has been deemed ethically and morally acceptable to use in appropriate situations (Bruce, Hendrix, & Gentry, 2006). The hospice medical director sometimes calls upon the hospice pharmacist to assist in selecting appropriate drugs or doses in patients who have unrelenting symptoms despite high doses of palliative medications or doses that are causing toxic effects. The drugs and doses used in palliative sedation therapy are sometimes similar to those that might be used for euthanasia or physician-assisted suicide (PAS), but the intent is entirely different. PAS is now legal here in Washington State, although under a very strict protocol.

Our hospice does not participate in PAS for ethical and philosophical reasons. We will not abandon a patient who chooses to participate, but by policy our staff members cannot be present if and when a patient chooses to initiate the process. During the campaign to enact PAS in Washington, some of the proponents of PAS attempted to compare PAS with PST, asserting that "PST is nothing more than slow euthanasia." This argument is of course invalid, as both the intent and outcome of the two are different (Bruce et al., 1997).

Intractable Suffering

The goal of palliative care is to relieve suffering but maintain as much function as possible. Occasionally patients who are near death will experience extreme suffering (pain, delirium, anxiety, nausea, vomiting, shortness of breath) that does not respond to aggressive dosing of palliative medications, or patients experience intolerable side effects from high doses of these medications such as nausea, hallucinations, dysphoria, myoclonus, or hyperalgesia (a phenomenon that is associated with paradoxical worsening of pain intensity with increasing doses of opioid) (Teutebert, 2005). When symptoms become intractable despite aggressive treatment, hospice clinicians must sometimes consider the use of PST. It is not appropriate to attempt to sedate the patient by simply increasing the dose of the opioid, as this would not only be ineffective but could lead to opioid toxicity (dysphoria, myoclonus, seizures, or hyperalgesia). However, opioids should be maintained when initiating PST at the level necessary to control pain or shortness of breath, and if opioid toxicity occurs, patients should be rotated to an appropriate alternative opioid as described elsewhere in this chapter (Johanson, 2006).

PST uses additional pharmacological armamentarium, including several drugs used in general anesthesia. The goal is to titrate these agents to the point where symptoms are relieved even if the patient becomes unconscious or unresponsive. PST is considered in our agency only when a patient is within hours or days of dying. The term "proportionate palliative sedation" is sometimes used to demonstrate that the intent of this procedure is to provide the minimal amount of sedation required to control symptoms. This can range from the patient being in a sleepy but arousable state to total unconsciousness and unresponsiveness. Patients receiving PST do not need to have routine vital signs taken, as these can be intrusive and defeat the purpose of comfort care. Patients should be monitored according to a protocol for responsiveness to interventions. If there is concern over the level of sedation, a downward titration of dose by 25% to 50% may be warranted, but patients should be closely monitored for return of unrelenting symptoms (Johanson, 2006).

Patients who are rendered totally unresponsive by this therapy would be unable to take nourishment or fluids unless administered parenterally or by feeding tube. For this reason, in our hospice patients and families must be counseled about the option to begin artificial nutrition and hydration as part of the informed consent process for PST. They should be counseled on the goals, the risks, and the benefits, and the patient must have an advance directive and "do not resuscitate" status. Hospices who administer PST should have written guidelines and protocols, and all interdisciplinary staff involved should be thoroughly familiar with the protocols. This includes medical directors and other involved physicians, pharmacists, chaplains, volunteers, nurses, and social workers. It is helpful to have input from an ethics committee to review the protocol and address any issues with patients, family, and staff that may occur. The protocol should include a teaching module for staff; a background of the moral, legal, and ethical principles guiding this therapy; procedures and forms for informed consent; references of drugs used and dosage ranges; and possibly provisions for team members to ask for an ethics consult or to opt out if they have a conscientious objection to the procedure. The National Hospice and Palliative Care Organization (NHPCO) has an excellent position paper available that addresses PST (Kirk & Mahon, 2010).

It is possible that PST could hasten death in a patient who is sedated to unconsciousness, even though this is not the intent. There are anecdotal reports that give credence to the contrary—that management of unrelenting symptoms may actually extend life. Physiologically, this makes sense when one considers that a patient who is experiencing intractable suffering may be writhing in pain, with very high blood pressure and rapid breathing and pulse with air hunger. His body's "fight or flight" mechanism is activated, leading to release of catecholamines such as epinephrine into his system that can worsen symptoms and potentially lead to a stroke or heart attack. But when symptoms are relieved with PST, the patient's breathing calms, the pulse normalizes, blood pressure drops, and the patient relaxes.

Unlike PAS, PST is reversible. In some cases patients may request to be awakened from their sedation, such as when waiting for a loved one to arrive in order to say goodbye. Occasionally patients may awaken on their own for short periods without the recurrence of their intractable symptoms, especially when lighter levels of sedation are used. When this occurs, it would be inappropriate to increase levels of sedation unless the intractable symptoms recur (Johanson, 2006).

A thorough review of the drugs and dosages used in PST is beyond the scope of this chapter. Teams who intend to utilize this therapy should have several members who have expertise in how to titrate these medications. Some of the medications utilized in PST include barbiturates (phenobarbital, pentobarbital, thiopental), benzodiazepines (midazolam, lorazepam, diazepam, and others), neuroleptics (haloperidol, chlorpromazine), and others such as ketamine and propofol. They are not all compatible with each other in an intravenous solution, so an infusion pharmacist with knowledge of drug admixture compatibilities should be consulted when more than one drug is used.

SUMMARY

The hospice IDT is exactly that: a team that relies on individual members from various disciplines working together for the benefit of the patient while complying with regulations. The team performs optimally when all members are working toward the same goal. The pharmacist is a crucial member of the team. Pharmacists are required to consider ethical principles in many of their roles on the team. Recommendations to abandon nonpalliative therapies when the goals shift toward comfort care require consideration of autonomy, patient preference, and justice. Formulary decisions require weighing beneficence, stewardship, futility, and patient preferences. Therapies such as palliative sedation require weighing those same ethical principles as well as autonomy, decisional capacity, nonmaleficence, and informed consent. The pharmacist can provide guidance to the team, the patient, and caregivers on the use of antibiotics, fluid and nutritional supplements, and aggressive therapies in cases where benefits no longer exceed the burden to the patient or caregivers.

ACKNOWLEDGMENTS

The author thanks Alan Abrams, ARNP, and Deborah Meyers, MD, for their assistance in preparing and reviewing the chapter.

REFERENCES

Arnold, R., & Weissman, D. E. (2005, July). #36: Calculating opioid dose conversions, 2nd edition. *Fast Facts and Concepts*. Retrieved May 2014 from http://www.eperc.mcw.edu/EPERC/FastFactsIndex/ff_036.htm.

Beers, M. H. (1997). Explicit criteria for determining potentially inappropriate medication use by the elderly. *Archives of Internal Medicine, 157*(14), 1531–1536.

Birks, J. (2006). Cholinesterase inhibitors for Alzheimer's disease. *Cochrane Database of Systematic Reviews,* CD005593.

Bonica, J. J. (1990). *The management of pain* (2nd ed.). Philadelphia, PA: Lea & Febiger.

Bruce, S. D., Hendrix, C. C., & Gentry, J. H. (2006). Palliative sedation in end-of-life care: The doctrine of double effect and principle of proportionality. *Journal of Hospice and Palliative Nursing, 8*(6), 320–327.

Centers for Medicare and Medicaid Services. (2013). *Conditions for coverage and conditions of participation.* Retrieved April 2014, from https://www.cms.gov/CFCsAndCoPs/05_Hospice.asp.

Christo, P., & Magloomdoost, D. (2008). Cancer pain and analgesia. *Annals of the New York Academy of Sciences, 1138,* 278–298.

Cruzan v. Director, Missouri Department of Health, 497 US 261 (1990).

Dahl, J. L. (1996). Effective pain management in terminal care. *Clinics in Geriatric Medicine, 12*(2), 279–300.

Gill, S. S., Anderson, G. M., Fischer, H. D., Bell, C. M., Li, P. Normand, S. T., & Rochon, P. A. (2009). Syncope and its consequences in patients with dementia receiving cholinesterase inhibitors: A population-based cohort study. *Archives of Internal Medicine, 169*(9), 867–873.

Johanson, G. A. (2006). *Clinicians handbook of symptom relief in palliative care* (5th ed.). Santa Rosa, CA: Sonoma County Academic Foundation for Excellence in Medicine.

Kirk, T. W., & Mahon, M. M. (2010). National Hospice and Palliative Care Organization (NHPCO) position statement and commentary on the use of palliative sedation in imminently dying terminally ill patients. *Journal of Pain and Symptom Management, 39*(5), 914–923.

McPherson, M. L. (2009) *Demystifying opioid conversion calculations: A guide to effective dosing.* Bethesda, MD: American Society of Health System Pharmacists.

Mercande, S. (1998). Pathophysiology and treatment of opioid-related myoclonus in cancer patients. *Pain, 74*(1), 5–9.

New Hampshire Hospice and Palliative Care Organization (NHHPCO). (2009). *Opioid use guidelines.* Retrieved April 2014, from http://www.nhhpco.org/opioid.htm.

Overshot, R., & Burns, A. (2005). Treatment of dementia. *Journal of Neurology, Neurosurgery and Psychiatry, 76*(Suppl), 53–59.

Rubin, S. B. (2007). If we think it's futile, can't we just say no? *HEC Forum, 19*(1), 45–65.

Teutebert, W. G. (2005, September). #142: Opioid-induced hyperalgesia. *Fast Facts and Concepts.* Retrieved May 2014 from http://www.eperc.mcw.edu/EPERC/FastFactsIndex/ff_142.htm.

Weissman, D. E. (2006, July). #68: Is it pain or addiction? (2nd ed.). *Fast Facts and Concepts.* Retrieved May 2014 from http://www.eperc.mcw.edu/EPERC/FastFactsIndex/ff_068.htm.

Wrede-Seaman, L. (1999). Symptom management algorithms for palliative care. *American Journal of Hospice and Palliative Care, 16*(3), 517–524.

Wrede-Seaman, L. (2005). *Pediatric pain and symptom algorithms for palliative care.* Yakima, WA: Intellicard.

Wrede-Seaman, L. (2009). *Symptom management algorithms—A handbook for palliative care* (3rd ed.). Yakima, WA: Intellicard.

CHAPTER 4

The Continually Evolving Role of the Hospice Medical Director

JOAN HARROLD

Hospice patients and families coping with end-of-life issues have a myriad of needs. The role of the medical director varies according to the situation, the needs of the patient and family, and the skills of other team members. In addition to complying with applicable laws and regulations, the medical director advocates for the patient, facilitates physical diagnosis, participates in analyses of emotional and spiritual issues, promotes best clinical practices, supports staff to maintain healthy boundaries, and limits risk for the hospice organization. The medical director is a clinician, a member of the interdisciplinary team, and a participant in the organizational leadership. Ethical principles guide the physician to honor the different relationships that constitute the role of medical director and manage the opportunities and tensions that can arise when advocating for patients, supporting team members, fulfilling obligations to hospice programs, and complying with regulations.

As a clinician, the medical director is guided by a synthesis of beneficence, nonmaleficence, and respect for patient autonomy. As a member of the team, the prevailing principles include beneficence, professional integrity, patient safety, and the functional health of the team. As an organizational leader, the medical director complies with legal and regulatory requirements, helps maintain institutional financial health, and supports the overall mission to serve all patients and families—a combination of stewardship and distributive justice.

Although physicians should not impose distributive justice at the bedside of individual patients, the medical director often utilizes this ethical principle in decision making at the level of organizational policy and practice in her role as an administrator. The medical director has a substantial role in helping a hospice discern how to use its resources for the provision of hospice and palliative care in accord with the best practices of the field and, often, the expectations of the community. While payment structures may change, the typical per diem nature of payments to hospices is likely to continue. Thus, the distributive justice issues that most physicians can avoid in their clinical practice are nonetheless important ethical concerns for all hospice administrators, including the medical director.

ADMISSION, TREATMENT, AND DISCHARGE
DECISIONS: REGULATORY ISSUES

Given the age of the typical hospice patient and the reliance of most hospices on Medicare funding, determining eligibility for hospice services often means determining eligibility for Medicare coverage of hospice services. According to the Medicare conditions of participation (CoPs), a patient must be certified, "based on the physician's or medical director's clinical judgment regarding the normal course of the individual's illness" to have a prognosis "6 months or less if the terminal illness runs its normal course" (Center for Medicare and Medicaid Services [CMS], n.d., §418.22).

Although the CoPs specify "clinical judgment" as the basis of determining prognosis, payers have adopted policies detailing factors upon which clinical judgment should be exercised and Medicare payments made. Most of these policies include demonstrable decline, weight loss, and disease-based guidelines originally developed to help identify patients eligible for hospice care with diagnoses other than cancer (Stuart et al., 1996).[1] If the physician determines that a patient has a prognosis of 6 months or less despite not meeting the guidelines, the physician has an ethical and regulatory obligation to substantiate clinical judgment with reference to clinical circumstances, published studies, accepted prognostic algorithms, professional expertise and experience, and other relevant data.

This substantiation can be provided in the required "brief narrative explanation of the clinical findings that supports a life expectancy of 6 months or less" (CMS, n.d.). The narrative should not merely summarize the patient's clinical history or list the patient's myriad diagnoses; it should emphasize clinical data that justify the medical judgment of a prognosis of 6 months of less. The physician typically needs to write only a sentence or two. Some patients have diagnoses with inherently poor prognoses; others clearly meet the disease-based guidelines. But when the guidelines are not specifically met, the physician has an ethical obligation to support the prognosis more vigorously.

Determining, certifying, and documenting eligibility draws upon several key ethical obligations related to the various roles played by a medical director. As a clinician, beneficence and respect for autonomy necessitate justification of eligibility, enabling the patient to receive hospice care as desired if it can benefit the patient and is consistent with the patient and family's goals of care. As a member of the interdisciplinary team (IDT), thorough, timely, and informed documentation of the patient's medical eligibility for hospice care gives the team important information necessary to collaborate with the patient and family to develop a plan of care. As an administrator, stewardship for the organization's financial resources promotes thorough and consistent documentation of eligibility, maximizing the organization's position to receive reimbursement from payers for each patient care day at the appropriate level of care. Distributive justice requires preserving the financial ability of the hospice to serve all patients and families by helping to design and promote procedures that meet quality standards for ensuring and monitoring effective assessment and documentation of eligibility for all patients served by the organization.

When eligibility is more ambiguous, the medical director has ethical obligations to care for the patient while upholding regulatory requirements and financial practices that maintain the ability of the hospice program to serve others.

Although overall life expectancies and trajectories of cancer may be changed by chemotherapies and radiation, end-stage signs and symptoms characteristically progress rather predictably. Eligibility for patients with noncancer diagnoses may be more ambiguous. Patients with heart failure, advanced lung disease, chronic kidney disease, and dementia often have periodic symptom exacerbations interrupting daily frailty and debility. A prognosis of hours to days may be easy to assess during acute decompensation. But overall prognosis may be quite poor for months, even years (Christakis & Lamont, 2000).

Some hospice patients outlive the initial 6-month prognosis. The mere fact of outliving a prognosis, however, does not mean that the estimated prognosis should have been longer. It is difficult to know, for example, whether hospice care itself contributes to longer life with frequent nursing visits, provision and oversight of medications, and emotional and spiritual support for patient and caregivers. Moreover, using best clinical judgment, the patient may continue to have a prognosis of 6 months or less.

Beneficence, nonmaleficence, and respect for patient autonomy dictate that the hospice medical director provide the best care possible, consistent with a plan of care shaped by the goals of the family and patient. If the physician and hospice team believe that a patient has a prognosis of 6 months or less and should be certified for benefits, the medical director should work assiduously to justify that eligibility.

Certification of eligibility may be challenged, usually in the form of review and nonpayment by Medicare intermediaries or other third-party payers. Since ultimate decisions regarding Medicare eligibility rest with Medicare and its contracted reviewers, medical directors should collaborate with their hospices to determine how to reconcile clinical determinations of eligibility and ongoing provision of services with recurring nonpayment due to a patient being deemed ineligible by the payer.

Alternatively, the life expectancy of some patients may improve and extend beyond 6 months. In such cases, medical directors can work with team members to ensure that families receive adequate notice of a change in eligibility and careful, compassionate explanation of the likelihood that the patient may have to be discharged. Some patients and families may realize that prognosis has improved and understand the eligibility implications of this change. Others may be desperate for services and feel bereft or betrayed at the thought of losing hospice services—services perhaps not otherwise available to them, especially if they live at home, have no needs to justify home health services, and do not have the resources to pay for hospice care out of pocket.

Honoring beneficence and autonomy requires that discharge planning be a collaborative process between the team, the patient, and the patient's family. The process should be driven by the patient's goals as well as the duty to maximize benefit and minimize harm. As such, it should include provision of ongoing care and support by available resources for which the patient qualifies. As a clinician and IDT member, medical directors should be attuned to, and provide critical support for, such processes. Stewardship and distributive justice dictate that the medical director not harm the program by failing to comply with regulations or obligate the hospice to provide care for which it is unlikely to be reimbursed as expected. As an administrator, the medical director needs to carefully balance the aforementioned obligations to the patient with her duties to protect the accreditation and financial health of the organization. Ensuring that eligibility and discharge planning processes are clear, well-developed via organizational policy, and efficiently executed is one way to honor both sets of obligations.

When Hospice Eligibility Is Not Medicare Eligibility

Although hospices in the United States are overwhelmingly supported by Medicare (CMS, 2009), patients may have other forms of insurance, have no insurance, or pay privately for their health care. They may also choose not to utilize their Medicare benefits in order to pursue interventions not provided by the hospice. Individual hospice programs determine how they assess eligibility and provide care to patients not utilizing Medicare to pay for hospice services (CMS, n.d., §418.54).[2] Each medical director should know how to assess eligibility and provide care apart from Medicare requirements.

Patients may become ineligible for continued hospice care due to clinical improvement. A patient admitted following a stroke may unexpectedly recover swallowing ability, markedly extending her prognosis. An elderly patient admitted with rapid weight loss and functional decline may improve following interventions for his complicated grief and depression. In these cases, discharge planning may be simplified by clinical improvement and change in treatment focus.

However, actual improvement may not be so clear. A patient may appear to improve because symptoms are better managed or because side effects from discontinued interventions are resolving. In these situations, "improvement" does not alter the disease-based prognosis. The prognosis and the eligibility are based on the natural history of the underlying condition.

A patient admitted with a diagnosis marked by fluctuations may be admitted during a period of exacerbation when the prognosis looks particularly poor, only to stabilize or appear to improve. Team members may be conflicted about the patient's continued eligibility but reluctant to withdraw services clearly benefitting the patient and family. In a meticulous review of overall prognosis, the physician should help the team discern whether hospice care itself was contributing to the appearance of a prolonged prognosis. One way to accomplish that is to have a careful balance between weaning of services and ongoing assessment of clinical status.

The abrupt discontinuation of support services from a hospice patient could potentially unmask symptoms or lead to sudden clinical decline in patients whose prognoses were artificially inflated by ongoing care, clinical oversight, and emotional and spiritual support. While potentially dramatic, such scenarios are neither kind nor necessary. Instead, the physician can help identify services that support the patient in a way that could simulate improvement in prognosis. The team might provide decreasing assistance with personal care and medication preparation to the level that will occur after discharge. Fans might be used to help a patient who will not qualify for home oxygen therapy but has intermittent shortness of breath. Patients might be encouraged to visit their physician in the office instead of depending on the hospice nurse to relay information. Such maneuvers may clarify discharge planning needs, supporting the patient, family, and hospice team to feel confident that good care is in place. Conversely, these maneuvers may uncover clinical issues that lead to reassessment of plans or prognosis—preventing harm from untimely discharge.

It should be noted that this approach is a sincere effort to confirm prognosis while identifying postdischarge needs. It should not be confused with withholding services that are clearly needed in an attempt to provoke decline only to justify prognosis and eligibility. The physician should help the team develop a plan for downward titration of services that is meaningful in clarifying prognosis and safe for the patient and caregivers.

The Risk of "Automatic" Revocations

Once a hospice chooses to admit a Medicare beneficiary, it may not automatically or routinely discharge the beneficiary at its discretion, even if the care promises to be costly or inconvenient, or the State allows for discharge under State requirements. The election of the hospice benefit is the beneficiary's choice rather than the hospice's choice, and the hospice cannot revoke the beneficiary's election. Neither should the hospice request or demand that the patient revoke his/her election. (CMS, 2012, §20.2.1)

Once a patient has elected to use the Medicare hospice benefit, there are four ways to be discharged alive from hospice care: extended prognosis, transfer out of the hospice area of service, discharge for cause, and revocation. Transfer out of the service area is self-explanatory. Extended prognosis and discharge for cause are discussed elsewhere in this chapter. Revocation occurs at request of the patient (or proxy) and may be requested for a variety of reasons.

The regulations are very clear: Hospices cannot demand that a patient revoke the Medicare hospice benefit. This is one way in which patient autonomy is embedded into the federal regulations themselves. However, there are practices that, if adopted by a hospice, could intimate that revocations are expected. To promote good care for patients, provide support for the hospice team, and comply with regulations, the medical director should be alert to any erroneous assumptions that a patient or family's desire for certain interventions automatically leads to revocation.

Patients and families may desire tests, treatments, or medications that a hospice does not provide. Beneficence, nonmaleficence, and autonomy require that the team, including the medical director, be able to discuss these interventions with patients and families and, when appropriate, explain why the hospice will or will not pay for them as part of the hospice benefit. Otherwise patients may not only fail in exercising autonomous decision making but also be financially burdened, as Medicare instructs patients that "all care that you get for your terminal illness must be given by or arranged by the hospice team" or the patient "might have to pay the entire cost" (CMS, 2013, p. 7). Note, however, that explaining a decision to not cover a particular intervention as part of the hospice benefit is not equivalent to, or always concurrent with, discharge. Patients may remain on service while exploring other care options, and in cases where patients and families find other means to pay for or obtain treatments not included in the hospice plan of care, hospice organizations should be prospectively clear—both internally and with patients and families— about if, why, and under what conditions such arrangements would lead to a recommendation of revocation and how that recommendation might be communicated in a way that honors ethical obligations and regulatory requirements.

The hospice may have a variety of reasons for not providing specific interventions, including ineffectiveness in late-stage disease, greater discomfort than benefit, or lack of meaningful contribution to determining the plan of care. The consideration of expanded diagnostic testing, sophisticated treatments, or atypical interventions should prompt a conversation about patient and family goals of care and concurrence with hospice philosophy. Are the goals focused on symptom management, supportive care, and treatment of reversible complications? Or are they more focused on state-of-the-art disease management, life prolongation, and interventions that offer diminishing likelihood of benefit?

Hospices may consider some interventions incompatible with their philosophies, outside their usual areas of expertise, or beyond their capacity to manage. There may even need to be a conversation as to whether the hospice has the financial wherewithal to pay for very expensive tests or interventions. Beneficence dictates clarification of the patient's and family's goals as opposed to reflexively referring to a list of noncovered interventions. Although it may be tempting to state simply, "We don't pay for that," beneficence also dictates that the physician help the hospice team develop skills and words to explain why the intervention is not part of the hospice plan of care. The patient may still choose to revoke hospice benefits to pursue the intervention, but not because the hospice insinuated that revocation was the expectation.

Discharge for Cause

A hospice may discharge a patient if...the patient's (or other persons in the patient's home) behavior is disruptive, abusive, or uncooperative to the extent that delivery of care to the patient or the ability of the hospice to operate effectively is seriously impaired. (CMS, n.d., §418.26)

Before discharging a patient for cause, the hospice must advise the patient that discharge is being considered, make a serious effort to resolve the problems, ascertain that the proposed discharge is not due to the patient's use of necessary hospice services, and document the problems and efforts made to resolve them in the medical record. This is not only a regulatory requirement but also the most beneficent and nonmaleficent process as well.

The role of the medical director may vary depending on the circumstances leading to this rare and extreme response. If the behavior of the patient is leading to discharge, however, the physician should consider medical reasons leading to disruptive behaviors, including neurologic injury, substance abuse, delirium, and mental health diagnoses. While competent patients may decline intervention for any or all of these, medical assessment and intervention should be offered when appropriate. If the caregivers, other members of the household, or visitors are the source of the disruptive behaviors, medical evaluation can be recommended and support offered. But neither the hospice team nor the medical director has consent to treat anyone other than the patient.

Hospices may make extraordinary attempts to manage disruptive behaviors—placing "lock boxes" in the home to eliminate medication diversion, making joint visits to provide a "buddy system" for staff, developing contracts for acceptable behaviors by patient or caregivers, and even calling ahead to give patients and families notice to remove threatening people or items prior to a visit. The medical director may be helpful not only in contributing to developing the plan of care but also in helping the hospice team maintain healthy boundaries while simultaneously investing additional time and effort into delivering care. The medical director may also promote the safety and integrity of clinical staff by advocating for discharge when abuse of staff and disruptions of care cannot be mitigated by the measures attempted by the hospice.

If the behaviors include repeated use of medical services that are unknown or unauthorized by the hospice, this could also be considered disruptive to care. Any decision to use this as justification for possible discharge for cause, however, should include conversation with the medical director about medical necessity for the services obtained, options for including them in the plan of care (when reasonable to do so), and creative options for delivering hospice care that might reduce or eliminate the need for the unauthorized services.

ADMISSION, TREATMENT, AND DISCHARGE DECISIONS: PHILOSOPHICAL AND FINANCIAL ISSUES

Clinical effectiveness, cost effectiveness, and the responsibility to honor patients' wishes—beneficence, stewardship and distributive justice, and respect for autonomy—must all be considered when determining the interventions that the hospice can provide.

> [D]rugs and biologicals related to the palliation and management of the terminal illness and related conditions, as identified in the hospice plan of care, must be provided by the hospice while the patient is under hospice care. (CMS, n.d., §418.106)
>
> Only drugs...which are used primarily for the relief of pain and symptom control related to the individual's terminal illness are covered. (CMS, n.d., §418.202)
>
> *Palliative care* means patient and family-centered care that optimizes quality of life by anticipating, preventing, and treating suffering. Palliative care throughout the continuum of illness involves addressing physical, intellectual, emotional, social, and spiritual needs and to facilitate patient autonomy, access to information, and choice. (CMS, n.d., §418.3)

The CoPs note that hospices provide palliative rather than curative care (CMS, n.d., §418.24). Palliative care includes symptom management and support for improved quality of life and is "applicable early in the course of illness, in conjunction with other therapies that are intended to prolong life" (WHO, 2002, p. 84). But the distinction between life prolongation and symptom management blurs when interventions are employed in an attempt to modify disease to control symptoms and prolong life. When utilized with conventional measures to manage symptoms, it can be impossible to differentiate the effects of disease-modifying therapies and standard hospice medications.

From a clinical viewpoint, this is not problematic. Medications and treatments can be utilized while effective and discontinued when they become ineffective, harmful, or burdensome. The provision of all possible interventions could make it easy to avoid issues surrounding limited prognosis, impending death, and cost. But from a strict disease-management perspective, there are few impediments to the idea of providing palliative care and life-prolonging care simultaneously.

Hospices, however, have significant dilemmas with the differentiation, or lack thereof, between palliative and curative interventions—between the intent to manage symptoms or to extend life expectancy. If an intervention has no reasonable expectation of promoting cure, then is it, by definition, palliative? Is the hospice obligated to provide any interventions and medications that are palliative under this definition? Or is an intervention palliative when it is reasonable and necessary to prevent or alleviate suffering, typically by palliating specific symptoms?

Philosophically, a hospice's primary mission may be to alleviate pain and symptoms. Staff may find it easier to determine that anticancer interventions are primarily disease modifying with minimal potential of reducing symptoms. But they may struggle to discriminate between disease modification and symptom management when considering cardiac, pulmonary, and neurologic medications. The medical director should not only understand the individual hospice's philosophy regarding disease-modifying treatments but also bring knowledge of pharmacology and pathophysiology to bear on those decisions in order to provide the best care and symptom management to patients.

Financially, the difficulties are often more complex. Interventions such as chemotherapy, inotropic support, and total parenteral nutrition are usually too costly to continue when effectiveness is in doubt. The medical director may be called upon to determine whether such interventions are achieving the expected benefits, help the staff prepare to explain why interventions are not indicated or helpful anymore, and visit patients and families to discuss goals of care.

Conflict can arise at numerous points. The attending physician, hospice staff, patient, and family may have very different assessments as to the actual or expected benefits of continuing an intervention or medication. The hospice may not be willing to pay for high-cost interventions yielding little benefit but not want to anger the attending physician who wants to continue them. Hospice staff may believe that a patient will struggle for lack of support after opting to revoke the hospice benefit to pursue these interventions, but they may be reluctant to remind the patient and family of their financial responsibility for interventions not coordinated by the hospice. There may also be a concern that donors would not approve of spending charitable donations to pay for costly interventions for a very few patients.

The medical director is not likely to be the one and only arbiter of these conflicts. However, the medical director should expect to be involved, especially if the determination of clinical benefit needs to be defined, discussed, and included in decisions about the hospice plan of care.

Admitting a Patient Receiving Interventions Not Typically Provided by the Hospice

When a patient is referred to hospice with unusual, high-cost, or high-complexity interventions in place, more than philosophy and finances are involved. There are also issues of habit, familiarity, and trust. Patients may be accustomed to structuring their lives around regular clinic appointments, blood tests, and other tests and interventions. They have often come to know and feel supported by the medical personnel associated with these interventions. They may not have previous experience with the hospice in which they enroll—or any hospice. Therefore, patients may not be ready to let go of everything and everyone that has gotten them to this point and trust a team they do not know.

Advising a patient to relinquish medications, testing, or interventions that he has come to see as essential to living may be difficult. Successfully advising a patient you do not know may be fraught with distrust and fear that death will be hastened. After all, he may believe that these are the very things that kept him alive this long—that stopping them up is tantamount to "giving up," even if they have lost effectiveness.

While the interventions may be unnecessary (even harmful), refusing admission to the patient until the interventions are no longer desired may deprive the patient and family of the very help they need to acknowledge that the interventions are no longer useful. If the hospice staff can manage the complexity of the care, the medical director may be able to help the patient, family, and hospice team structure a plan that builds trust. By agreeing to make incremental changes and assess the effects of those changes, patients and families can develop trust with the hospice team and simultaneously better evaluate the benefits and burdens of the interventions.

For example, a patient may have become accustomed to having blood counts checked weekly, even though transfusions have only been needed every 6–8 weeks. The hospice may propose to reduce routine surveillance studies when symptoms are not occurring. The medical director can help the staff develop and explain a plan to incrementally decrease testing, assess for subtle symptoms before they become severe, and reduce the burden on the patient and family.

If interventions are more complex, then the hospice will have to determine whether increased education or adjustments to visit schedules would increase the ability of the hospice team to serve the patient and family. The medical director can help the hospice determine whether such interventions are becoming a standard of care in the community and should be included in hospice services or whether they are unusual and likely to remain outliers.

Although hospice organizations are not to base admission, certification, or discharge decisions on the costs of care, providing some interventions may be financially intimidating. (These interventions are often life prolonging or highly complex, making cost only one of the issues.) Some may be excluded from a hospice plan of care due to creating financial hardship. Medical directors may need to advocate for the inclusion of some higher cost interventions, however, if they are effective at managing symptoms.

Hospices should also determine how they will provide care to patients eligible for hospice but not choosing to elect their hospice benefits in favor of continuing interventions beyond the hospice's ability to provide. Medical directors should be familiar with how these decisions are made in their hospices and what services are available to these patients and families. As hospice staff may find it difficult to tell patients and families that hospice services will not include some interventions, even those previously considered routine, medical directors should also help hospice staff learn the skills and words to explain these decisions to patients and families.

Initiating Interventions Not Typically Provided by the Hospice

Questions about interventions may arise in the midst of care. A patient feeling better after symptoms are controlled may become interested in starting or resuming interventions that had been previously offered or discontinued. A patient may also experience a clinical complication that could require advanced, but costly or complex, interventions. By staying abreast of advances or changes in standard medical interventions, the medical director can help her organization balance the indications for, and expected effectiveness of, such interventions with the hospice's philosophy and financial capabilities.

The medical director may also help establish the parameters for a *time-limited trial* of an intervention with uncertain effectiveness or possible intolerable side effects. This could include a course of antibiotics to determine whether an infection is reversible, inotropic therapy to see whether cardiac symptoms improve, or chemotherapy to see whether the medication is tolerated. The results of the trial would then dictate whether the intervention is continued. If the intervention is beneficial to the point of extending life expectancy, eligibility can be re-evaluated.

Determining Which Interventions a Hospice Covers: Effectiveness, Cost, and "Relatedness"

Medicare covers...[d]rugs for symptom control or pain relief [and] [a]ny other Medicare-covered services needed to manage your pain and other symptoms related to your terminal illness, as recommended by your hospice team. (CMS, 2013, p. 6)

Hospices are charged with providing coverage for pain and symptom management medications, but there is neither consensus about, nor guidelines defining, which medications are included in that directive. As previously noted, the advent of interventions that modify diseases in an attempt to both prolong life and control symptoms has clouded the distinction between curative therapies, palliative (noncurative) management of diseases, and palliation of symptoms. Furthermore, the intersections of various diseases can make it nearly impossible to determine how related a symptom is to one diagnosis compared to another. And the causes of a terminal condition may arguably be "related" differently to that condition as compared to the resulting symptoms of the condition. Therefore, the role of the medical director may include not only the assessment of effectiveness but also the determination of "relatedness."

"Relatedness" can be particularly daunting when conditions are intertwined physiologically, but common sense dictates that they are too distinct to consider them related from a treatment standpoint. For example, heart and lung diseases are often related due to pathology and reciprocal effects. While hospices provide "services needed to manage your pain and other symptoms related to your terminal illness" (CMS, 2013, p. 6), it stretches credulity to think that a hospice program should routinely cover long-acting beta agonists and steroids for shortness of breath due to chronic obstructive lung disease when a patient is admitted with cardiomyopathy and heart failure.

It can be even more difficult to reconcile "relatedness" when considering the causes of a diagnosis and the resulting symptoms of a diagnosis. Does "palliation and management of the terminal illness and related conditions" and treatments "used primarily for the relief of pain and symptom control related to the individual's terminal illness" imply that hospices should cover surgical repair of all hip fractures, treatment of urinary tract infections, and wound care equally? Is "relatedness" so global that almost all interventions are covered for this broad diagnosis? Or are some diagnoses related but sufficiently distinct such that it changes the responsibility of the hospice to manage them?

Hospices answer these questions differently depending on their philosophies, resources, staff expertise, community standards, and interpretation of federal and state regulations. The medical director has a pivotal role in helping to delineate clinical effectiveness, cost effectiveness, "relatedness," and need for staff education.

If a hospice determines that an intervention is not covered as part of the hospice plan of care, hospice staff must explain to a patient why it is not covered and what options the patient has. The patient may opt to revoke, perhaps choosing to pay privately for hospice care. The patient may also opt to pay for the intervention and continue hospice benefits. Regardless of the patient's choice, these conversations can be difficult for hospice staff. Hospice staff may be reluctant to tell a patient or family that hospice services do not include all the interventions they desire. The physician should help the hospice team develop skills and language to be more comfortable having these conversations.

When a hospice determines that an intervention is not covered as part of the hospice plan of care, a patient may opt to revoke to continue traditional treatments. This decision should be part of an overall plan to pursue a different direction of care. Hospices should not discharge patients or encourage them to revoke to pay for a prescription or procedure, only to re-elect hospice benefits in a day or two. Medical directors can help the hospice team review the overall direction of care and make certain that the hospice is in full compliance with the spirit of the regulations.

ADMISSION, TREATMENT, AND DISCHARGE DECISIONS: CLINICAL ISSUES

Admitting a Patient With Complex Needs

Family Conflict

Although the members of the hospice team are usually quite skilled in helping to resolve a variety of conflicts, the medical director may need to participate in family meetings about goals of care, prognostication, interventions, and medications. The medical director may also be able to help the team maintain perspective about the difference between problems that can be solved and problems resulting from years of coping and communication styles in a family.

Physical Abuse and Neglect

There are legal requirements regarding the reporting of abuse and neglect, which hospice social workers are likely to know well. The medical director may need to visit a patient to evaluate and document potential injuries. Some local social service agencies rely on hospices to help resolve or monitor situations in which a hospice patient is the subject of abuse and/or neglect. In addition to participating in team discussions about physical care and safety, the medical director may also be able to help the team members discern whether they are being drawn into a more custodial role than is appropriate.

Symptoms Requiring Multidrug Regimens, High-Dose Opioids, or Parenteral Medications

Patients requiring high-dose opioids also require meticulous monitoring of pain levels, medication side effects, toxicities, and need for adjustments. Although the patient's attending physician may perform these tasks, it is increasingly expected that the hospice medical director will assist with, or even assume full responsibility for, managing complicated medication regimens, high-dose opioids, and parenteral medications. In addition to providing medical oversight, the medical director may also need to educate the team about these modalities.

Drug Misuse, Abuse, or Diversion

When there is medication mismanagement by the patient or family, the medical director may help set expectations and limits to manage symptoms while limiting the risk of misuse, abuse, or diversion. When misuse by the patient is a concern, the medical director may be able to assess the symptoms and prescribe a regimen that addresses them more effectively. For example, a patient who is using increasing does of opioids to manage anxiety may benefit from a change in medication as well as more intensive emotional or spiritual support. Concerns about abuse or diversion may require more secure storage of medications, once-a-day medication that is administered in the presence of hospice staff, contracts for safe use, and an agreement among all treating physicians that only one will prescribe controlled substances. The medical director can help the team develop care plans that manage symptoms as effectively as possible within legal and regulatory constraints.

Resuscitation

Some patients may want hospice care while also desiring resuscitation—or feeling unable to decline resuscitation. The medical director may discuss goals of care, explain expected outcomes on interventions, and document patient preferences. The medical director may also encourage hospice staff to find satisfaction in honoring a patient's wishes if they become disheartened at the continued desire for resuscitative measures.

Honoring Patient and Family Goals That Seem Unsafe, Unattainable, or Unwise

Hospice teams usually excel in providing care within the context of the values and preferences of patients and families. However, they encounter challenges and frustration when these values and preferences result in inadequate symptom management, support, safety, or achievement of goals. The medical director can help create the best plan allowed by the patient and family while protecting vulnerable patients from abuse and neglect and supporting the team.

For example, a patient who allows less than optimal symptom control may not only suffer physical distress but also engender feelings of failure in family and hospice caregivers. This could be the patient who takes subtherapeutic doses of pain medication or declines diuretics despite massive edema. The medical director can support patient autonomy and praise others for doing the same while concurrently acknowledging and addressing the team's sense of inadequacy that can arise from not being allowed to do more. The medical director may be also able to help the team develop an approach to talking with the patient about treatment concerns, benefits and side effects of alternative regimens, and the suffering of family members.

Sometimes a patient will opt for a plan that appears to be unsafe, such as living alone or in unsanitary conditions. The medical director should help determine whether the patient has the capacity to make such decisions. If decision-making capacity is intact, then the hospice team must determine how much support it can, and is willing to, provide to maintain the plan. Are there additional financial or staff resources that can be utilized to help the patient? Is the hospice willing to dedicate these resources to a plan that appears destined to fail in the name of patient autonomy? Or are these resources scarce, making it harder to justify their use in a futile effort to sustain one patient's plan a little longer? The medical director helps the team analyze the answers to these questions. The medical director can also help the hospice organization develop an overall approach to assessing the medical, ethical, and legal aspects of these situations.

In some circumstances, hospice team members may have objections to the care desired by patients or families. For example, someone may object to providing care to patients with illnesses that are not typically seen as terminal or that appear to be treatable. The hospice team may struggle with providing care to a young patient with refractory anorexia nervosa because of the patient's youth and the mental health diagnosis as the etiology of a terminal condition. The medical director must explain the medical aspects of the disease to the team, support the team members who provide care, and help the organization address the concerns of those who request to not be involved in the care of the patient.

CARE IN AN INPATIENT HOSPICE UNIT

There are times when patients require care in an inpatient hospice. One of the challenges in this setting is to maintain the interdisciplinary aspect of hospice care even as the patient is in need of increased medical care to maintain comfort. Physicians play a pivotal role in such inpatient care—assessing, diagnosing, treating, and documenting. But the medical director must discourage the evolution of a physician-based hierarchy that focuses on medical care to the point of diminishing the roles of the other team members. Patients and families should be able to depend on the whole team for information and support without perceiving the care as dependent on the presence of the physician. The hospice team should also maintain its balance of disciplines to avoid becoming overly reliant on the physician for assessment of the patient, communication with the patient or family, and planning for return to home.

Medical Direction: Balancing the Needs of Inpatients and Patients at Home

When the hospice medical director oversees medical care in both an inpatient and home hospice settings, it is necessary to address needs of the patients and staff in those areas simultaneously. For the good of patient care and team cohesion, the medical director must ensure that hospice physicians serve patients in both care environments, without favoring one or the other, while facilitating communication between teams in both settings. For example, home hospice teams may think that the inpatient team has a poor understanding of the significant limitations in care that can be delivered in some patients' homes. Questions about why a patient requires inpatient care or plans to return the patient home sooner than expected may imply to the home hospice team that the inpatient stay was unnecessary. The medical director can remind the home hospice team that the questions prior to inpatient admission do not constitute criticism. Instead, they may help preserve continuity for the patient and family and speed symptom management by reducing the likelihood of duplicating previous therapeutic interventions.

Conversely, inpatient staff may wonder why a patient transferred from home with symptoms became comfortable with minimal intervention. The medical director can point out that entering a calm atmosphere with around-the-clock support and professional hospice care can reduce anxiety, soothe fears, and allow interventions to work that had been thwarted by the stress and anxiety in the home environment.

COMBINING MEDICAL DIRECTION AND INTERDISCIPLINARY TEAMWORK

The medical director is a member of the interdisciplinary team and, according to the CoPs, is also responsible for certification, recertification, and oversight of the medical plan of care. Thus, some tasks are shared with the team while others are not. It is important to keep these in perspective.

Certification Is Not a Team Decision

It is the responsibility of the medical director to certify a hospice patient. Information from the team is critical in assessing symptoms,

functional status, and goals of care. But the determination of prognosis and subsequent certification is a decision reserved for the medical
director. Consensus is valuable when it can be achieved, but it is not
required. If the hospice team believes that a patient should be certified
and the medical director disagrees, then they must discuss these dispa-
rate assessments. The medical director may not be aware of information
that changes the prognostic estimate. The team may be leery of not certifying the patient due to the level of need and the complexity of services
required. The patient may appear frail but not have a diagnosis that supports a limited prognosis. The medical director must weigh these issues
and determine eligibility for certification. He or she cannot cede the
decision to the team.

The opposite situation can also occur. A team may not think that certification is indicated, perhaps because decline is not persistent or because
impairments appear to be chronic. If the medical director believes that the
physical assessment, medical literature, and other clinical factors support a
prognosis of 6 months or less, this information should be shared with the
team and certification provided.

Plan of Care Is Not a Medical Decision

The medical director has responsibility for oversight of the medical plan of
care. But the overall plan of care is developed by the hospice team. When
the medical director and the team are weighing the benefits and burdens of
medical care options vis-à-vis other goals, preferences, obligations, or limitations of the patient and family, the medical director does not have greater
authority than other members of the team. In fact, the medical issues may
be superseded by a variety of emotional, spiritual, social, financial, and
even legal issues. It behooves the medical director to maintain some humil-
ity about his or her role in the development of the comprehensive care plan
while supporting the team in working to their highest standards.

CONCLUSION

The role of the medical director has evolved to include direct medical care
of patients, medical oversight of all patient care, regulatory compliance,
staff training and support, and, in many hospices, organizational leadership. Beneficence and nonmaleficence dictate good care and support of the
patient, family, interdisciplinary team, and hospice organization. Patient

autonomy is to be respected in treatment decisions and support for choices. Distributive justice demands that the medical director maintain regulatory compliance and fiscal awareness so that the organization is able to serve the needs of all patients and families. The medical director must participate in decision making and provision of care that upholds the highest ethical standards in all of these practices.

NOTES

1. These guidelines were intended to be inclusionary; patients who met the guidelines were deemed to have a prognosis of 6 months or less if the disease ran its usual course. Developed in 1995 and refined in 1996 through review and consensus by hospice and palliative medicine clinicians, there were few studies available at the time elucidating how to best estimate prognoses in conditions such as advanced heart failure, chronic lung disease, end-stage liver disease, and chronic renal failure.
2. See also the final rule with comments as published in the 2008 *Federal Register* (73[109], pp. 32088–32220): "Since election requirement is particular to the Medicare and Medicaid hospice benefits, hospices are free to establish a similar starting point for non-Medicare and Medicaid patients in their own policies, based on the needs of the hospice, its community, and any applicable State and local laws and regulations" (p. 32102).

REFERENCES

Christakis, N. A., & Lamont, E. B. (2000). Extent and determinants of error in doctors' prognoses in terminally ill patients: Prospective cohort study. *British Medical Journal, 320*(7233), 469–472.

Centers for Medicare and Medicaid Services (CMS). (2009). *Hospice data: 1998-2008*. Retrieved April 2014, from http://www.cms.gov/Medicare/Medicare-Fee-for-Service-Payment/Hospice/Downloads/Hospice_Data_1998-2008.zip.

Centers for Medicare and Medicaid Services (CMS). (2012). Coverage of hospice services under hospital insurance. In *Medicare Benefit Policy Manual* (Rev. 156, Ch. 9, § 20.2.1). Retrieved April 2014, from http://www.cms.gov/Regulations-and-Guidance/Guidance/Manuals/Downloads/bp102c09.pdf.

Centers for Medicare and Medicaid Services (CMS). (2013). *Medicare hospice benefits* (CMS Product 02154). Baltimore, MD: Centers for Medicare and Medicaid Services. Retrieved April 2014, from http://www.medicare.gov/Pubs/pdf/02154.pdf.

Centers for Medicare and Medicaid Services (CMS). (n.d.). *CMS Hospice conditions for coverage and conditions of participation*. Retrieved April 2014, from https://www.cms.gov/CFCsAndCoPs/05_Hospice.asp.

Stuart, B., Alexander, C., Arenella, C., Connor, S., Herbst, L., Jones, D., et al. on behalf of the NHO Standards and Accreditation Committee. (1996). *Medical guidelines for determining prognosis in selected non-cancer diseases* (2nd ed.). Arlington, VA: National Hospice Organization.

World Health Organization (WHO). (2002). *National cancer control programmes: Policies and managerial guidelines* (2nd ed.). Geneva, Switzerland: World Health Organization.

CHAPTER 5

The Interdisciplinary Team—Integrating Moral Reflection and Deliberation

TERRY ALTILIO AND NESSA COYLE

They don't ease the transition from a former life to a dying life—they don't pay enough attention to the transition—as if the person did not have a life before. They are fine when you are actually dying but [show] a rigidity beforehand. They seem to really care about you when you are dying.

—A bereaved wife, 10 days after the death of her husband

This chapter focuses on moral reflection and deliberation as core processes in the work of an interdisciplinary team. These core processes allow us to examine and reflect on the work of the team from the perspective of our practice—as individuals, as part of a team, as part of an institution, and as part of multiple cultures.

Palliative and hospice teams are challenged to balance the varied cultures, values, and communication styles that converge within the team itself as well as between team, patient and family. Paying attention to the systems in which teams practice is necessary in order to ensure that unspoken and unconscious forces do not cause iatrogenic suffering to the patient and family and within the team itself. Care and service to patients and families are impacted on a day-by-day basis by forces beyond the team dynamics and that of individual members. Palliative consult services may, for example, be implicitly or explicitly coerced by hospital pressures such as facilitating early discharges, "getting the DNR (do not resuscitate order)," and rapid transition to hospice. Time frames may be based on institutional priorities rather than the readiness of patients and their families. Hospice teams may be driven to set expectations for patients and families that mirror the philosophical or economic boundaries of the organization rather than providing services that acknowledge and reflect an acceptance of the wide range of choices and possibilities open to individuals as life draws to an end.

As a consequence, teams may be "quietly shaped" and reshaped by external forces that go unrecognized. Over time, some can become frozen, building walls to preserve a comfort with the familiar. Others recognize and relish the creative tension that comes from a changing environment and the balance between harmony and disharmony. Through reflection and thoughtful deliberation, we have the potential to create a safe space to examine our work and process, recognize and be energized by the need to change or adapt, or perhaps recommit to current values and practice.

This chapter also reviews some of the tensions and opportunities created by societal, political, and institutional changes, as well as rapid advances in science, medicine, and technology as they impact the work of the team. The purpose throughout is to use this chapter to model a process of reflection and deliberation. Rather than providing answers, the intent is to isolate select aspects of the changing practice milieu and their potential to impact the individual and team values of authenticity, competence, and fidelity. Implicit is a shared responsibility to keep patients' interests primary, maintain mutual trust and confidence, and carry out commitments with faithful attention (Davenport, 1997). Implicit also is the mandate to explore our collaborations, compliance, and complicity and to "do no harm" whether to self, patient and family or to colleagues, within the team and beyond. Through reflection and deliberation team function can be enhanced and the impact of institutional forces or unspoken beliefs and fears can be brought into the open, reflected upon, and their influence explored and actions considered.

MORAL REFLECTION AND DELIBERATION

Moral reflection and deliberation are processes that can infuse thinking, dialogue, and decision making at varying levels in the work of hospice and palliative care. We may reflect on the team itself—the value judgments that permeate our process, the power balances, voices loud and soft or the values that inform decisions with patients, families, or their intimate network. We may reflect on external processes and forces that subtly or blatantly influence our direction. Hermsen and Ten Have (2005) integrate the concept of reflexivity as a significant aspect of effective teams.

A concept particularly relevant to reflectivity in hospice and palliative teams is "reflexivity." West, relates reflexivity to the group's overt reflection and communication about "objectives, strategies and processes, adapting them to current or anticipated circumstances" (West, 2000, p. 296). While "reflexivity" has many definitions, the description by Opie (1997) relates well to the focus of this chapter. Opie describes reflexivity as a "meta-process involving a conscious critique of the way members think about the process of their work" (p. 265). Moral reflection and deliberation are processes that inform this "conscious critique."

Hermsen and Ten have describe the moral dimensions of reflexivity as a focus on value judgments. This is an especially intricate aspect of teamwork in palliative and hospice care, as the values of team members, patients, families, and institutions converge around decisions and goals that are often full of uncertainties and provoke complex emotions. In the setting of decisions that are value laden and informed by the boundaries and uncertainty of medical knowledge, patients and families and colleagues need to be able to count on a full and transparent team process of reflection and deliberate care planning.

Deliberation is described as a path to reflect upon that eventually leads to shared interprofessional decisions which are balanced and prudent (Gracia, 2001, 2002; Hermsen & Ten Have, 2005). The deliberation process at its best and most challenging is a dialectic that invites different perspectives for analysis and critique in an environment of listening and mutual respect. "Moral deliberation is grounded in the assumption that good care gets defined and re-defined in concrete situations" where a dialogue occurs between ethical principles, professional standards, constraints, and the unique circumstances of each narrative (Abma, Molewijk, & Widdershoven, 2009, p. 222).

While many deliberation processes are led by formally trained leaders and follow specific models, the process advocated here is one of shared responsibility for questioning and learning in a setting of respect and psychological safety (Edmondson, 2008). In this manner, new meanings, perspectives, and behaviors are explored—perhaps to the end of mediating suffering in clinicians as well as the patients and families they care for. Where respect and psychological safety are absent, this process is not appropriate and can create disharmony and an assault to fundamental beliefs. This may occur in the absence of a "holding environment" that supports and sustains as beliefs, values, emotions, and behaviors are explored. It is assumed that "flash points," or points of dissension during the evolution and daily work of a team, may be sparked by internal dynamics, as represented by the narrative that follows, or by external mandates that impact team and individual equilibrium, as exemplified by the second narrative. Reflection and deliberation offer an opportunity to deconstruct such flash points.

Narrative: "This is just wrong—I won't be part of it"

A young physician from a different continent and culture was accepted into a palliative care fellowship program. The patient population he encountered was varied, and his training involved not only pain and symptom management but also goals of care discussions, including options and choices. Part of this spectrum was guidance and support to patients, families, and staff when discontinuing life support, including ventilator support, was the plan of care.

The palliative care team experienced such cases to be challenging and emotionally difficult, but at the same time they supported the rights of patients or their surrogates to make these decisions. The team was unaware of this fellow's strongly held views on discontinuing life supports until they became abundantly clear when the palliative care staff was reviewing a recent patient's terminal extubation. This team review was a normal process to give the involved staff an opportunity to debrief the experience as well as the process. With obvious strong emotion the fellow who had not been involved in the terminal extubation described it as "morally wrong," "pulling the plug," and something he could neither condone nor be part of. The fellow's explosive and unexpected outburst was startling and upsetting to the team. Representative of many different cultures and belief systems—and usually a source of support for each other—they became quiet and felt under attack.

Analysis

Using a model of reflection and deliberation, the team leader, with support from the social worker and chaplain, asked the team members to consider their own cultures and spiritual beliefs and tensions they might experience when end-of-life choices caused internal conflict or confusion. The need to be true to oneself and to recognize one's own moral stance and sense of personal integrity and how that affected interactions with patients and families was explored. For example, would personal views affect a trainee's or staff member's ability to counsel about the full range of options and choices around this aspect of end-of-life care? Did all disciplines have similar conflicts or did the difference in roles and responsibilities influence the degree and direction of moral conflict? Did physicians who order or perform an extubation have a unique response because of the quality of their participation? And what of the suffering or moral conflict of nurses, whose roles often involve long and intimate relationships with patients and their families, including providing direct physical care?

The fellow concerned could not reconcile his moral convictions with the practice of terminal extubation and consequently felt unable to counsel and support patients and families around this choice. While respecting the rights of the fellow to hold personal values, the team reflected on whether these values could be accommodated within the team or the specialty, so that harm to self and others was minimized and patient care and autonomy uncompromised. They discussed the place of conscientious objection and explored whether clinician autonomy and personal moral conviction are truly respected when they are expected to seek another to provide the "morally objectionable" service. The need for openness was the strong message, yet important questions emerged. To what degree does palliative care training assume acceptance of certain beliefs and values and expect allegiance? What is the range of therapeutic options expected to be available within the skill set of palliative care specialists? What is the risk to team members when they raise issues of a complex moral and ethical nature or question whether teams can truly be egalitarian when roles and culpability may be so different; when some bear the responsibility to act and others to provide a supportive presence and bear witness to what is happening?

Most training programs in hospice and palliative care are in tertiary settings and, consequently, this particular situation may be less likely in home hospice. However, as norms of society change, parallel situations may evolve in the home setting. For example, the choice to elect physician-assisted death (variously termed aid in dying, physician-assisted suicide, death with dignity, etc.) has brought similar challenges to the values, beliefs, and practices of teams in the states where it has been legalized.

Reflection and deliberation are a way of talking "together" rather than talking "about." They are different. The process of reflection and deliberation described earlier explored individual cultural, spiritual, and moral values and how these values affected patient care, leading to greater awareness of forces that may be "bubbling under the surface." The *individual* psychic and spiritual lives of team members present opportunities for connection—as well as risks for disconnection—between team members that can affect the ability of the team to function well and offer integrated, effective palliative care. Teams also have a *collective* psychic and spiritual life, which was called into question in this instance. Engaging in reflection and deliberation revealed to this team the importance of exploring the assumed values that may or may not inform this collective psychic and spiritual life. The team process generated by the emotion and conflict of the individual fellow was followed by discussions, mentoring, and counseling of the fellow by

the service chief. This fellow eventually redirected his training from palliative and end-of-life care to pain management—a specialty that allowed him
to treat the suffering of patients and families in a less conflicted manner.

We began our discussion of reflection and deliberation with a narrative
describing the distress of an individual morally unable to participate in a
specific intervention—withdrawal of respiratory support at end of life—
requested by the family. The following narrative exemplifies moral distress
consequent to a change in agency structure and regulation. This created
feelings of helplessness in team members, perhaps mimicking the sense of
powerlessness we sometimes see in patients and families.

Narrative: "This is not what I signed up for"

A small not-for-profit home hospice program had a change of leadership reflecting a
mandate to grow revenue by significantly increasing the patient census. The program
rapidly increased in size, the nurses' case loads expanded, and nurses were unable to
spend as much time with patients as in the past. Many clinicians experienced this
change as a profound personal loss, and they believed that the integrity of the care they
were able to provide was compromised. Concurrently, the roles of each discipline within
the team became more clearly delineated. Nurses, for example, who saw their role as providing comprehensive total patient care, were asked to take on more task-specific functions. Concomitantly, the change in the Medicare Conditions of Participation (CoPs)
required that physicians or nurse practitioners make specifically timed visits to "recer-
tify" patients as still being hospice eligible, rather than visiting the patient based on an
identified unmet need. These internal and external forces disrupted the team structure
and equilibrium. Individual clinicians felt their personal and professional motivation
for choosing to work in hospice and palliative care was challenged, and their sense of
personal fulfillment diminished.

Analysis

Such external (e.g., CoPs) and institutional challenges to the structure, cohesion, and leadership of a team can create disequilibrium and a need for reor-
ganization. These dynamics often go unnamed and unrecognized, creating
smoldering emotions that can erupt at times of stress. The sequence of exter-
nal/institutional challenges→unrecognized disequilibrium→smoldering emotions may contribute to demoralization or moral distress, as team members
engage in the profound and personal work of palliative and hospice care and

struggle to consider a response that weighs both professional and personal risk and benefit. Demoralization can be described as an expression of existential distress exemplified by hopelessness, loss of meaning, and a subjective sense of incompetence (Connor & Walton, 2011). Moral distress, on the other hand, may include the physical and emotional suffering that is experienced when constraints, either internal or external, prevent the clinician from following the course of action that he or she believes is right (Hamric, Davis, & Childress, 2006). Reflection and deliberation in a case such as this one can be extremely helpful. Individual team members may invite discussion of the impact on their work and brainstorm to make suggestions or adapt practice patterns based on the identified common goals and values that connect both practitioners and administrators. Such common goals and values might include patient satisfaction or diminishing the moral distress of practitioners, thereby enhancing the well-being of staff and minimizing turnover. Reflection and deliberation do not end in conversation. Often action is necessary to mediate the suffering of staff and the suffering of patients and families.

WHO GETS WHAT AND WHEN? WHEN IS "MORE" LESS AND "LESS" MORE? THE IMPACT OF BUSINESS, POLITICS, AND ECONOMICS ON THE TEAM, PATIENT AND FAMILY

Since the inception of hospice in the United States, programs have proliferated. Patients and families transitioning from acute or chronic care environments into hospice care can be faced with complex and emotionally infused decisions about resuscitation, artificial hydration and nutrition, dialysis, or (dis)continuing expensive medications that may not be covered by the hospice benefit. Economic pressures are pervasive. Clinicians and systems struggle to meet changing needs in the setting of a broken health care system without a shared vision and mission. Hospitals are pressured to discharge quickly and to move patients to the most "appropriate setting."

The following narrative reflects one patient's interpretation of the competing forces that have "crept like a fog" into the US health care system.

Narrative: The "Safety" of Competing Motivations

Mr. C, a 64-year-old African American educator diagnosed with pancreatic cancer, has been asked about resuscitation and urged to consider care in a hospice residence. He understands that he is coming to the end of his life but does not want that process

hastened and believes that resuscitation may extend his life in a manner that is acceptable to him. He is ambivalent about hospice and worries that his death may be hastened
because potentially reversible situations will not be aggressively treated. As he ponders
the forces that influence his life, he weighs his worry about hospice and his perspective
about insurance companies, their values and motivations. He says that the hospice residence will want to keep their bed filled, and this need will counterbalance the benefit his
death would bring to the insurance company, who would prefer not to continue to pay for
his care. He is hopeful that these opposing forces will converge to protect him.

Analysis

Mr. C's focus on the ways that the economic interests of others affect his
prospects for getting care may strike some as cynical. In the view of others
this narrative reflects a poignant and honest perspective, especially given
the historical treatment of African Americans by the medical system and
the vulnerability of those living with serious illness.

How care organizations have integrated responses to changing economic
pressures into their approaches to care of patients potentially impacts the
integrity of the institution *and* the integrity of teams that plan and provide
care to patients and families. Do teams inadvertently support a belief system in which the ability to persuade patients to sign a DNR order is considered an important clinical competency, and the percentage of patients on
a care service with signed DNR orders is an indicator of care quality? If so,
have these teams become unreflectively complicit in cost-saving measures
contributing to the financial health of their care organizations?

Alternately, do hospice program efforts to remove barriers to accessing
hospice care by implementing "open access" policies and enrolling patients
who still wish to receive resuscitation and artificial hydration and nutrition indicate that we have strayed from our mission of embracing dying as
a normal, natural process at the end of life? Or do such policies reflect an
increasing awareness that hard and fast rules are often incongruous with
the evolving science, experience, and process of individuals from different
cultural and spiritual beliefs as they approach the end of life?

Many changes in hospice intake guidelines are designed to remove
barriers so that more patients are served and length of stay is extended.
This has potential benefits for the patients and families and for the business model. Yet clinicians and teams may be confused by a mission that
has become "diluted" by extending end-of-life care to those who choose
to receive life-prolonging treatments during the last phase of life. In this

setting of complex economic, clinical, and political forces hospice care has become an industry—and is referred to as that—whether for profit or not for profit. The term "industry" is jarring to some, as it emphasizes the business aspects of care delivery, while, for most, hospice at its core is about relationship and personhood.

The convergence of a multiplicity of forces arising from phenomena like financial performance targets, ever-evolving regulatory requirements, and shifting economic and political winds in health care "marketplaces" can produce insidious effects within organizations. These effects may influence not only the organizational environment in which teams practice, but even the microenvironments within the teams themselves. Teams that are able to attune themselves to these forces create another kind of opportunity for reflection and deliberation, one that identifies openings for reciprocal influence and opportunities for advocacy on behalf of patients and colleagues alike. The insight and action arising from this process can, in turn, prevent the slow erosion of a team's sense of integrity and "soul."

For example, hospices often vary in what they will and will not cover as part of a patient's hospice benefit. "Medical appropriateness" and a seamless transition for the particular patient are not always the bases upon which decisions are made. Although the request to continue an expensive medication may be reasonable in the medical or emotional sense, the financial resources may not be there to pay for the medication. A resolute philosophy of care may dictate that a certain treatment, such as hydration, be strongly discouraged. An example might be a patient who is on a very expensive anticoagulant as a preventive measure. Trusted clinicians may have stressed the importance of this drug as a means to minimize the risk of clots and a stroke. When proceeding through the admissions process, the patient may be told that the hospice will not pay for her current anticoagulant, but it will pay for a generic alternative that will offer similar benefit. Maintaining a semblance of stability in the setting of changing care providers may be an important therapeutic goal. Medication may have symbolic meaning. While an alternative cheaper medication may have a similar benefit, the impact of changing the medication at a time of transition to new providers, before the patient feels "safe" in his or her new environment, requires thought. Patient, family, and the admissions nurse may all experience distress at what they perceive to be a tension between (a) adhering to a hospice drug formulary conceived, in part, as a way to reduce pharmaceutical expenditures and (b) the therapeutic goal of maintaining clinical stability as trust develops in a new team of caregivers.

Authenticity and building trust with patients and families mandate that these kinds of issues be deliberated within the team, and that the organization as a whole be given an opportunity to reflect and deliberate upon how its limited resources are allocated. These conversations may be arduous and, at times, contentious, yet they are necessary to honor and respect the integrity of the patients, staff members, and the organization itself. Focusing on what is possible (a) with the resources available and (b) consistent with the organization's guiding philosophy then becomes the shared work of patient, family, and team from which decisions flow and choices are made. This may sometimes result in some patients deciding to change their service provider. Such a result may, however, not be a failure but a success if it means that all parties were able to honor the values most important to them.

CONTINUITY OF CARE ACROSS THE ILLNESS TRAJECTORY

Advances in science and medicine are part of the landscape within which hospice and palliative programs have proliferated. Rapidly fatal diseases have become chronic, slowly progressive illnesses for many, and costs have skyrocketed. By the time a hospice team enters the life of a patient and his or her family, the patient may have received care for long periods of time from specialty teams—cardiology, pulmonology, oncology—as well as multiple disciplines within these teams, including physicians, nurses, social workers, and chaplains. In addition to primary services, there is increasing access to interdisciplinary palliative care teams who focus beyond the disease or organ system and orchestrate a care plan created to meet the needs of this particular patient and his or her family as a whole. Thus, coordination and continuity becomes particularly meaningful as patients move toward end of life and their emotional and financial resources may have become exhausted by the long and evolving illness. These interacting variables invite reflection and deliberation lest we ignore the consequences and miss opportunities to adapt and enhance our clinical response.

The longer trajectory of illness challenges programs and practitioners to consider the effect not only on patients but also on their families and caregivers. Within the hospice system, where family has become at one and the same time both caregiver and the recipient of care, how have teams accommodated service? Can we adapt services and expectations based on an ethic of accommodation wherein team and agency responses and plans of care emanate from the unique circumstances and best interests of a particular patient and family, and family caregiver (Levine & Zuckerman, 1999)? Or do we expect all patients and families to elect our package of services, play by our rules, and consent to our management of their care?

For some, an ethic of accommodation means a clinical decision to provide hydration during the last weeks of life to ease anxiety and distress, or to correct electrolyte imbalance with the hope of recovering alertness and lucidity—a state valued by most patients and families. For others, an ethic of accommodation means that we have identified those who wish to protect the integrity of "home" by avoiding, whenever possible, the placement of medical equipment such as semielectric beds and commodes.

What are some additional consequences that flow from longer trajectories of illness associated with advances in science and medicine? Hospice programs admit patients and families who may have long and meaningful relationships with their earlier clinicians. They have shared a journey of uncertainty, joys, and sadness. In some instances ties to previous providers are abruptly ended when palliative or hospice care is initiated, while in other instances, possibly as a recognition of a long or brief but intense trajectory of illness, a "sharing" relationship with prior providers is purposefully built into the treatment plan. Perhaps this latter example reflects an expanding understanding of fidelity and "nonabandonment." As we consider a broadened view of nonabandonment, how are relational histories with prior clinicians recognized, nurtured, and respected as teams design plans of care? Might we be mandated to expand our definition of "team" to include prior clinicians, so that we do not add additional loss to the lives of patients and their families? And what of the loss to clinicians who may experience an abrupt disconnect from the patient, and with it the opportunity to know, emotionally and cognitively, how their work impacted the death of the patient and the experience of the family. Whether this impact was positive or negative, we have much to learn from both situations. Is it possible in our pressured health care system to sustain connection to prior clinicians until and if they naturally fade in importance?

As we reflect and deliberate on the challenges and potential benefits in linking clinicians along the continuum of illness, the emergence of technology creates limitless possibilities. We might imagine meta-teams meetings, where teams or individual clinicians are connected via teleconference or conference call, with or without patients and families, to enhance continuity and reflect on the care plan for patients as well as the nature and potential in their collaboration.

TEAM IS AT THE HEART OF HOSPICE WORK

Team is at the heart of hospice work. Many would say that it is the vehicle through which clinicians and staff actualize their commitment to create plans of care. Implicit in the work are shared ethical values such as non-abandonment, beneficence, respect for persons, and social justice. As noted earlier, the team is also a nexus where philosophical, administrative, political, regulatory, and financial forces converge, creating covert influences and tensions that may go unrecognized and unexplored. How teams interface with that tension is reflective of their philosophy, courage, beliefs, and values—individually and collectively. Team communication may be infused with language such as "dignified death," "a natural death," and "family as the unit of care" and/or "part of the team." These phrases suggest certain values and an ethic of care, a common understanding, and a set of expectations. Yet they may be unexamined as to their meaning and applicability to the unique narrative of a specific patient, family, or team member.

How do we create safe team environments that invite examination of our language and allow exploration of both internal and external influences and assumptions? What is the nature of a setting that accepts and encourages curiosity, questions, disagreement, and emotion? Can a milieu be created that supports members as they move from reaction to thought, accepting both as ingredients of critical thinking? Recognizing that thoughts, emotions, beliefs, and cultures might be very different among team members, "touching the third wire" or team "nerve" may not be uncommon, and it needs to be recognized, expected, and treated with humor, compassion, and inquiry. To "do no harm," leaders, whether of institutions or discrete teams, must assure that there are team members who have the maturity and experience to create and maintain such an atmosphere. While opportunities to weave patient narratives together with the unique perspectives, values, and thoughts of team members exist day to day, this may only happen in a context which accepts that such narratives can be vehicles to shared learning, team exploration, and moral discernment.

Setting-specific factors influence the manner in which teams might choose to integrate reflection and deliberation into their shared processes. Teams with stable membership from week to week and a large patient census may create a separate meeting that is a protected time to attend to their own processes. In academic centers where training is a primary goal, teams may have members who anchor the group from week to week while training clinicians rotate into the team for specific periods. The leaders of the training program would have to prioritize reflection and deliberation as essential learning just as they do the palliative care curriculum that focuses on patients and family needs. The commitment to create opportunities for moral reflection and deliberation can be established within an institution or within the group itself—teams do not need permission. The modality can be as unique as creating a monthly meeting that applies a format of "civic reflection" to the central questions of the work of palliative care and hospice. This modality, currently being studied by a group at Valparaiso University, uses short pieces of literature, images, audio, or video to promote dialogue (Center for Civic Reflection, 2012).

The invitation to reflection and deliberation can be as simple as asking the "unasked question": What factors impact team members as they consider the risk and benefit of moral inquiry? The concept of psychological safety, as described by Edmondson (2008), implies an assessment of the degree of risk one takes in asking, seeking help, or providing feedback. This risk is described both internally, within the cognitive or emotional life of the individual, and externally in the environment. For example, an internal risk might relate to the degree to which we "impression manage" a process that can be conscious or unconscious. Some clinicians may fear displeasing others or being humiliated and thus tread very carefully to control how they interface within their team. They consequently manage the impression that they make on others for emotional reasons. Some manage their impression for the purpose of instrumental benefit as they seek a raise in salary or a promotion within their agency and would not risk displeasing those in power. Some self-protect, fearing failure or sanction or being thought of as disruptive, negative, or ill informed. Others fear success and the concurrent responsibilities that success may imply. External risks and benefits rest in the environment of team and agency, which may be accepting, inclusive, and nonjudgmental or punitive and demeaning of its members. Internal and external risk do not obviate the responsibility of clinicians who chose to care for vulnerable people, to weigh the risk in their unique team and institutional culture, to accept the shared responsibility of advocating for patients and families, and to find options within organizational constraints (Abma, Molewijk, & Widdershoven, 2009).

CONCLUSION

We have touched on a few concerns that have, over time, entered the profound and rich work that we share. On a daily basis many clinicians and teams are practicing with wisdom, skill, and thoughtfulness. Others practice according to a philosophy or mandate that goes unquestioned and is powerfully influenced by forces that are neither acknowledged nor explored. Still others recognize the limitations, barriers, and struggles yet believe that they can, and do, make a difference within these constraints. As teams are challenged by such options as assisted death, the requested removal of ventilatory support, or artifical nutrition in an alert patient, the complexity—medical, ethical, spiritual, emotional, economic, and political—of the interplay of forces shaping the space in which care is given and received must be made transparent and open to scrutiny. More simply, our assumptions about such concepts as the "good death" and the responsibilities of families need to be replaced with a respect for, and a willingness to honor, difference—molding systems to the needs of persons rather than forcing persons to fit rigid constructs. Pervasive silence around these topics leaves patients, families, and clinicians to worry in isolation, as they struggle with the many poignant aspects of living with life-threatening illness.

To counteract this silence and its ensuing negative effects on the health and effectiveness of care teams, we have put forward a process model of moral reflection and deliberation. In our combined several decades of experience as members of palliative care teams, we have found that our teams—and the care given by those teams—was at its best when opportunities for reflection and deliberation were identified and teams thoughtfully engaged in this process. Similarly, when teams practiced in care environments wherein opportunities for reflection and deliberation were not created and these processes not engaged, teams suffered from the lack of insight, shared understanding, and clarity of purpose that reflection and deliberation can help provide. This, in turn, made it much more challenging for the team to identify effectively the sources and presence of patient suffering and offer well-integrated interdisciplinary care to alleviate that suffering.

Moral reflection, deliberation, and humble inquiry are essential to the work we do as hospice teams. Given the vulnerability of the patients and families we serve, we have a fiduciary responsibility to ensure that our teams are performing at their highest levels. Attunement to the collective psychic and spiritual lives of teams reduces the risk that complicated internal and external forces that influence the team's ability to thrive go undetected and unaddressed. What we have attempted to do in this chapter through proposing a process of reflection and deliberation is to open up one way to begin to "clear the fog" and get back to "personal legend" (Coelho, 1993).

REFERENCES

Abma, T. A., Molewijk, B., & Widdershoven, G. A. M. (2009). Good care in ongoing dialogue. Improving the quality of care through moral deliberation and responsive evaluation. *Health Care Analysis, 17*(3), 217–235.

Center for Civic Reflection. (2012). *Civic reflection with hospice and palliative care teams*. Retrieved from http://civicreflection.org/search/search&keywords=palliative+care/.

Coelho, P. (1993). *The alchemist*. New York, NY: Harper Collins.

Connor, M. H., & Walton, J. A. (2011). Demoralization and re-moralization: A review of these constructs in the healthcare literature. *Nursing, 18*(1), 2–11.

Davenport, J. (1997). Ethical principles in clinical practice. *The Permanante Journal, 1*(1), 21–24.

Edmondson, A. C. (2008). Managing the risk of learning: Psychological safety in work teams. In M. A.West, D. Tjosvold, & K. G. Smith (Eds.), *International handbook of organizational teamwork and cooperative working* (pp. 255–276). Chichester, UK: Wiley.

Gracia, D. (2001). Moral deliberation: The role of methodologies in clinical ethics. *Medicine, Health Care and Philosophy, 4*(2), 223–232.

Gracia, D. (2002). From conviction to responsibility in palliative care ethics. In H. Ten Have & D. Clark (Eds.), *The ethics of palliative care: European perspectives* (pp. 87–105). Buckingham, UK: Open University Press.

Hamric, A. B., Davis, W. S., & Childress, M. D. (2006). Moral distress in health care professionals: What it is and what we can do about it. *The Pharos, 69*(1), 17–23.

Hermsen, M. A., & Ten Have, H. A. M. J. (2005). Palliative care teams: Effective through moral reflection. *Journal of Interdisciplinary Care, 19*(6), 561–568.

Levine, C., & Zuckerman, C. (1999). The trouble with families: Toward an ethic of accommodation. *Annals of Internal Medicine, 130*(2), 148–152.

Opie, A. (1997). Thinking teams thinking clients: Issues of discourse and representation in the work of health care teams. *Sociology of Health and Illness, 19*(3), 259–280.

West, M. A. (2000). Reflexivity, revolution and innovation in work teams. In M. M. Beyerlein, D. A. Johnson & S. T. Beyerlein (Eds.), *Product development teams. Advances in interdisciplinary studies of work teams* (pp. 1–29). Stamford, CT: JAI Press.

Organizational and Policy Ethics in Hospice

CHAPTER 6

Ethical Issues in the Care of Infants, Children, and Adolescents

MARCIA LEVETOWN AND STACY ORLOFF

In this chapter, we will argue that societal denial of childhood illness and death has led to ethically problematic outcomes in the delivery of pediatric hospice and palliative care (PHPC), including the following:

- A lack of evidence-based treatments to prevent or relieve suffering for infants, children, and adolescents
- A dearth of sufficiently trained personnel to provide effective and efficient PHPC
- Few programs willing to render comprehensive care to these desperate families
- Willingness to subject children to treatments that the majority of adults reject for themselves
- Regulations, reimbursement schemata, and laws that subject seriously ill children and their families to unnecessary emotional, physical, and financial burdens

BARRIERS TO HOSPICE CARE FOR CHILDREN

Societal Denial of Child Illness and Death

Despite the fact that over 440,000 infants (<1 year of age), children (1–14 years of age), and adolescents (14–18 years of age) in the United

States are living with serious, chronic, and life-threatening conditions (Feudtner, Christakis, & Connell, 2000), there remains a public perception that all children are healthy and destined to live a long, full life. Even among acute care pediatric health care providers, a commonly held attitude prevails that sufficient will, effort, money, and technology can render all illness reversible. This construct has damaging consequences, ranging from insufficient allocation of research resources to determine the causes of and effective interventions for chronic pediatric conditions to poor reimbursement for supportive, rehabilitative, palliative, and hospice care for children (Hewitt, Weiner, & Simone, 2003).

Wide Variability of Life-Threatening Conditions

There are many causes of chronic and life-threatening conditions among children, and they are often ill defined (Feudtner, Christakis, & Connell, 2000). Most adults who die non-injury-related deaths, however, have one of six problems: cardiovascular disease, cancer, stroke, chronic lung disease, diabetes, or a neurodegenerative condition (NCHS, 2011). In contrast, children who may live most, if not all, of their lives with serious illness may have one of hundreds of defined and still-to-be-determined metabolic or enzyme deficiencies (e.g., muscular dystrophy, cystic fibrosis, Pearson's syndrome); chromosomal and other genetic anomalies (e.g., Trisomy 5, 13, 18, Rett's syndrome); developmental defects (problems with cell migration and maturation during the fetal development, including anencephaly and hypoplastic left heart syndrome); complications of prematurity and other forms of maternal/fetal incompatibility; perinatal infections; severe brain injury, whether cerebrovascular (e.g., stroke), hypoxic (e.g., "near-drowning"), metabolic (e.g., sepsis syndrome), or traumatic (e.g., motor vehicle crash or child abuse); or other childhood-onset illness (e.g., cancer) (Kochanek, Kirmeyer, Martin, Strobino, & Guyer, 2012; Newacheck & Halfon, 1998; Newacheck et al., 1998). Fortunately, relatively few children are affected by each of these conditions. As a result, children with serious conditions most often receive their care at one of approximately 250 children's hospitals in North America ("Concurrent care for children implementation toolkit," 2009), frequently located hundreds of miles from their home and families, leading to financial sacrifice and social separation at the most stressful times of these families' lives. In addition, the smaller number of affected children for each condition results in a lack of a critical mass for research investment and study. When attempted, research studies on serious pediatric conditions are by necessity multi-institutional and often multinational, increasing the difficulty of funding and execution. Due to the relatively poor "return on investment" for these expensive undertakings, children with serious and rare conditions are therefore often "therapeutic orphans."

Drug Dilemmas

Most drug trials have historically included only adults. Unlike children, large numbers of adults suffer from the same illness process, physiology is more uniform, and most can consent to participate in studies. Children were routinely excluded from drug trials until the voluntary pediatric exclusivity provision of the Food and Drug Administration (FDA) Modernization Act of 1997 (FDAMA), reauthorized as the Best Pharmaceuticals for Children Act (BPCA, 2002), provided 6 additional months of patent exclusivity, allowing for substantial profit in exchange for pediatric testing. Further, the 2003 Pediatric Research Equity Act (PREA) allows the FDA to require pediatric drug studies to gain drug approval. Few medications are approved each year, however; thus, the vast majority of medications remain "off label" for children, not having been tested for efficacy or safety in that population (Kimland & Odlind, 2012; Rowell & Zlotkin, 1997). The effect and metabolism of drugs differ based on the patient's illness, body composition, and enzymatic activity, all of which vary substantially over the phases of neonatal, infant, child, and adolescent development. This fact complicates drug testing in children further, adding to the expense; additionally, there are few children who will use such medications, so the volume of sales will not offset the price of testing. Once medications' patents expire, there is minimal profit to be made on their sales. Thus, there is no financial incentive for the research infrastructure or companies to test such drugs for safety and efficacy. Some medications most commonly used in hospice, such as morphine, may be ineffective or even dangerous to children but will never be studied in this population.

Reluctance to Provide Care

In our experience, many hospice care providers are drawn to the field to relieve the suffering of fellow human beings. They are concerned that health care has historically not focused on the personal and family experience of illness, including not only the physical manifestations but also the spiritual, psychosocial, and emotional elements. Hospice care fills that void. Nevertheless, few hospice workers volunteer to care for children, saying, "That would be too sad for me," "I don't know enough about it," or "They scare me." The personal need of the health care provider to avoid the burden of learning about pediatric care and to avoid emotional pain seem to outweigh the need to address and ameliorate the suffering of the child and family. Little if any thought is given to the fact that, in the absence of community-based care options, these children are relegated to remain far from home in a tertiary care center, separated from siblings, friends, pets, and familiar surroundings, often subjected to marginally beneficial, invasive, and/or painful medical interventions in the final phases of their lives. Additionally, little attention is paid in many of these tertiary care centers to the suffering of the child or that of the family members, especially those who are not physically present (Aschenbrenner et al., 2011).

Hospice clinicians' reluctance to care for children can be reinforced by a similar reluctance of hospice administrators, as it is expensive to provide pediatric palliative care. Well considered or not, efforts to overcome the child's illness often persist, even as death nears. Throughout the illness, however, even from the time of diagnosis, children and their families benefit from the minimization of suffering. This duality of goals of care, to both limit suffering and to continue with disease-directed interventions, has been allowed by many private payers, but it was not consistent with the structure and reimbursement of the Medicaid hospice care benefit until the concurrent care benefit passed as part of the Patient Protection and Affordable Care Act of 2010 (PPACA, 2010). This benefit has not been implemented in every state. Nevertheless, the lack of willingness and training of hospice providers to care for children remains a barrier (Davies et al., 2008).

Even when a child is truly receiving exclusively palliative interventions, such interventions can be quite costly and even technically challenging. As an example, the most common pediatric cancer is hematologic cancer (affecting the blood cells). Children with these disorders are frequently tired, dyspneic, and in pain from profound anemia. Red blood cell transfusion can restore their quality of life by providing them energy to play and engage with family and peers while relieving pain and breathlessness. However, in our experience, transfusions are infrequently provided in hospice care due to expense and practical considerations.

Some children who die each year have been receiving mechanical ventilation in the home setting. As can easily be imagined, the family is unlikely to welcome hospice into their lives and shut off the ventilator on the same day, yet the emotional, spiritual, and practical support from trusted care providers and the need for bereavement support may be best managed by hospice personnel. Some of the larger pediatric hospice programs have begun admitting children receiving mechanical ventilation, often following a palliative care consult. The decision regarding whether to admit ventilator-dependent children is not always based on philosophical or financial factors; there are significant practical barriers as well, including the perceived need to staff these cases 24/7. In the absence of the capacity to provide this support, the family may have to increase their responsibility for ventilator care from 8–16 hours a day to 24. Some hospices may admit ventilator-dependent children with the understanding that discontinuation of mechanical ventilation will occur within hours, days, or, rarely, weeks.

Some pediatric hospice candidates are severely brain damaged and may be receiving medically provided (artificial) nutrition and hydration (ANH). In addition to the ethical, legal, and emotional issues associated with decisions regarding ANH (discussed later), the practical issue of the cost of enteral tube and intravenous nutritional supplementation creates a barrier to the acceptance of hospice care for these children. The cost of ANH may be reimbursed by routine Medicaid, but will likely exceed the per diem rate paid under the Medicaid hospice benefit.

The Role of Hope

Children who are terminally ill and their parents have had to face a seemingly impossible choice, too often made without the assistance of a palliative care team, to keep treating with (most often an unrealistic) hope for a cure or to cease all disease-directed care and be admitted into hospice care. As a result, fewer than 5% of US children who die each year die while receiving hospice care (NHPCO, 2007); it will be interesting to see how the PPACA impacts the use of hospice among child patients. Many children who could be cared for in hospice have rare disorders leading to uncertainty in prognosticating life expectancy and disease trajectory, resulting in difficulty identifying when disease-directed interventions are unduly burdensome relative to their potential benefits. It is easy to understand, then, why parents find it so difficult to "give up hope." When a physician cannot provide concrete guidance and the hospice program is "required" to ascertain the patient has a life expectancy of 6 months or less, meeting criteria to receive hospice care is difficult (Davies et al., 2008; Docherty, Miles, & Brandon, 2007). Finally, parents often say the hardest part of agreeing to a hospice admission is "giving up their sense of hope," an attitudinal problem that may persist, as the term "hospice" is often conflated with death itself.

In a recent study by Reder and Serwint (2009), bereaved parents understood hope as an essential aspect of parenting a child who might die. While health care professionals tend to perceive a tension between hope and accepting the reality of the prognosis, parents in this study understood these as mutually compatible and necessary for coping with their child's illness. Unfortunately, some standard hospice regulations ignore this need, requiring the parent (and child) to stop all disease-directed care, thus abandoning any "hope" for cure. Treatments with a goal of palliation may continue; however, hospices differ in their willingness to provide some palliative treatments that may also prolong life, such as transfusions for a child with leukemia or expensive antibiotics that help a child with cystic fibrosis to breathe comfortably. Hope for a comfortable death and trust that the child's quality of life is the hospice's highest priority are compromised in these cases.

Without access to palliative care early in the illness trajectory, many parents and children are unable to make the decision to forgo disease-directed interventions until the child is very close to death, as can be inferred from the low proportion of pediatric deaths attended by hospice care, and the low median lengths of stay for those pediatric patients who do die on hospice care. The child's physician is instrumental in facilitating this shift in goals of care (Mack et al., 2007). While no amount of information or counseling reduces the family's feelings of sadness and loss, compassionate guidance and clear information enable the achievement of successful, family-centered care planning, including earlier referral to hospice. Families who access hospice or palliative care well before the child's death are better able to balance hope with the reality of their child's prognosis, thus limiting the use of treatments with little chance of success (Kreicbergs, Valdimarsdóttir, Onelöv, Henter, & Steineck, 2004; Surkan, Dickman, Steineck, Onelöv, & Kreicbergs, 2006). Parents can have the dual goals of hope for cure, while accepting its diminished likelihood, and hope for the maximal quality of life more easily than most health care providers (Mack et al., 2007). Access to pediatric hospice staff assists terminally ill children and their families to transform the object of their hope to be realistic outcomes, such as to survive to achieve milestones: a particular holiday, birthday, or event (Miller, 2007). Feudtner (2005) asserts that hope is increased when the expectation for a desired goal seems attainable. Hospice can help parents focus hope on retaining their capacity to be loving parents and finding ways to make the most of each and every day, lowering the risk of regret after their child's death (Kreicbergs et al., 2004).

Several states have developed innovative processes to increase access to PHPC (Armstrong-Dailey & Zarbock, 2009). Recognizing the difficulty of forgoing disease-directed measures, Florida, Colorado, and California submitted pediatric hospice care demonstration waivers, reallocating the funds designated for terminally ill pediatric Medicaid patients to enable the provision of concurrent disease-directed and palliative care. The Patient Protection and Affordable Care Act of 2010 provides an opportunity for national implementation of this model within Medicaid.

"Informed Consent" and the Research Imperative

Another barrier to referral to hospice care is the research "imperative" in pediatric specialty hospitals, especially within pediatric oncology programs. Attending physicians in specialty hospitals are often both clinicians and investigators. As such, their enthusiasm for experimental treatment to advance science (and their careers) can influence parents to enroll their children, sometimes without the knowing child's input, in trials rather than opt for hospice care, perceiving the trials as one "last hope" for a cure. Confusing the boundaries between treatment and research can challenge the integrity of the informed consent process.

Informed consent is an elusive construct, even for adult patients who are relatively healthy (Appelbaum, Lidz, & Klitzman, 2009). In the context of impending death and its associated highly wrought emotions, decision making regarding research on terminally ill children is complicated. Truly informed parental permission and child assent can be difficult to achieve. Given the high potential for suffering, it is imperative that all reasonable efforts are directed to ensuring that parents and children understand all of their options—including the option of hospice care—and that the knowing child is given a voice in these decisions (Alderson, Sutcliffe, & Curtis, 2006; Bluebond-Langner, Decicco, & Belasco, 2005; Kodish, 2003).

True informed consent for research participation includes the following:

- An adequate understanding of the current condition or situation
- An appreciation (on the part of the staff, investigative team, family, and child) of the concept of the null hypothesis and the randomization process relevant to the current research study
- The alternatives for ongoing management, including the following:
  i. The likelihood of the hoped-for and anticipatable short- and long-term benefits of each alternative
  ii. The likelihood and severity of the anticipatable short- and long-term burdens of each alternative

iii. A clear understanding of the goals of each management alternative, including how "response to treatment" is defined and how that translates into the patient experience (i.e., Is "response" clinically or merely statistically relevant in terms of improvement in symptom distress, quality, and length of life?)

- A viable choice not to participate or to later choose to stop participating, without penalty
- Lack of coercion, including the lack of emotional coercion (e.g., "We have tried so hard to help him so far—please just give us one more chance!"; "You owe it to the children who sacrificed for him!"; "It is his only chance for cure!"; "There is nothing else to do")
- Reasonable alternatives for care when declining to participate in the research protocol, including promises of nonabandonment. (Appelbaum, 2007; Freyer, 2004)

Numerous studies conducted in the aftermath of death have found that bereaved parents often regret the additional suffering to which treatment decisions subjected their dying children in the blind hope of being able to restore health and prolong life (Rosenberg, Baker, Syrjala, & Wolfe, 2012). Our job as ethical health care providers is to prevent unnecessary suffering and regret for the child and the family, while enabling informed and voluntary participation in studies. Participation in research studies can lead to the satisfaction of a legacy of altruism and the advancement of science. These goals are important, but they do not trump informed consent.

A parent's job, above all else, is to protect his or her children (Keene-Reder & Serwint, 2009)—most especially from death. As a result, parents will grasp at any alternative that is promoted as holding the potential for cure or life prolongation. They ask few if any questions and can be blind to their child's suffering (Bluebond-Langner, 1978) in the pursuit of a "cure" for an incurable problem. In the absence of a long-term relationship with a trusted advisor who is able to assist parents to consider the relative benefits and burdens of ongoing disease-directed intervention or even experimental treatments through the lens of their values, parents very often agree to more "treatment." PHPC services, integrated with disease-directed clinical care starting near the time of diagnosis, can promote the well-being of the child and family throughout the illness and especially when the decisions become more difficult (Baker et al., 2008; Golan et al., 2008; Mack & Grier, 2004; Mack & Wolfe, 2006; Wolfe et al., 2000).

While the pressure to enroll children in research protocols for new disease-focused treatments can be a barrier to accessing hospice care, there is also a lack of research validating and developing new palliative interventions for children (Steele et al., 2008); such research is desperately needed. Until recently, many institutional review boards (IRBs), bodies that approve research proposals after ensuring appropriate human subjects protections, rejected PHPC investigations outright or made the conditions so onerous as to prevent sufficient enrollment (AAP Committee on Bioethics, 1995; Hinds, Burghen, & Pritchard, 2007). This was done to "protect" the children; by contrast, disease-directed investigations are routinely approved with minimal hesitation, even when proposed for these same vulnerable children. The provision of unproven and therefore potentially harmful or at least suboptimal care should also be of concern to IRBs when considering how best to protect children's safety (Hinds et al., 2007). Few studies have looked at the experience of the child in participating in research, regardless of its goals. Participation in research on pediatric palliative care has proven beneficial for bereaved parents, however (Dyregrov, 2004).

Lack of Clinical Expertise and Experience

Insufficient training in the provision of PHPC is an issue for hospital-based as well as hospice care providers. Attending physicians who have had little formal training in palliative and end-of-life (EOL) care are often uncomfortable discussing shifting the goals of care from cure to exclusive goals of palliation with children and their families, creating the first of many barriers to hospice care (Davies et al., 2008; Hilden et al., 2001). Care transitions are not clearly identified, resulting in children being referred very late or not at all to hospice (Hinds et al., 2007).

In a 2006 study, Fowler et al. surveyed pediatric oncologists (N = 632) and found that in the previous year, only 38% of respondents had any patient die at home. Respondents believed that hospice providers in their area were not experienced in providing care to children. With few child referrals, it is not cost efficient for the hospice to hire specialized pediatric staff. This is clearly a circular problem. Additional reasons oncologists infrequently referred to hospice were as follows:

- Ongoing use of disease-directed intervention (57%)
- Limited access to needed resources within hospice care (43%)
- Uncertain or extended prognosis beyond 6 months (38%). (Fowler et al., 2006)

The same study demonstrated that pediatric oncologists were most comfortable referring to hospice:

- Late in the disease course (44%)
- When death was imminent (20%)
- When there were no disease-directed options available (26%). (Fowler et al., 2006)

Sadly, only 2.5% of all surveyed oncologists referred to hospice at the time of relapse, waiting instead for imminent death, perpetuating the perception that hospice referral is tantamount to a death sentence and ensuring a length of stay too short for the child and his or her family to reap the benefits of the counseling and treatments available in a hospice program (Fowler et al., 2006).

Sixty-four percent of parents surveyed in a more recent study stated they would consider changing treatment goals if they believed their child was suffering, and 43% acknowledged being influenced by their child's physician's estimated prognosis (Michelson et al., 2009). Additional challenges for health care providers in providing PPC and referral to hospice are lack of experience providing such care, prognostic uncertainty, and the personal existential pain of providing EOL care to children (Sahler, Frager, Levetown, Cohn, & Lipson, 2000). Given these barriers, it is no wonder that few children are referred to hospice.

Another study queried hospital staff regarding their comfort in providing hospital-based PHPC (Contro, Larson, Scofield, Sourkes, & Cohen, 2004). The investigators found that staff expressed discomfort in four categories:

- Communication with families
  i. Challenges communicating with patients and patients' families regarding EOL issues and limitations of resuscitative measures
- Pain management
  i. Attending physicians (43%) and residents (56%) felt inexperienced regarding pain management
  ii. Fifty percent of nurses felt inexperienced managing non-pain symptoms and 30% felt inexperienced managing pain
- Support for the professional
  i. Lack of designated time to debrief after a child's death
  ii. Desire for ongoing support and education regarding EOL care
- Consequences of insufficient training
  i. Overall felt less competent and more susceptible to "burnout." (Contro et al., 2004)

Other disciplines have also identified PHPC learning needs. Social workers have developed PHPC competencies (Bosma et al., 2010). When asked about their educational needs related to EOL care, social workers from the National Association of Social Workers (N = 1,100) stated they needed additional information about the following:

- Psychological and social needs of child patients and their families
- Psychosocial interventions to reduce stress
- The effect of death on family dynamics
- Assessment of the complex needs of patients and families
- Effective communication of patient and family psychosocial needs to other interdisciplinary team members. (Bosma et al., 2010)

Fifty-four percent noted this content was not regularly offered as part of their graduate training. Csikai and Raymer (2005) found that only 28% of social workers in their sample (N = 391) had field placements where EOL care was a central focus.

The impact of education on patient referrals to hospice is illustrated by the fact that Florida nurses participating in the state's pediatric hospice Medicaid waiver demonstration program have a higher rate of referring children for EOL care than nurses without PHPC experience (Knapp, Madden, et al., 2009).

Hospice staff must have the appropriate skills and knowledge to meet the care needs of children, their extended families, and members of the community affected by the child's illness and death; the current lack of such staff is yet another barrier to hospice care for children. Many parents in northern California identified these clinical concerns regarding their hospice providers (Contro et al., 2004), noting they were unable to manage the logistics of caring for their children, staff were inadequately trained, shift care scheduling was poorly done, and temporary hospice staff were inadequately trained prior to placement in a dying child's home. Parents noted a specific deficit in pain management training (Contro, Larson, Scofield, Sourkes, & Cohen, 2002).

Hospice care is directed to the prevention and relief of suffering; hospice care teams achieve these goals, at least to some extent, for all patients, regardless of age or condition. While clinical care is always imperfect, all providers should "pursue perfection" (http://www.IHI.org); with continued education, outcomes measurement, and dedication to ongoing improvement, the care for patients of all ages and diagnoses can improve. The gap between ideal and current states of clinical care is particularly wide in PHPC. This does not mean that hospice care for children is not beneficial; it merely means there is still work to be done to improve it. In the meantime, it is important for hospices to develop collaborative relationships with other providers who can help fill the gaps and mentor their improved capacity to provide effective PHPC. This may mean having a close relationship with the palliative care team at the referral hospital; it may mean having a statewide, regional, or even telemedicine PHPC team, including experts in pediatric nursing, medicine, pharmacology, spiritual care, and psychosocial care, that can be accessed for education, direct care provision, and remote advice, as well as the development of policies and procedures that better address the needs of terminally ill infants, children, and adolescents and their families.

Regulatory Barriers and Poor Reimbursement

Regulatory barriers can result in reimbursement challenges for pediatric hospice care, as insurance regulations often stipulate who can be admitted into hospice and for how long, dictating payment streams. Recent efforts to change this restrictive environment include the aforementioned pediatric hospice Medicaid demonstration programs. The goal of such programs is to explore the hypothesis that cost savings and quality of care increase when children have earlier access to hospice and palliative care (Lowe et al., 2009).

The most progressive and well-funded hospices attempt to limit suffering by providing open access to patients of all ages who can benefit from hospice care, regardless of ability to pay or projected time until death. However, most public and private health care benefit plans currently limit hospice eligibility to the projected last 6 months of life. Yet research in adult and pediatric EOL care has shown that earlier access to hospice and palliative care facilitates an improved quality of life of the final months, an increased likelihood of achieving life closure and appropriate goodbyes, and often reduces overall health care costs (Gans et al., 2012). While hospices may be willing to care for children with a life expectancy of greater than 6 months, few funding streams support the substantial cost of interventions still valued by families at that point, including chemotherapy, transfusions, intravenous feeding, expensive antibiotics, and sometimes mechanical ventilation or even intensive care unit stays. Unfortunately, this reimbursement challenge even applies to some pediatric hospice patients who are expected to die within 6 months, whose parents are comforted by their long-standing routines and treatments. Hospices' per diem payment per patient is expected to cover all costs associated with the terminal diagnosis. The per diem payment, however, rarely covers the cost of care for pediatric patients, creating financial risk in taking children on service, constituting yet another barrier to pediatric hospice care.

At least 15% of children in the United States do not have any public or private health care insurance (Friebert, 2009). This is in stark contrast to adults receiving hospice care, the majority of whom are Medicare beneficiaries eligible for hospice benefits. Few hospices can afford to admit children into their programs without any expectation of compensation, particularly given the increased costs of care associated with PHPC. Although the number of uninsured children is expected to decrease due to the PPACA (2010), it is unknown how, if at all, this legislation will impact access to pediatric palliative and hospice care.

In 2009, Knapp et al. investigated pediatric hospice users in the state of Florida and the factors that affect the costs associated with their care (Knapp, Shenkman, Marcu, Madden, & Terza, 2009). Their findings suggest that the optimal time for the initiation of hospice care, in terms of the balance of expenditure and reimbursement, is at least 2–3 months prior to the child's death, perhaps due to less frequent use of expensive care interventions once hospice becomes involved. Since most children are referred to hospice much later in the disease trajectory, the hospice is financially disadvantaged by a constant per diem in the face of extraordinary care costs at enrollment, which then taper over weeks. Initial costs include organizing medication needs and durable medical equipment and managing parental and child distress, requiring intensive team time and resources. Similarly, costs rise immediately prior to death, as symptom distress and social distress escalate. A longer length of stay allows the hospice provider to "bank" the per diem reimbursement during the more stable and less costly days to compensate for the resource-intensive days. Late referrals, often in the midst of a crisis, and lengths of stay on program lasting hours to days, contribute to hospices' reluctance to care for pediatric patients.

Several states have certificate of need requirements for hospice care, creating a large geographic monopoly of hospice services. In these systems, with larger numbers of patients per organization, lower cost patients offset the expenses of higher cost patients. Such larger hospices (mostly found in metropolitan or urban areas) also may have associated grants and foundations and *may* therefore even be able to admit children without any health insurance. Another advantage of larger hospices is that they have volumes of service that may allow for the maintenance of staff with pediatric expertise. Children in rural areas or in cities with multiple hospice providers often have virtually no hope of gaining access to pediatric hospice care (Davies et al., 2008). Alternative solutions noted earlier, such as regional pediatric palliative care consortia, with telemedicine approaches and multistate reach, have yet to be designed and implemented, though they are a potential (yet complex) solution to this problem.

PHPC usually includes services beyond the core adult-oriented hospice services identified by the US Congress in 1983. The hospice per diem payment is based upon these designated core services, leaving many programs willing to serve children to do it substantially at their own cost. The highest performing pediatric programs provide care to a much broader circle than the nuclear family, such as school classmates, service groups (e.g., Boy/Girls Scouts), and faith youth groups, none of which is compensated under existing models of hospice care. In our experience, bereavement follow-up for the family of pediatric patients typically requires care well beyond the 13 months required by Medicaid and Medicare.

Criminal Investigation of Expected Home Death

There is no federal mandate that exempts a hospice death from being investigated as a potential crime. Many states do allow for some type of hospice exemption, but not all. Therefore, in some states, law enforcement officials must be called when a child dies.

At one end of the spectrum, Florida law recognizes a hospice patient death as an attended death, obviating the need to contact the Medical Examiner's office unless the cause of death is unexpected or otherwise suspicious. The Medical Examiner must also be called when the child's terminal condition is due to an accident (e.g., a car accident or post drowning) or criminal activity (e.g., child abuse), regardless of how long ago the inciting event occurred. Law enforcement officials usually acknowledge the hospice staff at the child's home and understand the child was expected to die. Nevertheless, survivors are unnecessarily traumatized by the implication that they have done something wrong or illegal when a uniformed officer comes to their home at one of the most devastating and vulnerable moments of their lives. Furthermore, even without flashing lights, neighbors may become suspicious of wrongdoing, and any privacy the family had hoped for surrounding the event of the death is lost.

At the other end of the spectrum, Massachusetts law requires all home deaths of a child under the age of 18 to be investigated, regardless of cause or whether the death was expected. The specter of this type of investigation may cause some families to choose the hospital as the site of the child's death, despite patient or family's preference for a home surrounded by extended family members and family pets, comfortable in their own beds, in a safe secure environment. State laws requiring investigations of child deaths regardless of circumstance constitute another barrier to pediatric home hospice care.

The Child's Involvement in Decision Making

The law often defines minimal thresholds for societal rules. In the case of contracts and consent, 18 years of age has been arbitrarily chosen as a threshold conferring capacity for autonomous decision making and consent for most individuals. However, most clinicians (and parents of "adult" children) would attest that the 18th birthday does not seem to confer any great wisdom or maturity, nor does being younger than 18 guarantee a lack of either capacity or maturity (AAP Committee on Bioethics, 1995; King & Cross, 1989; Leikin, 1989; Nitschke, Caldwell, & Jay, 1986).

Capacity for decision making is defined as being able to do the following:

- Understand the situation
- Understand the options and their likely outcomes, good and bad, short and long term
- Apply a consistent set of (long-held) values
- Understand the irreversibility of death, in the case of life and death decisions

Capacity for some individuals precedes the 18th birthday by many years; for others, it never manifests. Children who have lived with illness over time often become disproportionately mature with regard to their illness and its management, even if not in other areas of their lives. Those who have endured long-term treatments begin to be able to weigh their benefits and burdens, having directly experienced many of the burdens. The benefits must be clearly emphasized to the child as well, when they exist, as delayed gratification is a sophisticated construct, foreign to immature beings. Nevertheless, children are often capable of engaging in this exercise. Unfortunately, despite the uniformity of the conclusions of research on the topic, children are still often not asked their opinion regarding goals of care and care plans, even when they are relatively well (Young, Dixon-Woods, Windridge, & Heney, 2003). In many cases, when children are allowed to express an opinion, it is ignored in deference to the needs of the adults around them, whether parents, clinicians, or researchers, even if these needs diametrically oppose those of the child. When asked, terminally ill children generally express a preference to return home to die (Surkan, Dickman, Steineck, Onelöv, & Kreicbergs, 2006).

Some studies (e.g., Siden et al., 2008) demonstrate that with advance care planning (ACP) preventing panicked decision making, children die at home about 50% of the time. ACP in these studies probably incorporated, but did not necessarily emphasize, the child's preferences. Of course, infants cannot express a preference. Leuthner et al. demonstrated that in Wisconsin, in part due to the legal climate, there are virtually no home-based programs that will accept infants for hospice care and therefore virtually all infants who die do so in the hospital setting (Leuthner, Boldt, & Kirby, 2004).

Withholding Information and Collusion

Children often feel abandoned and unloved when they are not provided information about their condition (Bluebond-Langner, 1978). When included in the conversation, both children and their parents feel better. Bereaved parents often cite their child's participation in decision making as one reason why they can cope with their loss (Kreicbergs et al., 2004; Sharman, Meert, & Sarnaik, 2005). Nitschke et al. (1982) challenged the status quo of not including children in decision making for Phase I trials. Prior to this intervention, clinical researchers did not discuss options with the involved child, instead only requesting permission from their grieving, desperate parents. Not surprisingly, he and others had extraordinarily high rates of participation in clinical trials, to their professional and economic benefit. When Nitchske included the child patients from the beginning of their illnesses in briefings regarding the disease process, their capacity grew. When asked, two thirds of these patients rejected participation in Phase I clinical trials when they entered the terminal phase of illness, in preference to achieving their final personal goals or maintaining social ties. Given these and subsequent data, it is difficult to justify the ongoing withholding of information, especially under the pretense of "protecting" the child.

Many health care personnel recognize parents' legal right to withhold information as well as the potential for surviving parents to bring legal action, but three important constructs should contribute to the decision to engage in collusion:

1. Even while respecting and providing family-centered care, our foremost responsibility is to the patient and his or her well-being.
2. To have a successful legal action, one must be able to prove direct culpability and damages. In this instance, the risk is quite small.
3. Sometimes what is legally correct is not necessarily ethically correct.

Adults are afforded the opportunity to forgo unwanted attempts at resuscitation in the outpatient/nonhospital setting if they are terminally ill. The mechanism to notify the emergency medical services (EMS) system not to intervene is called an "out of hospital DNR" or "DNRO." Children with special health care needs typically have an individualized health care plan (IHCP); this plan could easily include DNRO status (National Association of School Nurses, 2012). Attending school is a critical part of a child's social and developmental experience; it allows the child to have important closure with school friends and teachers (who often also benefit from the opportunity), supports a sense of normalcy, and even sustains an important sense of hope. No uniform policy regarding acceptance of a child's DNRO status at school exists, although the American Academy of Pediatrics (AAP) published a policy on this matter in 2010 (AAP Council on School Health and Committee on Bioethics, 2010). Seriously ill children with signed DNROs who wish to attend school must be aware that their school might override their choices, contact EMS, and begin unwanted, invasive treatment. If schools do not honor DNROs, many children who are capable of, and would benefit from, returning to school face a powerful disincentive to doing so.

Little assessment exists about state laws or school policies. A 2005 review found that over 80% of prominent school districts did not have policies, regulations, or protocols regarding DNROs (Kimberly, Forte, Carroll, & Feudtner, 2005a). Seventy-six percent of these same districts stated they would not honor a child's DNRO. The 20% that would honor a child's advance directive would require additional documentation beyond a fully executed DNRO, such as a physician's written order or court order (Kimberly, Forte, Carroll, & Feudtner, 2005b).

Some school administrators are concerned that their personnel might not respond to easily reversible problems or other situations that are not covered in the DNRO. Additionally, school administrators and school boards may fear liability in the event that an inexpert school staff member does not prevent a premature death (AAP Council on School Health and Committee on Bioethics, 2010). The DNRO is not directed at school staff; it is directed at EMS, who should be called (at the same time as the parents) to evaluate the child. A care plan should be in place that enables EMS to provide comfort care and to prevent transport when it is not consistent with the family's wishes and the child's condition. Children's hospitals and hospices can advocate on the local and state level to ensure that children cared for in a hospice program with completed advance care plans have the ability to attend school if they can still benefit from being there and can tolerate it socially, physically, and intellectually (AAP Council on School Health and Committee on Bioethics, 2010).

Forgoing Medically Provided Artificial Nutrition and Hydration: Social and Ethical Ramifications

In modern Western society, food is love. First dates and holidays often involve shared dinners, and special foods are often given as gifts. Infants and very young children depend on their caregivers for sustenance, including food and shelter. The emotional and biologic bond of a mother nursing her infant is undeniable.

Patients of all ages can become ill and incapable of eating or adequately ingesting sufficient calories to engage in the restorative, healing, or maintenance processes needed by their bodies. Medically provided nutrition and hydration—delivered intravenously or via a nasogastric, gastric, or jejunal tube—was developed as a bridge to health while waiting for a reversible gastrointestinal or neurologic process to resolve.

Medically provided nutrition and hydration, whether enteral or parenteral, is a medical treatment with clear indications. As with other medical treatments, artificial nutrition and hydration (ANH) has the potential for harms and benefits and, as with all other medical care, is best used when the benefits clearly outweigh the harms, regardless of the patient's age or condition.

As with adults, consideration of forgoing ANH in children is socially and emotionally challenging, primarily due to the conflation of "food" and love. However, having nutrients flow though a plastic catheter either directly onto the stomach or intestinal lining or directly into a blood vessel is nothing like the experience of sharing a holiday dinner—there is no tasting, chewing, swallowing, or sharing at the dinner table.

The main justification for forgoing ANH in terminally ill children is the greater harm than good that pertains to the individual. As recently summarized by the American Academy of Pediatrics, families of pediatric patients may choose to forgo ANH in four situations, all of which have parallels with adult patients:

- When initiating/continuing ANH exacerbates suffering
- In the face of imminent death
- In the setting of total intestinal failure
- In the face of profound, irreversible cognitive failure, such as persistent/permanent vegetative state. (Diekema & Botkin, 2009)

While ANH may be forgone in these settings, it is not required to withhold or withdraw ANH. Parents or guardians and, when possible, patients themselves must be involved in decision making regarding ANH. It is also critical that they receive support for their decisions from health care providers, as there is a high risk of being questioned and criticized by family, friends, and caregivers, regardless of their choice. The people most intensely impacted by the results of this decision are the patient, parents, and immediate family—thus, their concerns should be weighed most strongly in decisions regarding ANH.

CONCLUSION

In this chapter, we have argued that there are several ethically troubling impediments to the delivery of high-quality PHPC services in the United Sates. These barriers include the following:

- A lack of evidence-based treatments to prevent or relieve suffering for infants, children, and adolescents, due in part to the existing regulations and economic incentives
- A dearth of sufficiently trained personnel to provide effective and efficient PHPC, in part due to societal denial of the need for such training as well as myopic perspectives of some health care providers
- Few programs willing to render care to these desperate families, due to the reimbursement, structure, and organization of PHPC services
- A questionable willingness to subject children to treatments that a majority of adults reject for themselves
- Denial of children's terminal prognoses and treatment preferences
- Existing regulations, reimbursement schemata, and laws that subject seriously ill children and their families to unnecessary, even cruel, emotional, physical, and financial burdens

It will take a serious and multifaceted effort on the part of many to overcome these obstacles to effective and available pediatric palliative care, but the results will be worth it.

REFERENCES

Alderson, P., Sutcliffe, K., & Curtis, K. (2006). Children's competence to consent to medical treatment. *Hastings Center Report, 36*(6), 25–34.

American Academy of Pediatrics (AAP) Committee on Bioethics. (1995). Informed consent, parental permission, and assent in pediatric practice. *Pediatrics*, *95*(2), 314–317.

American Academy of Pediatrics (AAP) Council on School Health and Committee on Bioethics. (2010). Policy statement—Honoring do-not-attempt-resuscitation requests in schools. *Pediatrics*, *125*(5), 1073–1077.

Appelbaum, P. S. (2007). Assessment of patients' competence to consent to treatment. *New England Journal of Medicine*, *357*(18), 1834–1840.

Appelbaum, P. S., Lidz, C. W., & Klitzman, R. (2009). Voluntariness of consent to research: A preliminary empirical investigation. *IRB: Ethics and Human Research*, *31*(6), 10–14.

Armstrong-Dailey, A., & Zarbock, S. (Eds.). (2009). *Hospice care for children* (3rd ed). New York, NY: Oxford University Press.

Aschenbrenner, A. P., Winters, J. M., & Belknap, R. A. (2011). Integrative review: Parent perspectives on care of their child at the end of life. *Journal of Pediatric Nursing*, *27*(5), 514–522.

Baker, J. N., Hinds, P. S., Spunt, S. I., Barfield, R. C., Allen, C., Powell, B. C., ... Kane, J. R. (2008). Integration of palliative care principles into the ongoing care of children with cancer: Individualized care planning and coordination. *Pediatric Clinics of North America*, *55*(1), 223–250.

Best Pharmaceuticals for Children Act (BPCA), Public L. No. 107-109, 111 Stat. 2298 (2002).

Bluebond-Langner, M. (1978). *The private worlds of dying children*. Princeton, NJ: Princeton University Press.

Bluebond-Langner, M., Decicco, A., & Belasco, J. (2005). Involving children with life-shortening illness in the decision to participate in clinical research: A proposal for shuttle diplomacy and negotiation. In E. Kodish (Ed.), *Ethics and research with children* (pp. 323–343). New York, NY: Oxford University Press.

Bosma, H., Johnston, M., Cadell, S., Wainwright, W., Abernethy, N., Feron, A., ... Nelson, F. (2010). Creating social work competencies for practice in hospice palliative care. *Palliative Medicine*, *24*(1), 79–87.

Concurrent care for children implementation toolkit. (2009). Alexandria, VA: National Hospice & Palliative Care Organization/District of Columbia Pediatric Palliative Care Collaboration.

Contro, N., Larson, J., Scofield, S., Sourkes, B., & Cohen, H. (2002). Family perspectives on the quality of pediatric palliative care. *Archives of Pediatric and Adolescent Medicine*, *156*(1), 14–19.

Contro, N., Larson, J., Scofield, S., Sourkes, B., & Cohen, H. (2004). Hospital staff and family perspectives regarding quality of pediatric palliative care. *Pediatrics*, *114*(5), 1248–1252.

Csikai, E., & Raymer, M. (2005). Social workers' educational needs in end-of-life care. *Social Work in Health Care*, *4*(1), 53–72.

Davies, B., Sehring, S., Partridge, J. C., Cooper, B., Hughes, A., Philp, J., ... Kramer, R. (2008). Barriers to palliative care for children: Perceptions of pediatric health care providers. *Pediatrics*, *121*(2), 282–288.

Diekema, D. S., & Botkin, J. R. (2009). Forgoing medically provided nutrition and hydration in children. *Pediatrics*, *124*(2), 813–822.

Docherty, S. L., Miles M. S., & Brandon D. (2007). Searching for 'the dying point': Providers' experiences with palliative care in pediatric acute care. *Pediatric Nursing*, *33*(4), 335–341.

Dyregrov, K. (2004). Bereaved parents' experience of research participation. *Social Science and Medicine, 58*(2), 391–400.

Feudtner, C. (2005). Hope and the prospects of healing at the end of life. *Journal of Alternative and Complementary Medicine, 11*(Suppl. 1), S23–S30.

Feudtner, C., Christakis, D., & Connell, F. A. (2000). Pediatric deaths attributable to complex chronic conditions: A population-based study of Washington State, 1980-1997. *Pediatrics, 106*(1, Pt. 2), 205–209.

Food and Drug Administration Modernization Act of 1997 (FDAMA), Public L. No. 105-115, §111, 111 Stat. 2296 (1997).

Fowler, K., Poehling, K., Billheimer, D., Hamilton, R., Wu, H., Mulder, J., & Frangoul, H. (2006). Hospice referral practices for children with cancer: A survey of pediatric oncologists. *Journal of Clinical Oncology, 24*(7), 1099–1104.

Freyer, D. R. (2004). Care of the dying adolescent: Special considerations. *Pediatrics, 113*(2), 381–388.

Friebert, S. (2009). *NHPCO facts and figures: Pediatric palliative and hospice care in America.* Alexandria, VA: National Hospice and Palliative Care Organization.

Gans, D., Kominski, G. F., Roby, D. H., Diamant, A. L., Chen, X., Lin, W., & Hohe, N. (2012). *Better outcomes, lower costs: Palliative care program reduces stress, costs of care for children with life-threatening conditions.* Los Angeles, CA: UCLA Center for Health Policy Research.

Golan, H., Bielorai, B., Grebler, D., Izraeli, S., Rechavi, G., & Toren, A. (2008). Integration of a palliative and terminal care center into a comprehensive pediatric oncology department. *Pediatric Blood and Cancer, 50*(5), 949–955

Hewitt, M., Weiner, S. L., & Simone, J. V. (Eds.). (2003). *Childhood cancer survivorship: Improving care and quality of life.* Washington, DC: National Academies Press.

Hilden, J. M., Emanuel, E. J., Fairclough, D. L., Link, M. P., Foley, K. M., Clarridge, B. C.,...Mayer, R. J. (2001). Attitudes and practices among pediatric oncologists regarding end-of-life care: Results of the 1998 American Society of Clinical Oncology survey. *Journal of Clinical Oncology, 19*(1), 205–212.

Hinds, P. S., Burghen, E. A., & Pritchard, M. (2007). Conducting end-of-life studies in pediatric oncology. *Western Journal of Nursing Research, 29*(4), 448–465.

Keene-Reder, E., & Serwint, J. R. (2009). Until the last breath: Exploring the concept of hope for parents and health care professionals during a child's serious illness. *Archives of Pediatric and Adolescent Medicine, 163*(7), 653–657.

Kimberly, M., Forte, A., Carroll, J., & Feudtner, C. (2005a). Pediatric do-not-attempt-resuscitation orders and public schools: A national assessment of policies and laws. *American Journal of Bioethics, 5*(1), 59–65.

Kimberly, M., Forte, A., Carroll, J., & Feudtner, C. (2005b). A response to selected commentaries on "Pediatric do-not-attempt-resuscitation orders and public schools: A national assessment of policies and laws." *American Journal of Bioethics, 5*(1), W19–W21.

Kimland, E., & Odlind, V. (2012). Off-label drug use in pediatric patients. *Clinical Pharmacology and Therapeutics, 91*(5), 796–801.

King, N. M., & Cross, A. W. (1989). Children as decision makers: Guidelines for pediatricians. *Journal of Pediatrics, 115*(1), 10–16.

Knapp, C., Shenkman, E., Marcu, M., Madden, V., & Terza, J. (2009). Pediatric palliative care: Describing hospice users and identifying factors that affect hospice expenditures. *Journal of Palliative Medicine, 12*(3), 223–229.

Knapp, C., Madden, V., Wang, H., Kassing, K., Curtis, C., Sloyer, P., & Shenkman, E. (2009). Effect of a pediatric palliative care program on nurses' referral preferences. *Journal of Palliative Medicine, 12*(12), 1131–1136.

Kochanek, K. D., Kirmeyer, S. E., Martin, J. A., Strobino, D. M., & Guyer, B. (2012). Annual summary of vital statistics: 2009. *Pediatrics, 129*(2), 338–348.

Kodish, E. (2003). Pediatric ethics and early-phase childhood cancer research: Conflicted goals and the prospect of benefit. *Accountability in Research, 10*(1), 17–25.

Kreicbergs, U., Valdimarsdóttir, U., Onelöv, E, Henter, J-I., & Steineck, G. (2004). Talking about death with children who have severe malignant disease. *New England Journal of Medicine, 351*(12), 1175–1186.

Leikin, S. A. (1989). Proposal concerning decisions to forgo life-sustaining treatment for young people. *Journal of Pediatrics, 115*(1), 17–22.

Leuthner, S. R., Boldt, A. M., & Kirby, R. S. (2004). Where infants die: Examination of place of death and hospice/home health care options in the state of Wisconsin. *Journal of Palliative Medicine, 7*(2), 269–277.

Lowe, P., Curtis, C., Greffe, B., Knapp, C., Shenkman, E., & Sloyer, P. (2009). Children's Hospice International program for all-inclusive care for children and their families. In A. Armstrong-Dailey & S. Zarbock Goltzer (Eds.), *Hospice care for children* (3rd ed., pp. 398–438). New York, NY: Oxford University Press.

Mack, J. W., & Grier, H. (2004). The day one talk. *Journal of Clinical Oncology, 22*(3), 563–566.

Mack, J. W., & Wolfe, J. (2006). Early integration of pediatric palliative care: For some children, palliative care starts at diagnosis. *Current Opinion in Pediatrics, 18*(1), 10–14.

Mack, J., Wolfe, J., Cook, E., Grier, H., Cleary, P., & Weeks, J. (2007). Hope and prognostic disclosure. *Journal of Clinical Oncology, 25*(35), 5636–5642.

Michelson, K. N., Koogler, T., Sullivan, C., Del Pilar Ortega, M., Hall, E., & Frader, J. (2009). Parental views on withdrawing life-sustaining therapies in critically ill children. *Archives of Pediatric and Adolescent Medicine, 163*(11), 986–992.

Miller, J. (2007). Hope: A construct central to nursing. *Nursing Forum, 42*(1), 12–19.

National Association of School Nurses. (2014). Do not attempt resuscitation. Retrieved May 2014 from http://www.nasn.org/PolicyAdvocacy/PositionPapersand Reports/NASNPositionStatementsFullView/tabid/462/ArticleId/640 /Do-Not-Attempt-Resuscitation-DNAR-The-Role-of-the-School-Nurse-Adopted-January-2014.

National Center for Health Statistics (NCHS). (2011). *Health, United States, 2010: With special feature on death and dying* [DHHS Publication No. 2011-1232]. Washington, DC: US Government Printing Office.

National Hospice and Palliative Care Organization (NHPCO). (2007). *2006 national summary of hospice care: Statistics and trends from the 2006 national data set and 2006 NHPCO membership survey*. Alexandria, VA: NHPCO.

Newacheck, P. W., & Halfon, N. (1998). Prevalence and impact of disabling conditions of childhood. *American Journal of Public Health, 88*(4), 610–617.

Newacheck, P. W., Strickland, B., Shonkoff, J. P., Perrin, J. M., McPherson, M., McManus, M.,...Arango, P. (1998). An epidemiologic profile of children with special health care needs. *Pediatrics, 102*(1, Pt. 1), 117–123.

Nitschke, R., Caldwell, S., & Jay, S. (1986). Therapeutic choices in end-stage cancer. *Journal of Pediatrics, 108*(2), 330–331.

Nitschke, R., Humphrey, G. B., Sexauer, C. L., Catron, B., Wunder, S., & Jay, S. (1982). Therapeutic choices made by patients with end-stage cancer. *Journal of Pediatrics*, *101*(3), 471–476.

Patient Protection and Affordable Care Act (PPACA), Public L. No. 111-148, §2302, 124 Stat. 119 (2010).

Pediatric Research Equity Act of 2003 (PREA), Public L. No. 108-155, 117 Stat. 1936 (2003).

Reder, E. A., & Serwint, J. R. (2009). Until the last breath: Exploring the concept of hope for parents and health care professionals during a child's serious illness. *Archives of Pediatric and Adolescent Medicine*, *163*(7), 653–657.

Rosenberg, A. R., Baker, K. S., Syrjala, K., & Wolfe, J. (2012). Systematic review of psychosocial morbidities among bereaved parents of children with cancer. *Pediatric Blood and Cancer*, *58*(4), 503–512.

Rowell, M., & Zlotkin, S. (1997). The ethical boundaries of drug research in pediatrics. *Pediatric Clinics of North America*, *44*(1), 27–40.

Sahler, O., Frager, G., Levetown, M., Cohn, F., & Lipson, M. (2000). Medical education about end-of-life care in the pediatric setting: Principles, challenges, and opportunities. *Pediatrics*, *105*(3), 575–584.

Sharman, M., Meert, K. L., & Sarnaik, A. P. (2005). What influences parents' decisions to limit or withdraw life support? *Pediatric Critical Care Medicine*, *6*(5), 513–518.

Siden, H., Miller, M., Straatman, L., Omesi, L., Tucker, T., & Collins, J. J. (2008). A report on location of death in paediatric palliative care between home, hospice and hospital. *Palliative Medicine*, *22*(7), 831–834.

Steele, R., Bosma, H., Johnston, M. F., Cadell, S., Davies, B., Siden, H., & Straatman, L. (2008). Research priorities in pediatric palliative care: A Delphi study. *Journal of Palliative Care*, *24*(4), 229–239.

Surkan, P. J., Dickman, P. W., Steineck, G., Onelöv, E., & Kreicbergs, U. (2006). Home care of a child dying of a malignancy and parental awareness of a child's impending death. *Palliative Medicine*, *20*(3), 161–169.

Wolfe, J., Klar, N., Grier, H. E., Duncan, J., Salem-Schatz, S., Emanuel, E. J., & Weeks, J. C. (2000). Understanding of prognosis among parents of children who died of cancer: Impact on treatment goals and integration of palliative care. *Journal of the American Medical Association*, *284*(19), 2469–2475.

Young, B., Dixon-Woods, M., Windridge, K. C., & Heney, D. (2003). Managing communication with young people who have a potentially life threatening chronic illness: Qualitative study of patients and parents. *British Medical Journal*, *326*(7384), 305–30.

CHAPTER 7

The "Patient–Family Dyad" As an Interdependent Unit of Hospice Care

Toward an Ethical Justification

PATRICK T. SMITH

It is widely regarded in hospice philosophy that the patient and the patient's family together are the primary unit of care. This chapter seeks to provide exposition and justification for this approach to hospice health care that sees the patient–family dyad as an interdependent unit of care. It also highlights some of the ethical challenges that emerge with numerous levels and layers of relationships, both personal and professional. In the pages that follow I argue that the dyad model is an important and essential approach to accomplish the goals of effective hospice care despite its potential, though by no means inevitable, ethical burdens.

TOWARD A JUSTIFICATION FOR THE MODEL

The emphasis on the patient–family dyad as an interdependent unit of care in some ways is a departure from the trajectory of contemporary Western approaches to medicine. In view of the gradual deinstitutionalization of specifically end-of-life health care, many hospice professionals think the commitment to the patient–family dyad is justified. Moreover, they deem this obligation necessary in order to provide quality palliative care to gravely ill patients. The primary claim presented here can be summarized as follows. Holistic patient care is one of the aims of hospice care. Furthermore, treating patients holistically entails caring for their families in such a way that the family both gives and receives care. If so, then treating the family as an interdependent unit of care is a necessary condition for delivering high-quality hospice care.

This chapter attempts to draw together three broad features that converge into the unique context of hospice care. My contention is that the intersection of these features provides some justification for the commitment that hospices make to families when caring for their ill loved ones. The first feature is that hospice care emphasizes that patients are to be treated holistically as persons on two distinct levels, individually and in community. On one level, patients not only have physical needs but also psychological, emotional, and spiritual concerns that are exacerbated by the underlying illness. These spiritual and psychoemotional dimensions of sickness and disease can affect patients' overall health in ways just as significant as physical ailment from the illness. On another level, patients also belong to a broader social network of intimate relationships that necessarily affect the people involved in them in some way or other. Hence, the focus on patients as individuals should understood in a way that isolates them from the larger social-familial context in which they develop, are cared for, and express their humanity. A second feature that justifies the commitment that hospices make to families is that family members or relatives in hospice more prominently play a dual role in care for their loved ones than in other forms of health and palliative care in general. And third, benefits to the patients occur when certain needs of families are met while they serve in the role of primary informal caregivers. The following sections provide further expression to and exposition of each of these features in turn.

The Holistic Context of Hospice Care

To begin, the holistic context of hospice care is important to keep in mind when reflecting on the ethics of the hospice commitment to the patient–family dyad as an interdependent unit of care. Some have suggested that wholeness or overall well-being is a central pursuit of human existence (Randall & Downie, 1999, p. 22). Even though there may be multiple visions of exactly what constitutes wholeness, the search, nevertheless, appears to be endemic to humanity. Obviously, many things can and do go wrong in human life, most notably, the occurrence of incurable disease leading to death. The purpose of hospice palliative care, therefore, is to restore or preserve as much personal and interpersonal integrity or wholeness as possible "during the final stages of illness, the dying process, and the bereavement period" by providing compassionate care for the patient and family (Wilder, Parker Oliver, Demiris, & Washington, 2008, p. 313).

Part of what it means to provide compassionate care in the hospice setting is to alleviate, within ethical and legal bounds, the pain and suffering and to preserve the quality of life of those near the end of their lives. Though often mentioned together, "pain" and "suffering" are not synonymous. Pain is understood as a "complex phenomenon with physical, psychological, social, and spiritual components," whereas suffering is often described as a "highly personal experience that depends on the meaning an event such as illness or loss has for an individual" (Panke, 2003, p. 84). The experience of suffering stems from a wide range of sources, including "fear of or actual physical distress, fear of dying, changing self-perceptions, relationship concerns, the need to find meaning in any given life experience, and past experiences of witnessing another person's distress" (Panke, 2003, p. 84). This is the complex nexus, containing both individual and social dimensions, in which hospice professionals address pain and suffering. Both of these dimensions of holistic care should be kept in view when providing care to patients and their families.

The Patient As a Complex Individual

The hospice philosophy of care acknowledges that there are multiple fronts on which a care team needs to interact with patients on an individual level that include both physical and spiritual/psychoemotional elements. "Physical pain remains a major cause of human suffering and is the primary image formed by people when they think about suffering" (Cassell, 2004, p. 31). Therefore, it could perhaps go without saying that providing compassionate care to patients at the end of life in a hospice context involves employing the most effective means possible of controlling physical pain to relieve the suffering often caused by the illness. Patients and their families are often concerned about whether the patients' physical symptoms will be properly managed in the dying process. And this can be the source of some familial distress. Proper care in hospice necessarily includes caring for patients' physical needs well and fully.

Hospice must also take seriously the psychological or emotional/spiritual dimensions of human existence. Panke is correct when she states, "Although pharmacotherapy is the foundation of pain management, with opioids as the mainstay, attention to and intervention for the many aspects of pain and suffering are necessary to relieve pain" (Panke, 2003, p. 84). So there is much more to providing compassionate care for patients in hospice than managing physical symptoms only through pharmacological means.

It is also widely recognized that human needs concerning spirituality are a crucial aspect of hospice palliative care. As O'Connell highlights:

> The moral weight of spiritual interests gains special prominence in the realm of palliative care that focuses upon end of life. Despite its positive and supportive thrust, end of life care does evoke a sense of limitation and inevitable loss. As the proximity of death becomes palpably more present, spiritual interests naturally come to the fore. The impulse to seek meaning and the need to envision some form of transcendence are no strangers to those who regularly encounter terminally ill persons. (O'Connell, 2006, p. 27)

While notions of spirituality, however understood, may be profoundly personal, they are not necessarily private. These aspects of spiritual perspectives affect families of patients and the formal care team as well. To be sure, spirituality ought not be confused with religion in a formal sense, though it can certainly be compatible with it.

In very broad and general terms, "spirituality may be defined simply as the characteristics and qualities of one's relationship with the transcendent" (Sulmasy, 2006, pp. 103–104). Sulmasy proposes that everyone has a form of spirituality (and hence spiritual needs) even if it does not take the form of ritual or religious, theological belief. The questions of "spirituality" are profoundly human ones that are asked and answered in different ways by different people, in the religious and nonreligious. These questions tend to take on more prominence in the context of death and dying. When patients are confronted with the reality of their own mortality, their levels of emotional fears and spiritual anxiety are often raised.

These stressful situations in which some terminally ill patients and the imminently dying find themselves can be the source of suffering not only personally but *also can carry over to the entire family unit.* The adverse impact on the *family* from their ill loved one's negative experiences can serve as a *further source of suffering for the patient.* This also includes cases in which the suffering is a result of unresolved spiritual or existential questions that are unsettled and troubling in the minds of patients and their loved ones. This is important for hospice health care professionals since *dying patients can experience suffering* not only as a direct result from the underlying illness but also from the *effect of their sickness on those in their social network.* Given that hospice care attempts to address the many emotional fears and spiritual anxieties that encompass the broad range of human experience, these multifaceted aspects of suffering present challenges to a hospice care team in many ways. "By giving credence to this important [spiritual, emotional, psychological] dimension in our lives," notes Puchalski, "we open ourselves up to a type of healing that, while not necessarily curative, does restore us to a wholeness that is perhaps more significant than the cure of a physical illness" (Puchalski, 2006, p. x).

The Patient As a Social Being

Since our patients are social beings who are interconnected in meaningful ways, the patient and family must be viewed as an interdependent unit of care. Dyck provides an informative description of the moral bonds of community that is helpful in understanding the necessary interconnectedness of human beings by virtue of being human. He explains:

> A community is an affiliated and mutually beneficial network of interdependent human beings who, as human beings, share what is requisite for forming and sustaining such a network. A network of individuals or groups can be connected or affiliated in a variety of ways, including ties created or sustained by procreation, nurture, affection, culture, religion, politics, or economic exchange—or some combination of these. These affiliations are characteristically mediated by language, symbols, and artifacts. Individuals might be affiliated in their capacities as moral agents or as recipients of human agency, for example, while they are infants or seriously incapacitated. This means that affiliated individuals might not always perceive the benefits of affiliation or actively ensure the mutuality of such benefits. These benefits are not always moral, but each affiliative relation is sustained by moral elements. (Dyck, 2005, p. 95, emphasis added)

As social beings, humans are linked to other people within the moral bonds of community. Human beings can and do express themselves in various ways from one social network to another and are also part of multiple networks simultaneously. Hence, the hospice team should be sensitive to and mindful of these relational dynamics when providing care and remain flexible to the changing needs of those they serve.

The family is one of the more prominent social networks in which patients participate, and in the overwhelming majority of cases hospices interact with the patients they care for in the context of the family system, not in isolation from it (Connor, 2009, p. 7). Therefore, an important question in this discussion is who actually constitutes a patient's family? Traditionally, the family has been understood as those who were in some sort of biological and legal relation to one another. The *majority* of informal caregivers have some sort of blood and legal relationship with the patient for whom they are caring. Panke and Ferrell reflect this *general* observation in oncology when they write, "Studies in oncology related to the family have generally found that approximately 70% of primary family caregivers are spouses, approximately 20% are children (of which daughters and daughters-in-law are most predominant), and approximately 10% are friends or more distant relatives" (Panke & Ferrell, 2004, p. 985).

However, Panke and Ferrell note the family also includes those "persons identified by the patient as significant in their lives, intimately involved with the patient, who love the patient, and have frequent contact with the patient" (Panke & Ferrell, p. 985). So for the purposes of this chapter, what constitutes the family is to be understood as "those bonded to the patient by blood, [legal], or emotional ties, that is, the patient's most immediate attachment network" (Connor, 2009, p. 7). In other words, a broad understanding of family, including all those individuals considered as such by the patient, is most fitting in the context of hospice care.

The imprecision with respect to the referent of the term "family" in a health care context can become problematic. Take a scenario where a health care team is caring for an incapacitated patient. There arises a conflict concerning the direction of patient care. On one side of the dispute is someone who is close to the patient and also considered by the patient to be family but lacks legal recognition. On the other side is one who has some legal rights due to biological connections, but the relationship lacks the property of closeness. These scenarios notwithstanding, many in hospice appropriately seem to use the saying "the family is the patient." It is important that this statement be properly understood. It is not so much that the saying is wrong, as it is inexact. Certainly the idea behind the assertion can and ought to be affirmed. As stated, however, it does not quite capture the complex and diverse interpersonal relationships that exist in the family–patient dyad. Therefore, the phrase "interdependent unit of care" is preferred here to denote the fact that there is, in an important sense, a unity between the family, however delineated, and the patient within the moral bonds of community. Even so, a distinction must be acknowledged and maintained between the two entities. "The conflicts of interest, beliefs, and values among family members are often too real and run too deep to treat all members as the 'patient'" (Hardwig, 1990, p. 5). Nevertheless, both groups, when in close relationship with each other, are appropriate recipients of hospice care.

The model of the patient and family as an interdependent unit of care rightly acknowledges that the familial social network is affected by the major life decisions made by the member of the group who is seriously ill.

> There is no way to detach the lives of patients from the lives of those who are close to them. Indeed, the intertwining of lives is part of the very meaning of closeness. Consequently, there will be a broad spectrum of cases in which treatment options will have dramatic and different impacts within the patient's family. (Hardwig, 1990, p. 5)

Hardwig suggests that there are many connected and, in some cases, competing interests between patients and close members in the family system concerning significant medical decisions. He maintains that being part of a family system entails a moral requirement not to make only self-regarding decisions even among those who are in poor health. He acknowledges that seriously ill family members have a right to special consideration, but he maintains that these patients still have a moral obligation to the unit (Hardwig, 1990, p. 6).

Nonetheless, it must be emphasized that there are significant responsibilities incurred by family members to care for their ill loved ones in major ways. Intimate relationships, as are the case with many family situations, not only are a privilege people enjoy but also come with burdens of responsibilities from which its members are not easily absolved. Nelson and Nelson claim, "Just as intimate relationships themselves aren't always the result of 'free choice,' so the responsibilities that stem from them are often not freely chosen" (1995, p. 77). Not only are family members required to, but inevitably do, make sacrifices simply by virtue of being part of that social network. This seems to be more so the case when a member is gravely ill and especially vulnerable. Of course, there are limits to the kinds and levels of sacrifice that one is called to make in these relationships.

Ethical Issues

Taking the patient–family dyad as an interdependent unit of care includes seeing this group as having a significant stake in the decision-making process. This, at times, can be the source of greater levels of complexity in the professional relationship. As one hospice professional points out,

> given that most people do not want to discuss the end of life until they must, it is no wonder that making any decisions on behalf of a dying loved one has

become so overwhelming. Making decisions such as whether to maintain life support is difficult enough for an individual. The difficulty can readily be compounded when decisions must be made by "committee," or family. (Beckwith, 2005, p. 145)

Those who have spent any time involved in hospice care are well aware that conditions emerge in this context that can give rise to numerous professional difficulties. Conflicts of interest can arise within the complexity of multiple interested parties, adding to the volatility of family dynamics. The emotional needs; choices about care; beliefs about life; religious reflections on death, dying, and the afterlife; or the lack thereof are not always in accord among family members. Some close family members may not have come to terms with the pending death of their loved ones. The stressful circumstances surrounding an impending death can exacerbate unresolved issues in family relationships, which can frustrate the ability to make difficult decisions. Though many times unintended, these unfortunate situations have a detrimental effect on the ill loved one and can hinder the professional hospice care team from providing proper care.

Moreover, it is not always the case that "families function healthily, and have the best interests of their dying loved ones at heart" (Kirk, 2007, p. 26). There can be past hurts and broken relationships that have gone unresolved among close family members. As Hardwig observes, "'Closeness' does not...always mean care and abiding affection, nor need it be a positive experience—one can hate, resent, fear, or despise a mother or brother with an intensity not often directed toward strangers, acquaintances, or associates" (Hardwig, 1990, p. 5). Even if forgiveness and reconciliation are desired by those in strained relationships, achieving these goals is difficult. Conceptually and theoretically these notions are complex and elusive, and in practice, as Griswold has noted, "it may seem at the outset that the dream of reconciliation...cannot be fulfilled through forgiveness because forgiveness...aspire[s] to something impossible: knowingly to undo what has been done" (Griswold, 2007, pp. xiv–xv). Given these realities and difficulties, there may be human longings that are not easily fulfilled and past injuries that are not easily overcome. Regardless of whether patients committed these perceived offenses or whether harms were done to them, when left unresolved these hurts can lead to regrets and precarious relationships between family members. These situations can generate interpersonal conflicts and ethical challenges for the care team, patients, and their families to overcome.

Conflicts can be due to a misunderstanding of one or more parties involved in the plan of care, unrealistic expectations, or lack of education.

In such circumstances the conflict should be seen not as an ethical issue but an information issue. For example, family members may disagree with each other and/or the formal hospice care team concerning the level of medication that the dying patient is receiving. One family member may be afraid that her loved one will become addicted to morphine if too much is given. Another family member may not be afraid of the possibility of addiction, but instead does not want the prescribed dose as recommended by the care team to be given because the patient is not as alert when this is done. While the dying patient's pain does not seem to be unbearable, the care team is concerned about the situation from another vantage point. They worry about whether the patient's pain is being managed as well as it could in this situation. There are difficulties to address and conflicts to resolve in a scenario like this, yet many would agree that it does not seem to rise to the level of an ethical dilemma. It could easily turn into one, however.

Hospice professionals can aid in resolving some conflicts and can provide a tremendous service to families when they take the role of negotiator. Even so, it would be naïve to think that every emotionally deep, long-standing family conflict could be resolved to the full satisfaction of all involved parties. Regardless, when the hospice care team intervenes and uses its rich resources to help negotiate these difficulties, many of these situations can have more positive outcomes than would have occurred otherwise.

While the patient–family dyad as an interdependent unit of care is widely embraced by many in a hospice context, the approach is not without its strong critics. The problem is not that there are resources hospice professionals can employ to resolve conflicts these critics suggest, but that using these resources would obscure the real issue. In other words, the problem is not merely in the complexity of professional practice but instead is intrinsic to the family-centered care model in hospice. This seems to be the thrust of the criticisms of Randall and Downie regarding the hospice commitment to the patient–family dyad as an interdependent unit of care. They write:

> [T]he philosophy of palliative care dictates that the relatives of the patient are also part of the remit of care. They appear to be given equal importance to that of the patient. It is perhaps puzzling that there has been so little discussion of the ethical problems which must then arise when there is a conflict of interest between the patient and family. The question must surely arise as to "who comes first, patient or family?" when such a conflict occurs. Despite the fact that this question is unavoidable if family and patient are given equal priority, some writers either try to avoid it or write what appears to be conflicting statements on the issue. (Randall & Downie, 1999, p. 76)

The notion that for hospice both patient and family are a focus of care and concern does not mean that the patient's well-being should be subordinated. I would argue that the commitment in hospice to the family should never be practiced in a way that is actually *detrimental* to the dying patient. Randall and Downie seem to argue that not only will conflicts between patient and family interests emerge, but also that it follows from the holistic and contextual orientation of hospice and palliative care that such conflicts are mostly resolved in ways that are harmful to patients. I do not believe that these problems are as intractable as Randall and Downie suggest. Rather, understanding the patient in the context of family relationality can be protective of the patient because it gives caregivers a more sensitive and concrete understanding of what the patient's needs and interests are. This is not so much a matter of taking sides as it is a question of avoiding abstractions and stereotypes and meeting patients and families where they are rather than where caregivers presuppose they are or should be. Randall and Downie are concerned about who gets priority when a conflict occurs; in these situations they ask, "Who comes first, patient or family?" The phrasing of this question, nevertheless, reveals an unexamined presupposition. It seems to assume that the question can be answered in the abstract. If so, this appears dubious. Whenever ethical dilemmas emerge in hospice care, the particular details and circumstances of the context must be examined in order to answer the question appropriately. It is difficult and, perhaps, impossible to attempt an answer to their question apart from an examination of the factual elements of the case.

For example, consider the following scenario:

Phil is an 84-year-old male with end-stage cardiac disease and is currently on hospice care. He has been living alone caring for himself for many years since the death of his wife. He has two children, one daughter who lives with her family across the country, and one son who lives within 30 minutes of his house with his wife and three young children who are very active in extracurricular activities. Phil has started to show signs of fatigue and shortness of breath with minimal exertion. He is forgetful and often misses taking his medication. He is incontinent of his urine sometimes and will not wear a brief. His son manages his care and makes sure he has food in the house.

The formal hospice care team has been providing supportive care to Phil several times a week for a few hours and have supported Phil's son in caring for his father as well. The care team has voiced a concern that Phil is not safe to live alone. They entered the home this week to find that he had left the burner on after making his breakfast. The son and his wife also worry about some of the dangerous behavior exhibited by Phil like leaving the stove on. Phil wholeheartedly agrees that he is unable to take care of himself in his home any longer. But he is adamant that he will not go into a nursing or hospice care facility. He states that he will only move in with his son. He insists that his son has a duty to care for him as he cared for and raised his son. The son and his wife do not feel that they are able to care for Phil in their home, yet they deeply care about him and insist they will remain active in his care. They have verbalized that they are rarely home between their jobs and the kids' schedules.

What might the response be to the question "Who comes first, patient or family?" in this situation? If we simply say "the patient," how is this to work in practice? It would seem that the formal care team has an obligation to Phil, but his request in this situation cannot be fulfilled. The formal hospice care team would need to look for another more creative approach to resolve this kind of ethical conflict. Even if the son could be forced to take in Phil, would that be beneficial to Phil's overall care? It seems difficult to imagine how it would, all things being equal. This is a question that requires exploring the meaning of patient autonomy, and the connection of that autonomy to place of care, in a manner more nuanced than the dichotomous choice between "patient vs. family" is able to capture.

Of course, there are other times when the patient's request should get the most weight. For example, Phil's case could be modified in the following way. Say Phil wants to go into a care center or a nursing home instead of living with his son. Yet the son is adamant that his father should live out his remaining days with him and his family. Most would concur that the care team should assist this family in resolving the issue in a way that Phil is able to live out his remaining days where he wants, which is in a skilled nursing facility or a hospice care center, assuming availability. Some hospice professionals may have differing opinions and judgments on these matters for various reasons. Whatever the case may be, the point remains that to answer the question posed by these critics without considering the details of the case seems unwise.

Primary Role of Informal Caregivers

The second feature that provides justification for the hospice commitment to the patient–family dyad as a unit of care is that families often serve as primary informal caregivers. The important point to highlight is that *relatives are not only part of the unit of care; they are also part of the care team*. This is crucial in appreciating the emphasis on the patient–family dyad as the appropriate unit of hospice care. This dual role creates a dynamic that is often missing in some forms of health care. The patient–family dyad as an interdependent unit of care attempts to bring together once again two ancient systems of care for the vulnerable, namely, family and medicine. This model recognizes the important fact that "families have played a most important role in the history of medicine, tending to the sick when doctors were unavailable or unavailing. Medicine and the family…are in part shaped by the other and rely upon the other for certain kinds of help" (Nelson & Nelson, 2004, p. 875).

Dual Role of the Family

Hospice care continues to serve a high number of people who prefer to be cared for in their homes when possible, regardless of whether beds are available in a hospital or hospice care center. This is often the case even if the place of death of many hospice patients is somewhere other than in their homes. Therefore, hospices must rely on the ability of *informal* caregivers, who most often are not professionally trained in hospice care, to perform caregiving tasks. These informal caregivers are frequently composed of those members who are considered the family by the patient. In the home, the family serves as the primary caregivers for the patient. The formal hospice care team comes alongside the family not only to meet the needs of the dying person but also to support family members in a way that they are able to fulfill their responsibilities to their ill loved one.

The responsibilities taken on by informal caregivers are numerous, including assisting with both primary and instrumental activities of daily living and administering complicated medication schedules. These are the kinds of activities that many trained medical professionals engage in and, in home hospice care, these are the activities that become the responsibilities of informal caregivers. Family members, as the primary caregivers for the patient in hospice care should therefore be seen as being part of the care team. They need to be supported by the resources that a formal hospice care team is best suited to provide. In a hospital setting, family members are often in the role of concerned bystanders; in hospice they become anxious and crucial participants in the care of their loved one.

Informal caregivers can have anxieties that emerge specifically in home hospice settings. Consider some examples. First, there is the fear of the unknown. Relatives serving as informal caregivers may experience anxiety due to lack of professionals in the immediate proximity to explain symptoms that may emerge suddenly. Often family members are anxious about recognizing what actually represents a genuine emergency in the home and whether a formal care team member should be notified in such an event. Second, there is the concern of not being able to appropriately assist the patient with personal care and daily activities. Often relatives "report feeling very inadequate for the task of caring at home, not knowing how to make the patient comfortable, unsure how to lift or assist the patient, or help with bathing or feeding" (Doyle, 2004, p. 1102). In short, many relatives are afraid of hurting their loved ones. Third, and closely related to the prior point, there is anxiety that comes along with the fear of wrongly administering medications. Doyle describes the situation of many informal caregivers with some clarity when he writes:

> Medications are given by untrained people who cannot be expected to be as reliable in this matter as hospital nurses would be. Particularly in the case when liquid medications have to be measured. Relatives can be very anxious lest they are responsible for the deterioration or even the death of the patient as a result of their administering a prescribed drug. It is easy to forget that most terminally ill patients are on several drugs, said to be on average 4, but ranging from 0–11. (Doyle, 2004, p. 1102)

All of these fears and anxieties, along with many others not mentioned, can have a cumulative effect of inadequate symptom management for the patient. Therefore, the family needs to be adequately supported by the formal hospice care team in order for them to properly care for their dying loved one in the home. The frequency and intensity of anxieties that relatives have as informal caregivers are often minimized when patients are in hospice care centers as opposed to being in the home. Nevertheless, family members still need the support of the formal hospice team to effectively care for their dying loved ones whether they are located at inpatient facilities or in the home. Given the various kinds of resources needed for relatives to fulfill their caregiving role, the overall point that the family should be seen as simultaneously recipients of care and givers of care, is reinforced. Thus, the family needs are and ought to be included in the scope of professional care in a direct, and not merely tangential, way.

Ethical Issues

The commitment of hospice to the patient–family dyad as an interdependent unit of care and part of the care team does raise some interesting ethical questions. One question centers on the notion of confidentiality. Should the family be privy to certain information that may be necessary for the care of the ill patient even if the patient does not want them to know? How much information is needed for the family in order for them to effectively care for their dying loved one?

> Dolores is a 64-year-old female dying of metastatic lung cancer. She has large wounds on her sacrum. She is thin and weak and requires assistance bathing, dressing, and with wound care. Her dressings are saturated with blood and must be changed twice a day. She lives with her son Jack and his new wife, Jill. Jill has been the primary informal caregiver for Dolores for the 2 months she has lived with them, which includes handling of Dolores's bloody dressings and cleaning her wounds. Dolores also has advanced stages of AIDS and requests that her HIV status be kept private. Even though Dolores does not know her new daughter-in-law well, she really likes Jill and her being with Jack. Dolores fears that if Jill knew her HIV/AIDS status that Jill would not care for her any longer, or she would leave her son, or that Jill would encourage Jack to place her somewhere else. The formal hospice care team notices that Jill is often handling the dressings without wearing gloves. The care team becomes increasingly concerned about this situation.

This scenario highlights the tension between the ethical values of fidelity to the patient in the form of confidentiality and patient autonomy, on one hand, and protection of the common good, on the other. What are care team's moral obligations to Dolores in a situation like this? What about Jill? Some would think that Dolores's HIV/AIDS status would be important information for formal members of the professional hospice team to know if they were going into the home to provide care to her. If so, then should not the same be the case with Jill, who is also part of the care team as the primary informal caregiver?

Given the social stigmas that are connected with HIV/AIDS, one would need to be very careful not to disclose this information without sufficient warrant. Some may think the care team should encourage Jill to take universal precautions, and if she does she should be fine. But in the face of a very serious communicable disease like HIV/AIDS, others may think that there is a moral obligation on the part of the care team to go against the request of Dolores in a situation like this. After all, the value of confidentiality, while extremely important, is not absolute. There are conditions in which the breach of confidentiality is professionally appropriate and perhaps even morally obligatory. One such example is the moral and professional obligation of a psychiatrist to inform authorities of a patient who is threatening harm to a specific person. If the care team is unable to convince Dolores to inform her daughter-in-law of her condition, then given the severity of risk, a care team may be justified in informing Jill, especially since she is the primary informal caregiver.

The dual role that informal caregivers have, in that they are not only part of the unit of care but also part of the care team, complicates the meaning and practice of patient confidentiality in hospice care. Indeed, confidentiality is a paradigmatic example of how family-centered care creates a tension between ethics, law, and the philosophy and structure of hospice care. Proactive organizational policy can help clinicians navigate this tension. When patients have decision-making capacity, the admissions process should explicitly address the important role of family members in the delivery of care and clarify with patients what kinds of protected health information can be shared with which family members, in what conditions, and for what reasons. Absent decision-making capacity, this discussion should be had with patient-appointed agents or legally designated surrogates.

Professional hospice care teams have special duties and responsibilities to the family along with their duties and responsibilities to the ill or dying patient. In order for the aims of hospice to be accomplished, hospice providers must be concerned about the personal well-being of the family in the role of *primary* informal caregivers especially in a home care setting. Thus, "the hospice philosophy emphasizes supporting caregivers to give the best care possible to their dying loved ones" such that "hospice professionals incur moral obligations to both the dying patient and that patient's identified caregivers" (Kirk, p. 27).

Benefit to Patient in Meeting Family Needs

The last justification for the commitment to the family is that there appear to be some benefits to dying patients when the various needs of their informal caregivers are met.

Potential Negative Impact on Patient

Family members of a patient often have a difficult time with the condition of their loved one. There can be severe emotional distress on family members or informal caregivers who observe their ill loved ones experiencing unrelieved pain (Panke, 2003, p. 84). Observing their family members in distress can be a source of suffering for patients. Vachon notes that "the manner in which an individual's significant others respond to the person and his or her illness may, in part, determine the individual's response to the disease" (Vachon, 2004, p. 961). If so, then it is a proper aim for hospice health care to mitigate insofar as possible the circumstances that can have a negative impact on the family or relatives' well-being as informal caregivers if in fact these conditions can have deleterious affects on the dying patient.

Informal caregivers need to have support in order to fulfill their caregiving responsibilities while simultaneously dealing with the imminent death of a loved one and perhaps maintaining some other employment as well. If caregivers' well-being is significantly diminished and some of their personal needs go unmet due to the pressure and stress of caring for their dying loved ones, then there are some tangible consequences concerning the ability of family members to perform their duties as primary caregivers to the ill patient. Thus, the support structures in the home that are provided primarily by these informal caregivers may very well collapse, resulting in an overall lower quality of care (Wilder et al., 2008, p. 314).

Research suggests that "the quality of life of patient and caregiver is often linked directly and indirectly" such that "attention to caregiver quality of life is important for both the caregivers themselves and the patients under their care" (Wilder et al., 2008, p. 316). A 2008 study set out to examine the social, emotional, financial, and physical effects of informal caregiving on the quality of life of family members who were caring for patients in hospice (Wilder et al., 2008). The hypothesis was that the decrease of quality of life would be higher in hospice informal caregivers than the decrease in non-hospice caregivers. If the hypothesis was supported, researchers expected to find a greater correlation between the direct and indirect link on the quality of life of patient and caregiver in a hospice setting than in other contexts. Since the hospice informal caregiver can have a greater decline in quality of life than other informal caregivers, then the more vulnerable hospice patients are to this detrimental situation as well. Wilder and others concluded, "caregiving for a dying loved one is a uniquely demanding task. The informal caregiver role is both necessary for the provision of gold standard end-of-life care as well as an important target for support within the hospice philosophy" (Wilder et al., 2008, p. 329). They also stress that "hospice teams must strive to continually improve their clinical services with regard to caregivers' quality of life, especially in emotional and social domains" (Wilder et al., 2008, p. 329).

As the US population ages and demands on the overall health care system increase, it will become all the more important that the patient–family dyad be taken seriously in hospice care. In a real sense, meeting the needs of the family is simultaneously to meet the needs of the patient. It is from this vantage point that we can better understand Connor's statement concerning hospice philosophy that "often the family's needs are equal to or greater than the dying person's" (Connor, 2009, p. 7). In other words, it is a mistake to regard the family in hospice care as a mere sideshow, a means to an end for the hospice care team or the dying patient. Each family member serving as an informal caregiver has value and dignity in his or her own right and must be treated as such. Conversely, the patient's concerns and well-being should not be lost with the commitment to the patient–family dyad as an interdependent unit of care.

In many hospice contexts, there is a strong emphasis placed on the self-care of the formal staff in order to maintain quality care, avoid burnout, and preserve personal integrity in light of the professional and personal burdens that come along with hospice work. And resources are often provided to this end. As highlighted earlier, if the family plays the dual role of being part of the unit of care and part of the care team, then it can be equally apropos for resources to be provided for informal caregivers for many of the same reasons that it is deemed important for the professionally trained care team. Given these realities taken together, the emphasis on the patient–family dyad as an interdependent unit of care is warranted.

CONCLUSION

In order for hospice to be effective with respect to its stated purposes and approach to health care in all of these dimensions of human life, it must employ a wide range of resources. These surely must come from the ranks of social workers, chaplains of various stripes, hospice aides, nurses and nurse practitioners, medical doctors, counselors, volunteers, and many others to address the challenges that emerge in this context. Therefore, professional hospice care for the terminally ill and imminently dying is necessarily interdisciplinary and multilayered.

The patient–family dyad as an interdependent unit of care acknowledges that human beings are not easily extracted from a given communal context. So we must care for patients not merely as individuals but as social beings. The family-centered model of care in hospice captures this reality and seeks to traverse the complicated dynamics that come with this commitment. A further advantage of the model is that it takes into account the dual role that the families as informal primary caregivers have in these situations. This simply just is the case, and it is difficult to think that given this reality that a model of care in a specifically hospice context should be conceived otherwise. Moreover, at the end of the day the care that is extended to the family by hospice professionals does have an impact directly and indirectly on patient care. The patient–family dyad approach of hospice care attempts to incorporate the full scope of the difficult realities families and patients face together during the experience of death and dying.

REFERENCES

Beckwith, S. K. (2005). When families disagree: Family conflicts and decisions. In K. J. Doka, B. Jennings, & C. A. Corr (Eds.), *Living with grief: Ethical dilemmas at the end of life* (pp. 143–156). Washington, DC: Hospice Foundation of America.

Cassell, E. J. (2004). *The nature of suffering and the goals of medicine* (2nd ed.). New York, NY: Oxford University Press.

Connor, S. R. (2009). *Hospice and palliative care: The essential guide* (2nd ed.). New York, NY: Routledge.

Doyle, D. (2004). Palliative medicine in the home: An overview. In D. Doyle, G. Hanks, N. I. Cherny, & K. Calman (Eds.), *Oxford textbook of palliative medicine* (3rd ed., pp. 1097–1113). New York: Oxford University Press.

Dyck, A. J. (2005). *Rethinking rights and responsibilities: The moral bonds of community* (rev. ed.). Washington, DC: Georgetown University Press.

Griswold, C, L. (2007). *Forgiveness: A philosophical exploration.* New York, NY: Cambridge University Press.

Hardwig, J. (1990). What about the family? *Hastings Center Report, 20*(2), 5–10.

Kirk, T. W. (2007). Managing pain, managing ethics. *Pain Management Nursing, 8*(1), 25–34.

Nelson, H. L., & Nelson, J. L. (1995). *The patient in the family: An ethics of medicine and families.* New York, NY: Routledge.

Nelson, H. L., & Nelson, J. L. (2004). Family and family medicine. In S. G. Post (Ed.), *Encyclopedia of bioethics* (3rd ed., Vol. 2, p. 875). New York, NY: Macmillan Reference.

O'Connell, L. J. (2006). Spirituality in palliative care: An ethical imperative. In C. M. Puchalski (Ed.), *A time for listening and caring: Spirituality and the care of the chronically ill and dying* (pp. 27–38). New York, NY: Oxford University Press.

Panke, J. T. (2003). Difficulties in managing pain at the end of life. *Journal of Hospice and Palliative Nursing, 5*(2), 83–90.

Panke, J. T., & Ferrell, B. R. (2004). Emotional problems in the family. In D. Doyle, G. Hanks, N. I. Cherny, & K. Calman (Eds.), *Oxford textbook of palliative medicine* (3rd ed., pp. 985–991). New York, NY: Oxford University Press.

Puchalski, C. M. (Ed.). (2006). *A time for listening and caring: Spirituality and the care of the chronically ill and dying.* New York, NY: Oxford University Press.

Randall, F., & Downie, R. S. (1999). *Palliative care ethics: A companion for all specialties* (2nd ed.). New York, NY: Oxford University Press.

Sulmasy, D. P. (2006). The healthcare professional as a person: The spirituality of providing care at the end of life. In C. M. Puchalski (Ed.), *A time for listening and caring: Spirituality and the care of the chronically ill and dying* (pp. 101–114). New York, NY: Oxford University Press.

Vachon, V. L. (2004). The emotional problems of the patient in palliative medicine. In D. Doyle, G. Hanks, N. I. Cherny, & K. Calman (Eds.), *Oxford textbook of palliative medicine* (3rd ed., pp. 961–984). New York, NY: Oxford University Press.

Wilder, H. M., Parker Oliver, D., Demiris, G., & Washington, K. (2008). Informal hospice caregiving: The toll on quality of life. *Journal of Social Work in End-of-Life and Palliative Care*, 4(4), 312–332.

CHAPTER 8

Inpatient Hospice Care

Organizational and Ethical Considerations

TARA FRIEDMAN

A key feature of hospice, as described by the Medicare Hospice Benefit (MHB), is access to four levels of care intended to meet the needs of patients and their families (CMS, 2012, §40.1.5, §40.2.1, & §40.2.2). The level of care known as "inpatient hospice" may be required to manage uncontrolled symptoms and/or to support an actively dying hospice patient. However, the depth and breadth of inpatient-level hospice care vary considerably by hospice. Not all hospice recipients have the same access to inpatient level of care, and hospices may have limitations on the type of care they can deliver. Inpatient hospice care may be provided in contract bed arrangements, designated hospice units within other health care institutions, or in a free-standing setting. Access to physician services and diagnostic or therapeutic services in these settings varies. Hospice philosophy and unit policies may sometimes be in tension when units are hosted in health care facilities not run by the hospice organization. Furthermore, the provision of appropriate care may be complicated by patients who initially meet hospice inpatient guidelines but later request care that is outside the scope of care provided by inpatient hospice services.

This chapter will explore the ethical issues related to both administrative and clinical aspects of inpatient hospice care. The chapter is organized into two sections. The first offers readers a broad overview of the most common ways that hospice organizations offer inpatient level of care to their patients. In so doing, it highlights strengths and drawbacks of each operational setting as they inform ethical aspects of care. The second section explores four ways ethical challenges may be experienced in the inpatient hospice care setting, and it offers readers thoughts on how to reflect upon, and address, each in their own organization.

INPATIENT HOSPICE CARE: A BRIEF OVERVIEW

In 2011, an estimated 1.65 million Americans received hospice care from one of 5,300 hospice providers (NHPCO, 2012). More than 95% of this care was provided as "routine level of care" almost exclusively in the "home" setting (i.e., private home, boarding home, nursing home, assisted living facility, or other residential facility). However, over the course of the recipient's illness, pain or other acute and/or complex symptoms may not be effectively managed in the home setting. In such cases, the recipient may desire to leave the home setting to go to an inpatient environment. A growing number of hospice recipients in the United States receive "inpatient level of care" for uncontrolled pain or the management of acute and/or complex symptoms that cannot be managed in another setting, as outlined in Table 8.1.

While the majority of hospice patients strive to stay out of health care institutions, 2.2% of hospice care days provided in 2011 were in the form of "general inpatient care" (NHPCO, 2012). And while most Americans would wish to be cared for at home if they were terminally ill and dying (Gallup Organization, 1996), 26.1% of hospice deaths in 2011 occurred in an inpatient hospice unit, an increase from 19.2% in 2007 (NHPCO, 2008, 2012). Depending on the size of the hospice, its financial resources, the availability of skilled staff, availability of space within existing health care institutions, and the hospice's relationship with the community, how and where inpatient level of care is provided varies considerably.

Table 8.1. INDICATIONS FOR ADMISSION TO INPATIENT HOSPICE CARE

Uncontrolled pain

Intractable nausea, emesis, or other major gastrointestinal symptoms

Respiratory distress

Severe decubiti or other skin lesions/wounds

Any other symptom distress identified by the interdisciplinary team that cannot be sufficiently managed under a routine home care plan of care

Approximately one in five US hospices have a designated inpatient unit (NHPCO, 2012). Designated hospice units may be free-standing facilities that are owned and operated by the hospice or may be housed in distinct areas of acute or extended-care facilities, where space is typically leased by the hospice. These units are commonly operated by the hospice or operated jointly by the hospice and the host facility. Additionally, hospices may establish contractual relationships with hospitals and/or long-term care facilities to provide inpatient level of care within the facility's existing beds on an individual recipient basis. Commonly referred to as "contract beds," in such situations day-to-day care is usually provided by the host facility staff with additional support and oversight provided by the hospice interdisciplinary team.

As most patients begin hospice in the home setting, discussions about how inpatient level of care is typically provided may not be considered until the patient requires it. Finding out that inpatient care is not readily accessible, or is not as envisioned by the patient and family, can add additional stress to the situation. Review of how and where inpatient level of care can be provided is ideally discussed at the initial presentation of hospice services.

Designated Hospice Inpatient Units

Many consider designated hospice units ideal not only because care is provided by hospice-trained staff, expert in providing for the palliative care needs of each recipient, but also because they allow the care to be provided in a "home-like atmosphere" (Kinzbrunner, 2001). As outlined by the Centers for Medicare and Medicaid Services (CMS), a "home-like atmosphere" must include a private space for patients and visiting family members, accommodations for family members to stay with the patient overnight, and space for the family to convene privately after the patient's death (CFR 42 §418.110.E, 2010). Moreover, patients must be able to receive visitors of any age and at any hour. Patient rooms must be designed and equipped not only for nursing care but also to encourage "dignity, comfort and privacy" (CFR 42 §418.110.E, 2010). While not a regulatory requirement, requests for private rooms are to be accommodated whenever possible.

Free-standing facilities, while having the advantages of a home-like environment, may not be able to provide for complex medical needs such as high-flow oxygen and infusion therapies, thereby limiting access for some medically fragile recipients. The hospice interdisciplinary team may at times wish to consult with another specialist. In this author's experience, physician consultations are most commonly requested to psychiatry for depression, psychosis, or determination of decisional capacity; gastroenterology for malfunctioning percutaneous endoscopic gastrostomy (PEG) tubes; radiation therapy for palliative radiation; and interventional radiology for therapeutic paracentesis. Ancillary services may also be necessary to provide radiology, commonly related to assessment of post-fall injuries, or physical therapy. While such services may be easily accessible in a hospice inpatient unit situated within an acute care hospital, access to these services may not be readily available in free-standing units and recipients may need to be transported to other facilities to receive these services. If transportation is too burdensome for a hospice recipient, the recipient may not be able to access specialist services. Whether such services are beneficial for a recipient who is too fragile for transport is dependent on individual recipient circumstances. Thus, services that are readily available at one hospice unit may not be available in another.

When hospices lease space from a hospital or nursing care facility for a designated hospice unit, the hospice typically purchases access to host facility services (like linen, food and beverage, housekeeping, and security) and may have enhanced access to physician and ancillary services that are already housed in the host facility. Consideration of how and when these services will be requested may help the host facility plan for staffing. For example, an already understaffed host physical therapy department may not be able to respond to consultation requests for a group of hospice recipients who would benefit from bedside physical therapy. In such cases, the hospice may need to bring in additional outside physical therapy support. Relationships with consulting physicians are ideally arranged prior to opening a new unit, but changes in physician practices can lead to unanticipated gaps in service. For example, if a consulting psychiatrist retires, the hospice may not find a suitable consultant willing to replace her. The hospice may then lean on a rotating team of hospital-based psychiatrists, perhaps impeding continuity of care for the inpatient hospice community. It is important to anticipate patient needs to prevent delays and dissatisfaction in service caused by factors related to care given by nonhospice staff.

Facility-based inpatient units have many benefits (Kinzbrunner, 2001). However, both parties should carefully consider where host facilities' policies and procedures may be incongruent with hospice philosophy and/ or practices. For example, most hospital visitation policies specify visiting hours and limit the number and age of visitors. On the other hand, Medicare-certified inpatient hospice units are required to have open visiting hours, providing access for visitors of any age at any time. Hospital policies governing how and where certain medications can be used may need to be reconsidered for a hospice unit opened within the hospital. A hospice recipient requesting removal of ventilatory support may require a benzodiazepine infusion, but the host facility policy may disallow such infusions outside a monitored setting. Host facility infection control policies may prevent a patient with methicillin-resistant Staphylococcus aureus (MRSA)-positive nasal swabs from cohabitating with a MRSA-negative patient, even when both patients are nonambulatory and facing imminent death. Thus, a hospice inpatient unit that is required to strictly adhere to host facility policies may not be able to take the MRSA-positive recipient or may be unable to put another recipient in the same room. Such policies can be detrimental to both hospice patients and families and the overall management of the hospice unit.

The integration of host facility policies and procedures must take into account the unique characteristics and specific needs of hospice recipients and their families. Hospice practices should be discussed and detailed prior to establishing a unit within another facility to avoid conflict once the unit is established. When the host facility provides pharmacy services for the hospice unit, the hospice should work closely with the pharmacy to ensure that the necessary palliative therapies are available and unrestricted to meet the needs of the recipients on the hospice unit. For example, opioid agents may be restricted in dose or volume in other parts of the facility but will need to be available to hospice recipients without unnecessary obstacles.

"Contract" Scattered Inpatient Beds

Although all Medicare beneficiaries are entitled to hospice care and all Medicare-certified hospices must provide inpatient level of care, not all hospices have designated inpatient units. A patient requiring inpatient level of care whose hospice provider does not have a designated hospice unit will likely be placed in a nonhospice inpatient facility and have non-hospice nurses providing around-the-clock care overseen by the hospice team. Even if the hospice has a distinct hospice unit, the unit may not be equally accessible to all recipients being served by the hospice, particularly if the inpatient unit is not centrally situated in the hospice's geographic service area. Given the paucity of hospice units in the United States (NHPCO, 2012), there may not be an available bed in such a unit when the patient needs one.

Beyond the walls of a designated inpatient unit, inpatient level of care may be provided in what is commonly referred to as a "contract bed."

In contract bed arrangements, hospice organizations typically provide inpatient-level care by leasing individual beds in an all-inclusive arrangement with the host facility. For an agreed-upon per-diem fee, the host facility allows the hospice to house a hospice recipient who needs inpatient level of care. The host facility typically provides the ancillary and day-to-day bedside care required by patients eligible for inpatient hospice care. Hospice staff members visit daily, at minimum, and provide guidance to the plan of care. Contract beds have the benefit of flexible location, but they lack the home-like environment of an inpatient unit and are greatly influenced by the skills and attitudes of host facility staff, administration, and institutional culture. Palliative care expertise provided by hospice staff may be diluted if the host facility staff are not adequately trained and supported to provide for the around-the-clock needs of the hospice patient.

For example, if floor protocol is to check vital signs during each nursing shift, an imminently dying hospice patient on a contract bed may be woken for vitals, even if doing so is disruptive to patient comfort and not appropriate for the patient's plan of care. A more dramatic example is that of a patient on hospice with lung cancer and brain metastases who is admitted to a hospital contract bed for management of agitation. If the host facility staff has adequate experience working with hospice recipients, communicates regularly with the hospice staff, and is supported by a knowledgeable physician, the patient should receive appropriate comfort measures for uncontrolled agitation. Without it, the patient might be subjected to inadequate symptom management, extensive testing, or, in a potentially worst-case scenario, restraints. While hospices have the obligation to oversee the plan of care, in a contract bed arrangement hospice clinicians have little, if any, authority over those clinicians who are providing the day-to-day bedside care. While trying to educate and provide support, hospice clinicians are typically not privileged to provide hands-on clinical support (i.e., administering or ordering medications) to ensure that patients benefit from their expertise. Therefore, if the treating physician in the hospital is not comfortable with a hospice's recommendation, or if the staff nurse is not comfortable carrying out the hospice's recommendation, the hospice has no authority to enforce it. Additionally, there may not be an alternative physician to take over the case if the facility's attending physician is uncomfortable with the patient's request for palliative care. Yet the hospice is held responsible for the total care of this patient. The importance of close supervision, communication, and respect for the palliative care expertise of the hospice team is paramount.

One benefit of contract beds is that they are potentially unlimited, sometimes referred to as "the hospice unit without walls." Therefore, if a hospice can negotiate agreements with several facilities in its service area, it may be able to provide inpatient level of care in a facility not far from the patient's home. Pertinent limiting factors include the hospice's ability to forge productive relationships with medical facilities within its service area and the facility's interest in supporting the needs of hospice patients in its community. Thus, in contract bed arrangements there can be tremendous variability in how inpatient level of care is provided by a hospice organization and experienced by hospice recipients.

Finally, whether it be in a hospital, nursing home, or other facility, contract beds might be thought of as a rental agreement of the room/bed and routine facility services for an agreed-upon per-diem rate. The hospice interdisciplinary team will supplement and guide the plan of care but does not provide the care that is being contracted from the host facility. The hospital, in turn, usually accepts a per-diem payment from the hospice as payment in full. Contracts between hospices and facilities require hospice education for facility staff and should include education about the roles of each member of the team. Extenuating circumstances—the need for a specialty bed for an obese patient or a patient requiring frequent and intensive wound care—may result in hospitals requesting additional payment for some patients. Whether these items are billable beyond the contract should be negotiated in advance to avoid conflict. While the hospice is obliged to provide inpatient level of care, the reimbursement for such care is fixed by the insurance provider. So the hospice must negotiate a per-diem rate with the host facility that is equal to or less than the per diem it receives from third-party payers or accept a financial loss when providing inpatient care using contract beds. Since the per-diem rate paid to hospice for inpatient care does not approximate the usual reimbursement a hospital can expect to collect for an acute care day, hospitals with lean nursing staff ratios or a paucity of available beds may not be interested in facilitating contract bed arrangements.

Hospice "Residences"

Some hospice organizations have "residences" that provide patients (and sometimes families) residential care while on service. Such units can offer valuable options to patients and families who do not have the resources—personal or financial—to receive hospice care safely at home and who do not meet eligibility requirements for inpatient hospice care. Typically free-standing, these residential units are not certified by Medicare or subject to regulatory oversight. As such, they cannot substitute for dedicated inpatient units or scattered beds to provide the Medicare-required inpatient level of care explained in this chapter. Hospices and their patients should be very clear that such facilities do not constitute inpatient care per CMS regulatory standards.

Without insurance-driven revenue to offset the costs of providing room, board, and various levels of clinician support, many use charitable funds to support the cost of running a residential unit. Commonly, patients and families are expected to pay some portion of the costs associated with stays in noncertified units. The lack of regulatory oversight for such "residences" can be a cause of concern, resulting in highly variable quality in living arrangements and levels of clinical and psychosocial support. Residential units are mentioned in this chapter simply to emphasize that the kind of care offered in such units is not the same as the inpatient level of care offered in Medicare-certified inpatient hospice facilities.

This section of the chapter has explained the two most common arrangements through which hospices offer inpatient care: dedicated units (free-standing or in host facilities) and scattered contract beds. In so doing, it has also highlighted advantages and disadvantages of each kind of arrangement. The next section of the chapter explores risks and opportunities for delivering care that honors the ethical values of patients, families, clinicians, and hospice organizations in each model of inpatient care delivery.

ETHICAL CHALLENGES AND OPPORTUNITIES IN INPATIENT HOSPICE CARE

This section explores four ways in which inpatient hospice care gives rise to ethical opportunities and challenges in the delivery of care at the end of life.

Collaboration With Ethics Committees in Host Facilities

Inpatient level of care is typically reserved for the most gravely ill, symptomatic, and frail patients. Given the high emotional charge that frequently accompanies such patients and families, hospice units are common sites of ethical dilemmas. Hospices may or may not have their own ethics committees to support the inpatient unit. A hospice unit based in a hospital facility might rely on the host's ethics committee. Whether it is productive to bring hospice issues to a host hospital's ethics committee depends upon the experience and knowledge of the ethics committee members, the relationship between committee members and hospice clinicians, and the relationship between hospital administrators and the hospice organization's leaders.

Perhaps the most productive host–hospice relationships include hospice representation on the hospital ethics committee. It has been this author's experience that hospital ethics committees have encouraged hospice participation when hospice inpatient units are hosted in their hospital. In committee meetings, away from the emotional charge of bedside care, diverse opinions may be respected and valued differently. These discussions, and the relationships that can develop as a result, enhance a mutual understanding of clinical cultures, enhance the hospital's ability to utilize hospice expertise for a broader array of issues, and allow the hospice to engage others in the importance of addressing palliative care goals (i.e., symptom management, goals of care, and advanced care planning) long before hospital patients are in the final stages of their lives. For example, through ethics committee work, this author and colleagues have influenced a committee-wide effort to change an existing hospital do-not-resuscitate (DNR) form, forged a relationship with a chief surgeon that enhanced the surgical intensive care unit's understanding and acceptance of palliative care consultations by the hospital's own palliative care team, provided training for an administrative committee to become a clinically active ethics committee, and helped another hospital develop a brain death protocol.

All of these developments had mutually beneficial outcomes for the hospice unit and the host facility: Hospice patients benefitted from more situation-appropriate guidelines for resuscitation and withdrawal of life-sustaining therapies and hospital patients benefitted from care teams and ethics committees with increased capacity for prospectively identifying and addressing palliative needs.

Navigating the Space Between Autonomy and Beneficence: Resuscitation and Life-Sustaining Treatments

While it may seem counterintuitive, hospice recipients are not required to have a DNR order. Distress and disagreement about if, when, and how to provide resuscitation are, of course, not limited to inpatient care (see Chapter 10). However, the questions surrounding resuscitation in inpatient hospice can present themselves in especially complex ways—different than they present in home hospice care.

While attempting resuscitation may seem contrary to the focus on comfort that a hospice strives to provide, CMS regulations for Medicare-certified hospice programs prevent hospice organizations from refusing admission based on a patient's resuscitation preferences.[1] Depending on an organization's interpretation of applicable regulations, some hospices will admit patients requesting resuscitation to hospice but limit the care to the home setting. Strict interpretation of the regulations might suggest that admission to hospice may not be limited to any level of care based on the patient's desire for attempts at resuscitation (e.g., CFR 42 § 418.110.N.2(vii) requires clinical staff in Medicare-certified hospice inpatient units to be trained and certified in CPR). The tension between an emphasis on comfort care and full code status is likely to rise more frequently in the inpatient setting, since to be eligible for admission to inpatient care patients need to be symptomatic and/or closer to death. Conditions that give rise to this tension are also created by the hospice care philosophy itself, which, as explained in Chapter 2, places equal emphasis on preventing suffering and respecting moral agency.

Caring for patients and families who request resuscitation can place hospice caregivers in the uncomfortable situation of trying to provide comfort to a patient while acknowledging that unless the patient changes her code status, she faces a number of painful and likely fruitless procedures at the time of death. Such situations create conditions ripe for conflict. Recipients of home hospice care must usually have a family member or caregiver call 911 to receive resuscitative interventions. However, because inpatient units—even those with a "home-like atmosphere"—can be perceived by patients and families as having hospital-like qualities (many inpatient units are located within host facilities that are acute care hospitals), inpatients and their families often expect resuscitation to be a standard intervention offered in the same way it is in "regular" hospitals: by unit staff or on-site code teams.

While there are little data regarding the accessibility of on-site resuscitation services for inpatient hospice units in the United States, anecdotal reports suggest that approaches to this issue vary widely across different hospice organizations. If units do not offer on-site resuscitation—either by unit staff or via liaison arrangements with host facility code teams—hospice clinicians will need to either transport patients to the emergency department or call 911 and request that emergency medical service (EMS) providers respond to the unit if resuscitation is to be an option for patients who request it. The former option requires units that may already be at capacity to sacrifice staff members to accompany patients to the emergency department. The latter option is not always possible if units are located within host hospitals, depending on local practices governing whether EMS will respond to calls from within hospitals with emergency departments. This presents hospice inpatients who wish to be resuscitated with an added dilemma: If they have symptom distress requiring an inpatient level of care, they may have to forego attempts at resuscitation to receive that level of care.

Another challenging situation arises on the hospice inpatient unit when patients and/or family members waver in their desire to prioritize quality over quantity of life. For example, a patient is admitted for interdisciplinary support for terminal extubation but later changes his mind and no longer wants to be taken off the ventilator. Before admission to hospice, physicians and/or nurses typically engage in a detailed conversation with the patient and/or designated health care surrogate to discuss decisions to withdraw life support. Ideally, these conversations include discussion of the patient's current condition, his reasons for pursuing terminal extubation, and available alternatives. This conversation should also include information about how symptoms will likely be managed, and what the patient and family can expect in the pre-, peri-, and postextubation periods. However, conversations in advance of transfer do not ensure that a patient or designated surrogate will not change his or her mind after admission (this same point, it should be noted, applies to discussions and decisions about resuscitation, which are reversible if patient/surrogate preferences change). If the patient/family changes its mind because of dissatisfaction with service, unsubstantiated fears, or inadequate symptom management, the hospice is likely to be able to address concerns and work with the patient/family to meet their needs. However, if the patient/family truly no longer wishes for the patient to be extubated, the hospice may be faced with providing extended management of a ventilator-dependent patient, something most hospices are not prepared or willing to do.

With continued ventilatory support, some patients are no longer hospice appropriate. If, after individual issues are addressed, the patient and/ or surrogate decision maker still desires to continue with aggressive treatment in a manner that changes the patient's hospice eligibility, the hospice may need to help the patient re-enter the acute or chronic care setting. How this is accomplished will depend on the particular hospice inpatient unit and the circumstances of the individual patient (in this case whether the patient is already trached and needs access to a long-term ventilator facility or should be transferred to the nearest acute care hospital for tracheotomy). The immediate challenge revolves around the care the hospice will be providing while urgently seeking transfer for a patient who is on the hospice unit but no longer desires (or qualifies for) hospice care.

Hospice clinicians are experts in providing palliative care to patients with advanced illness, but they may be less comfortable caring for those who no longer prioritize comfort over life extension. In this author's practice, changes in goals of care, whether related to resuscitation or continuing life-sustaining therapies like ventilation, can present intense and urgent ethical challenges in inpatient hospice units. Respect for patient and family autonomy dictates that hospices explore changes in preferences and honor them when there is evidence that such changes are clear and genuine expressions of authentically held moral values (Beauchamp & Childress, 2012). Doing so also upholds the hospice commitment to restoring and respecting moral agency.

When patients and families make choices inconsistent with other components of the hospice philosophy (like relieving suffering), or choices that seem inconsistent with other widely recognized ethical principles, such as beneficence—providing care that maximizes benefit to patients—hospice clinicians can experience significant moral distress. While such distress is, in some situations, difficult to prevent, prospective planning via the terms of agreements with unit host facilities, the development of clear organizational policies and procedures, and well-established practices that support clinicians (see Chapter 5) can mitigate the intensity of this distress for care providers and maximize opportunities to provide care consistent with patient and family values.

The Intersection of Clinical and Organizational Ethics

Many patients access inpatient level of care for uncontrolled symptoms that, with the intervention of the hospice staff, stabilize over days or weeks. Most of these patients are then able to return to their prior residence. Some, however, cannot. If family members cannot provide the level of support needed in the home, or patients were previously residing in an assisted living or residential facility that is not comfortable supporting their increasing care needs, what can the hospice do for patients who remain hospice appropriate but no longer qualify for inpatient level of care?

In the past, Medicare guidelines were widely interpreted as permissive of inpatient stays for "family/system breakdown" (CFR 42 §418.202.E). This term for a breakdown or disruption in family dynamics describes situations in which family members are prevented from functioning as adequate caregivers for emotional or physical reasons. Clarification of Medicare guidelines in 2007, however, underscored that the inability of a caregiver to provide care for the patient does not substantiate inpatient level of care (CMS, 2007, p. 50220). Thus, patients may be ready for discharge from inpatient care but have no home to which to be discharged. Having successfully managed the patient's symptoms, the hospice may no longer bill Medicare for an inpatient level of care, though it is still required—legally and ethically—to provide hospice care. Lack of family support is not an indication to discharge for cause, and the hospice has made an ethical commitment in taking the patient on service, a commitment that forbids abandoning the patient.

Mrs. S was a prime example of this ethical challenge. An 89-year-old woman with advanced lung cancer, Mrs. S elected the hospice benefit for herself and requested the hospice inpatient unit for pain management. After several days in the hospice inpatient unit, her reversible symptoms were controlled. However, she remained weak, unable to get out of bed by herself, and became confused. She had no close family and distant cousins were unwilling to get involved in decision making. Increasing confusion resulted in loss of decisional capacity, and the hospice was faced with disposition planning for an incapacitated patient without a surrogate decision maker. Long-term care facilities were understandably hesitant to accept a patient without capacity who had no legal decision maker. During that time, the hospice's only option was to continue to provide care in the unit but bill Medicare for only routine level of care. During the lengthy, costly, and labor-intensive process of seeking a court-appointed guardian and decision maker, the patient became imminent and died. Having no access to the patient's financial resources, the hospice arranged for burial on the patient's behalf at the organization's expense.

While allowing Mrs. S to stay on the unit certainly upheld the ethical principles of beneficence and fidelity, her extended stay in the very busy unit raised concerns. Unit clinicians and administrators saw that her lengthy stay in the unit prevented admission of several home hospice patients who needed relief of complex symptom distress. On its surface, this case may appear to simply be one of complex discharge planning and a loss of decision-making capacity that was unforeseeable. However, many patients lose decision-making capacity in the days immediately preceding their deaths. As such, working collaboratively with patients to identify appropriate decision makers from the very first admission visit is one way to make prospective efforts to provide care consistent with patient values. In this case, the patient's presence on an inpatient unit intensified the hospice staff's sense of urgency for two reasons: The bed was unavailable to other patients in symptom distress, and there was considerable financial pressure to place the patient in another care facility because her reimbursement had switched to routine-level care.

Justice may be a helpful lens through which to consider the first concern. Distributive justice explores the allocation of resources in conditions of scarcity. In short, when there is not enough to go around, models of distributive justice attempt to offer a framework in which to determine the fairest way to distribute scarce resources (Beauchamp & Childress, 2012). The concern that Mrs. S occupied a bed that, after her symptoms were well managed, might more appropriately have been occupied by a patient who was in need of inpatient symptom management draws upon an assumption about what constitutes the just allocation of inpatient beds. In this case, the assumption seemed to be that inpatient beds should be given to those who *need* them most, with "need" being appraised in terms of the intensity of symptom distress. When there were other patients with unmanaged symptom distress in need of inpatient treatment, a bed being unavailable to one of those patients because it was occupied by a patient whose symptoms were well managed was seen as unjust.

Like many duties in health care ethics, distributive justice can only be meaningfully and appropriately applied in individual cases when there is a robust, transparent, and collectively embraced ethical framework at the level of organizational policy (Stretch, Hurst, & Danis, 2010). By its nature, distributive justice can only be assessed and addressed at the population level, for it seeks to distribute resources justly among groups, not to individuals. As such, while the staff's concerns about justice in the case of Mrs. S may make sense at an intuitive level, the way to address such concerns would be through the design and implementation of admission and discharge policies for the inpatient unit explicitly informed by a clearly explained and applied model of distributive justice.

The second concern in the case of Mrs. S—the financial pressure to place her elsewhere given the change in her reimbursement status—was not merely a business consideration absent ethical significance. The principle of stewardship addresses an organization's obligation to adhere to sound business practices and ensure that its capital and other resources are employed in a way that maximizes the ability to support its mission by creating and preserving fiscally sustainable operations (Magill & Prybil, 2004). Opening and running an inpatient unit presents new and complex challenges for hospice organizations whose previous experience is limited to home care and a few scattered contract beds. In addition to the operational complexities—which are significant, as in some ways a hospice inpatient unit functions as a mini-hospital—the financial expertise required to run an inpatient unit can be quite different from that required to manage a home hospice practice.

Inpatient units are typically not significant sources of net revenue for hospice organizations. Indeed, many run at a slight loss. A very small number of patients like Mrs. S can place not only the unit but also the entire hospice organization in financial peril. As with distributive justice, stewardship as an ethical duty is best approached at the level of organizational policy. So, while decisions that affect the finances of the organization are made at the level of individual patients every day, the financial health of the organization is not the responsibility of individual clinicians and administrators absent a policy framework in which to pursue that health.

The case of Mrs. S raises ethical issues that extend beyond clinical ethics and reach into the organization's duty and ability to distribute its resources, including its inpatient beds, fairly and operate with the stewardship required to continue to care for all of its patients by maintaining its financial health.

Collective Grief: Benefits and Harms Arising From Unit Environments

Beyond the expert bereavement support that hospice staff members offer patients and families, hospice inpatient units can be places for families going through similar experiences to support one another. It is not at all uncommon for families of one patient on a unit to offer comfort and concern for other families—families who, prior to admission, had been total strangers. Unlike recipients of home hospice care, who continue to reside in their homes and draw upon community sources of support that may have been cultivated over many years, patients and families in inpatient units are displaced from their normal home environments. As such, they often welcome the support of both unit staff and other families with loved ones on the unit when the support of their local friends and neighbors is not available.

Similarly, it is not unusual for patients to enjoy the company of a roommate; sometimes they ring call bells for each other and bond with each other's family. This author once cared for a patient who went home after a brief stay in the inpatient unit. After discharge, however, he returned daily for several weeks to visit with his inpatient roommate. Family members of the patient and the roommate told hospice staff members that their brief friendship and mutual support were very important to both having a meaningful dying experience.

However, for some patients and families, the close proximity of others' grief in an inpatient unit can feel like a burden, amplifying their own distress. Since each family grieves in its own way, some may even have uncomfortable experiences with other families in the hospice unit. For example, cultures that encourage large family gatherings at the bedside and multiple family members crying and physically demonstrating their grief may upset a more reserved family visiting another care recipient. Hospice respects the cultural norms of each patient and family, but it may need to limit visitors or make other restrictions on the unit to address behavior that aggravates the suffering of others.

Hospice units with semiprivate rooms should also consider the stress that the death of a roommate can cause patients already dealing with their own fears, loss, and grief. Mr. T, for example, experienced a prolonged inpatient hospice stay and asked to have his room changed after his third roommate died. He confided to clinicians on the unit that living with three consecutive patients who died just a few feet away from him—though all three died peacefully with symptoms controlled—was traumatic for him. Staff members readily arranged for him to move to a private room. A bereavement counselor met several times with Mr. T before he died 2 weeks later.

Nonmaleficence is an ethical principle that captures the dictum "first, do no harm" (Beauchamp & Childress, 2012). It is often paired with beneficence. And, while "doing good" may seem to logically imply doing no harm, this is not always the case. Indeed, most interventions in medicine achieve good via harm or the risk of harm. Surgery for an infected gall bladder, for example, can benefit patients greatly—in some cases saving their lives. In so doing, however, it also harms: It creates wounds, creates risk for inadvertent surgical injury and secondary acquired infections, and exposes patients to the risks of anesthesia. As long as such risks are necessary, and as long as the benefits of the procedure outweigh the risks, we consider beneficence and nonmaleficence to be honored.

As with any health care team, clinicians on inpatient hospice units strive to offer beneficial care to patients while simultaneously protecting them from unnecessary risk of harm. Identifying and addressing opportunities for benefit and risks for harm in an inpatient unit can require experience and expertise different from that gleaned in home care. In the case of Mr. T, having three roommates die during an unusually long stay on the unit resulted in psychological distress. Placing him in a private room, while incurring a small financial loss (he was not billed extra for the private room), was justified on grounds of nonmaleficence; the team believed this would mitigate any additional harm that might come from the death of future roommates and lessen the trauma of being in the same room where three had already died.

CONCLUSION

This chapter has explained several different models through which hospice organizations offer inpatient-level care, a Medicare requirement. It has also explored some opportunities and challenges to organizing and delivering inpatient care in a way that honors the ethical values and duties of everyone involved. Careful planning in the design and implementation of organizational policies and procedures governing inpatient care, combined with attunement to risks and opportunities like those addressed earlier, should place hospice organizations in a strong position from which to identify and address ethical issues imbedded in the delivery of inpatient care.

NOTES

1. The Patient Self-Determination Act (1994) prohibits any Medicare-certified health care provider from conditioning delivery of care on patients completing an advance directive. This includes conditioning the provision of care on patients stating a preference regarding any care option normally included in an advance directive. Thus, hospices cannot insist that patients accept do-not-resuscitate status—or, indeed, state any preference whatsoever regarding resuscitation—as a condition of admission.

REFERENCES

Beauchamp, T., & Childress, J. (2012). *Principles of biomedical ethics* (7th ed.). New York, NY: Oxford University Press.

Centers for Medicare and Medicaid Services (CMS). (2007). Medicare program: Hospice wage index for fiscal year 2008 [CMS Publication 1539-F]. *Federal Register*, 72(169), 50214–50249.

Centers for Medicare and Medicaid Services (CMS). (2012, June 1) Coverage of hospice services under hospital insurance. In *Medicare benefit policy manual* (rev. 156). Retrieved April 2014, from http://www.cms.gov/Regulations-and-Guidance/Guidance/Manuals/downloads/bp102c09.pdf.

Code of Federal Regulations 42 §418.110.E. (October 1, 2010).

Gallup Organization. (1996). *Knowledge and attitudes related to hospice care*. Arlington, VA: National Hospice Organization.

Kinzbrunner, B. M. (2001). How to help patients access end-of-life care. In B. M. Kinzbrunner, N. J. Weinreb, & J. S. Policzer (Eds.), *20 common problems in end-of-life care* (pp. 29–46). New York, NY: McGraw-Hill.

Magill, G., & Prybil, L. (2004). Stewardship and integrity in healthcare: A role for organizational ethics. *Journal of Business Ethics, 50*(3), 225–238.

National Hospice & Palliative Care Organization (NHPCO). (2008). *NHPCO facts and figures: Hospice care in America.* Alexandria, VA: NHPCO.

National Hospice & Palliative Care Organization (NHPCO). (2012). *NHPCO facts and figures: Hospice care in America.* Alexandria, VA: NHPCO.

Patient Self-Determination Act. Pub. L. No. 101-508, §4206 & §4751, 104 Stat. 1388 (1994).

Stretch, D., Hurst, S., & Danis, M. (2010). The role of ethics committees and ethics consultation in allocation decisions: A 4-stage process. *Medicare Care, 48*(9), 821–826.

CHAPTER 9

Ethical Issues Associated with Hospice in Nursing Homes and Assisted Living Communities

JEAN MUNN AND SHERYL ZIMMERMAN

Each year in the United States almost one quarter of the deaths of older adults occur in nursing homes (US Census Bureau, 2010), and in some states one third of deaths occur there (Miller, Teno, & Mor, 2004). Mortality rates range from 34% in the first year of residence to 24% thereafter (Kiely & Flacker, 2003). Assisted living communities are another site of death for older Americans, in which mortality rates range from 16% to 22% (Zimmerman et al., 2005). All told, almost one third of those who enter a long-term care setting will die there (Hanson, Henderson, & Rogman, 1999), and for older adults with dementia, these rates are even higher. In fact, the majority of cognitively impaired older adults (67%) die in a long-term care setting (Mitchell, Morris, Park, & Fries, 2004; Mitchell, Teno, Miller, & Mor, 2005). Furthermore, approximately one third of Medicare recipients who die in hospitals do so 3 days after being transferred from a nursing home (Smith, Kellerman, & Brown, 1995).

As staggering as these numbers are, they are expected to increase as the number of older adults in the United States doubles by the year 2030 and increases five-fold to 88.5 million adults in 2050. The fastest growing segment of the older adult population, those 85 years of age and older (US Census Bureau, 2010), happens to be the segment most likely to require nursing home care. Taken together, the preceding figures indicate that nursing homes and assisted living communities are and will continue to be critical in providing care for America's oldest and most vulnerable citizens during their dying days. Indeed, the frequency of death in these settings has made the end-of-life experience a common occurrence and established a sense of normalcy regarding death in nursing homes and assisted living communities (Munn et al., 2008).

Hospice services are seen as the gold standard of end-of-life care in many settings and existing studies support benefits to long-term care residents. Positive outcomes include fewer hospitalizations, alternative pain management, presence of advance directives, and nonmedical support (Munn, Hanson, Zimmerman, Sloane, & Mitchell, 2006; Murphy, Hanrahan, & Luchins, 1997). Indeed, hospice in long-term care can be seen as value added, as the hospice philosophy of care includes a focus on comfort rather than curative care (including pain relief and symptom management); defines the unit of care as patient and family; encourages care provision by a multidisciplinary team (e.g., nurses, volunteers, chaplains, therapists, social workers, bereavement counselors, and physicians); focuses on non-medical issues such as spiritual and psychosocial well-being; and provides bereavement support for families (Asch-Goodkin, 2002).

However, ethical challenges arise when the hospice philosophy of care and the existing long-term care culture are incongruent or perceived to be in conflict regarding what is best for the resident at the end of life. Another ethical issue arises around the need for the long-term care staff to care for many residents while meeting the intense needs of those who are dying, and whether hospice staff are available when care is needed. Finally, ethical challenges are raised when staff aim to promote resident self-determination for those with reduced cognitive capacity.

This chapter begins by describing long-term care, specifically nursing homes and assisted living communities, in the United States. The overview is followed by a discussion of complex issues that affect ethical decision making such as variability among those dying in these settings, a high prevalence of dementia and consequent ambiguity in decision-making capacity, and a regulatory environment that may make death and functional decline appear to be the result of poor care rather than a natural part of the life cycle. It then discusses the end of life in long-term care, followed by four critical points in time during which ethical dilemmas are most likely to arise in relation to the congruence between long-term care and hospice. In the final section, we propose a model of hospice for assisted living and long-term care residents that builds upon the strengths of hospice and mitigates some of the difficulties presented earlier in the chapter.

Nursing Homes

Nursing homes are by definition designed to care for persons who require ongoing nursing care in a residential setting; consequently, the function of a nursing home is both medical and supportive (Keay, Fredman, Taler, Datta, & Levenson, 1994). In 2008, 16,000 nursing homes were certified by the Centers for Medicare and Medicaid. This figure represents a 3% decrease from 2004, continuing a trend of decline from 18,000 in 1997. Most (43%) have between 100 and 199 beds, followed by those with 50–99 beds (36%). Small nursing homes, those with fewer than 50 beds (14%), showed the greatest decrease (13%) between 2004 and 2008. Of all settings, 67% are for profit (CMS, 2010) and, historically, 60% of those that are for profit are affiliated with a chain (Jones, 2002). Ownership of the remaining homes is largely nonprofit (27%) with 6% owned by the government (CMS, n. d.). Approximately one third are located in the South and another third in the Midwest. The largest portion (61%) is located in metropolitan areas. Occupancy rates vary with the lowest (67%) found in rural regions (Jones, 2002); however, overall occupancy rates have remained fairly stable between 2004 and 2008, averaging 84% (CMS, 2010). It is anticipated that these rates will rise as does the number of people over the age of 85 (Dumas & Ramadurai, 2009).

Resident Characteristics

There are an estimated 1.5 million nursing home residents in the United States (CMS, 2010). The majority (58%) are limited in three or more activities of daily living (ADLs) (e.g., bathing, dressing, toileting, eating, and transferring), compared to 7% of community-dwelling older adults who are similarly impaired. In fact, as more dependent older adults move to assisted living settings, the acuity and impairment of nursing home residents is increasing (Federal Interagency Forum on Aging Related Statistics [FIFARS], 2011). Further, 50% of new nursing admissions have dementia, and overall rates of cognitive impairment are estimated as high as 68% (Magaziner et al., 2000).

The nursing home population is largely White (83%) and female (66%) (CMS, 2010). The average age is 80 years old, and 37% are 85 years old or older. Medicaid, a needs-based medical assistance program, provides funding for 60% of nursing home residents. Residents are admitted to nursing homes from a variety of settings, with almost half (46%) being admitted from hospitals (CMS, 2010). Once admitted, the average length of stay for a resident is 2¼ years (CDC, 2011). Within this population there are some subgroups that differ from the population as a whole. A growing number of nursing home residents are admitted for short-stay rehabilitation. This group is younger and less frail than traditional long-term care residents.

While it might be assumed that all nursing home residents who are not admitted for rehabilitation are considered to be at the end of life, that assumption is simplistic—a point driven home by the statistic provided earlier that the average length of stay is 2¼ years (CDC, 2011). Determining who is dying has been the focus of both clinical and research studies, but they have not generated a definitive answer. For example, some researchers suggest that retrospective studies are appropriate for studying the end-of-life experience because it is impossible to determine, prospectively, whom to include in a study (Fowler, Coppola, & Teno, 1999). Consequently, many prospective end-of-life studies have been limited to including individuals who have diseases with a predictable trajectory, such as cancer. Persons with clinical and research backgrounds agree that identifying the dying role is problematic (Bern-Klug, Gessert, Crenner, Buenaver, & Skirchak, 2004) and that there is an ambiguous state between living and dying (Engle, 1998). Furthermore, these issues are more complex in long-term care as residents often have chronic conditions that worsen over years rather than days or months, and for whom the expectation of death is seldom clear prior to the residents' actively dying. Yet some residents die suddenly with no expectation of death by staff or family. These situations often result in limited end-of-life care and late referrals to hospice (Welch, Miller, Martin, & Nanda, 2008). A culture change movement to consider all long-term care residents as appropriate for end-of-life care has begun, but this is not yet typical of the long-term care environment (Bern-Klug, 2010; Schockett, Teno, Miller, & Stuart, 2005). Hence, difficulties establishing the expectation of death present an overarching ethical issue underlying many of the specific dilemmas noted in this chapter.

Despite the problems identified earlier, a small, important subgroup is composed of those 5% who are admitted specifically for end-of-life care— that is, with a life expectancy of less than 6 months upon admission. They are characterized as having symptoms congruent with dying (e.g., pain, incontinence, and dehydration) as well as diagnoses with predictable dying trajectories (e.g., cancer) or terminal status (e.g., chronic obstructive pulmonary disease, congestive heart failure) (Porock, Parker-Oliver, Zweig, Rantz, & Petroski, 2003). Of those admitted for end-of-life care, 59% are actually enrolled in hospice when admitted. They are more likely to be older,

White, and widowed (Buchanan, Choi, Wang, & Ju, 2004). Comparing hospice nursing home residents to hospice patients who live at home, those in nursing homes tend to be older; to be cognitively impaired; and to receive services related to nutrition, medication management, and physician care (Han, Tiggle, & Remsburg, 2008).

Regulatory Environment and Standards

Nursing homes represent the most institutional and highly regulated long-term care setting. These regulations are based on Section 1819(f)(6) (A-B) for Medicare and 1919(f)(6)(A-B) for Medicaid in the Social Security Act as amended by the Omnibus Budget Reconciliation Act (OBRA). OBRA intended to improve the quality of care and quality of life for nursing home residents by maximizing their independence and function (Department of Health and Human Services, 1989), consistent with the nursing home focus on curative or restorative models of medical care (Hodgson & Lehning, 2008). While there is no mention of hospice or palliative care within the regulatory requirements, OBRA did expand the Hospice Medicare benefit to nursing home residents (Stevenson & Bramson, 2009).

Nursing home services are provided within a federally designed, structured, and standardized protocol that includes conducting routine screening assessments and developing plans of care. Screening assessments involve completion of the federally mandated assessment tool, the Minimum Data Set (MDS), and those areas identified as problematic are more thoroughly assessed and then addressed by a plan of care. A registered nurse must oversee the screening, assessment, and care-planning process, and it is recommended, although not required, that an interdisciplinary team of clinicians be involved in the process.

The MDS is also used to determine Medicare reimbursement (CMS, 2010) and to derive quality indicators to evaluate the quality of care. Embedded in these indicators are principles of maintaining or improving resident function, but not indicators appropriate for optimal end-of-life care (Huskamp, Stevenson, Chernew, & Newhouse, 2010). Consequently, in some cases the quality indicators conflict with optimal care at the end of life (Shield, Wetle, Teno, Miller, & Welch, 2005), reflecting the view that physical, emotional, and mental decline are indicative of poor care (Hoffmann & Tarzian, 2005). This has somewhat been rectified with the introduction of the MDS Version 3.0 in 2011, which includes some items relevant to hospice or palliative care (e.g., pain assessment and management, shortness of breath), but the items are not extensive.

Another area that is not oriented toward the end-of-life experience in nursing homes is their structural arrangement. Despite the inverse relationship between the number of people in a room and resident quality of life, private rooms have not been the standard; instead, most use a model similar to hospitals with semiprivate rooms, beds side by side, and shared bathrooms (Zerzan, Stearns, & Hanson, 2000). Cost is the driving factor behind shared rooms, and Medicaid will not reimburse nursing homes for private rooms unless there are exceptional circumstances such as infection control issues related to individual residents (CMS, 2010).

Assisted Living

Assisted living grew rapidly as an alternate model of residential care that provides room, at least two meals a day, support for activities of daily living (ADLs), and 24-hour oversight (Mezey, Dubler, Mitty, & Brody, 2000; Zimmerman, Sloane, & Eckert, 2001). In 1998 there were an estimated 11,500 assisted living communities in the United States (Hawes, Phillips, Rose, Holan, & Sherman, 2003); by 2011 the number had grown to 31,100 settings, providing care for approximately 1 million older and dependent adults (Park-Lee et al., 2011). Assisted living originated as a consumer-driven response to older adults seeking alternatives to nursing home care (Mezey, Dubler, Mitty, & Brody, 2000; Zimmerman, Gruber-Baldini, et al., 2003).

The term "assisted living" is broad and nonspecific, and it applies to a variety of state-licensed settings also known as adult foster care, senior group homes, personal care homes, residential care, board and care, and domiciliary homes (Zimmerman, Munn, & Koenig, 2006). They range from high-rise buildings to small group homes (ALFA, 2011), and they offer services, including assistance in medication management, bathing, dressing, and transportation. Seventy-three percent of assisted living accommodations are in private rooms (Hawes et al., 2003).

The philosophy of assisted living is the provision of a homelike setting fostering independence, autonomy, and privacy (ALFA, 2011; Hawes, Rose & Phillips, 1999), including individualized care and continued involvement with the outside community. Consistent with this philosophy, health care should be administered as if the resident were in his or her own home. The fact that assisted living is state and not federally licensed has resulted in a wide variety of settings, not all of which necessarily subscribe to or implement this philosophy in daily practice (Frytak, Kane, Finch, Kane, & Maude-Griffin, 2001; Hawes et al., 1999; Morgan, Gruber-Baldini, & Magaziner, 2001).

Resident Characteristics

Almost 1 million persons live in assisted living communities, the majority of whom are older adults (ALFA, 2011). Almost two thirds (64%) of residents are over the age of 75 years and 33% are between 84 and 88 years of age (Phillips, Holan, Sherman, Spector, & Hawes, 2005). An estimated three quarters of assisted living residents are female, 82%–95% are White, and three quarters are widowed (Morgan et al., 2001); consequently, the typical assisted living resident is an 87-year-old White woman who requires some assistance with two to three ADLs (NCAL, n.d.). Only 14% of current assisted living residents require assistance with three or more ADLs (FIFARS, 2011).

Regulatory Environment and Standards

Unlike nursing homes, assisted living communities are regulated at the state level, meaning that the absence of an overarching federal regulatory template has resulted in a range of regulations that govern assisted living. In general, assisted living regulatory models are of four types: board and care (which sets standards for building requirements); new housing and services (which licenses both the setting and the services and emphasizes the assisted living philosophy of care; service (which licenses the service provider but not the building in which they are provided); and umbrella (regulations addressing multiple types of housing and services) (Mollica, 1998).

Staffing requirements also vary across states. All require awake staff 24 hours per day. In some states, there must be 24-hour registered nurse (RN) availability or the presence of an RN when medicines are administered or other nursing tasks are performed (Polzer, 2011). In fact, 23 states require licensed personnel to administer some medications, while 31 allow non-nurses to administer medications (Zimmerman et al., 2011). In terms of the number of overall staff, many states generally require that staffing be sufficient to meet the needs of the residents, allowing assisted living managers to determine this level and the complaint and survey process to assure that it is adequate (Hodlewsky, 2001).

One half of the states require some form of licensure, certification, or competency for staff, and training is variably specified in terms of its focus or number of required hours. However, the existence of state-based regulation should not be taken to assume homogeneity within states in reference to the living unit, the staff, the services, or any other component of assisted

living care. Assisted living is unique in that the criteria set forth by regulation set parameters for care, and providers have the latitude to structure,
administer, refuse, and provide care as they see fit within those guidelines.
Furthermore, state regulations continue to change (Polzer, 2011).

ETHICS IN LONG-TERM CARE

In its most basic form, and regardless of the setting, ethics relate to judging
what is right or wrong (Hicks, 2000). Predominantly in current Western
culture, medical ethics include an underlying respect for the patient or, in
the case of long-term care, a respect for a resident's self-determination.
That is, residents have the right to participate directly in medical decisions
and may refuse care or choose alternatives to life-sustaining treatment.
While these principles are not specific to long-term care, this emphasis
on self-determination is supported by seminal nursing home legislation
(Department of Health and Human Services, 1989). However, in long-term
care settings, uncertainty regarding a resident's ability to make decisions—
including those related to end-of-life medical treatments—is arguably
the most common ethical dilemma that arises (Fleming, 2007). Other
ethical concerns relate to access, such as the availability of resources for
adequate care; to policies, such as respecting resident autonomy and integrity (Solum, Slettebo, & Hauge, 2008); and to use of specific treatments,
such as termination of treatment or use of feeding tubes (Gjerberg, Forde,
Pedersen, & Bollig, 2010).

One tool that can support self-determination of residents is the use of
advance directives. Indeed, regulations require that nursing homes discuss advance directives at the time of admission (Department of Health
and Human Services, 1989). When properly drawn (while the resident is
competent, using directives that are durable in nature), advance directives
remain in effect even if the resident becomes unable to participate in later
decision making. Directives differ in many ways, though. For example,
some, such as do-not-resuscitate (DNR) orders, have specific contingen-
cies. Other, more general documents such as living wills present a philosophy of dying. More nuanced and comprehensive directives such as
physicians' orders for life-sustaining treatment (POLST) allow the resident, ideally in concert with his or her physician, to choose among alternatives regarding nutrition and medical interventions (http://www.POLST.
org). Directives also allow an individual to specify a health care surrogate,
who is then empowered to act in lieu of the resident if he or she is unable
to speak for himself or herself.

There are shortcomings to the use of advance directives, however, including lack of specificity or the inability to foresee specific circumstances. Indeed, current literature suggests that rather than simply signing documents, the optimal method of including resident input requires ongoing communication (Nelson, Schrader, & Eidsness, 2009) and adjustments related to changes in medical condition as well as cognitive status. Some literature suggests that in long-term care, this ongoing discussion does not occur. Rather, obligatory and sometimes apologetic (Ellershaw & Ward, 2003) discussions occur upon admission and such issues are not addressed again (Munn & Adorno, 2008).

There is great variability in how long-term care settings address ethical issues. Few nursing homes, and virtually no assisted living settings, have ethics committees or other mechanisms for methodically dealing with ethical dilemmas (Fleming, 2007). Rather, the staff who are confronted with these dilemmas tend to follow rules or guidelines set out by their individual professions, if such guidelines exist and if staff are aware of them. For example, the National Association of Social Workers (NASW) has established guidelines for palliative and end-of-life care, yet research indicates that less than half of NASW members are even aware these guidelines exist; notably, these same practitioners indicated the need for more education in order to attain competence in discussing end-of-life issues (Csikai & Bass, 2000). Similarly, nurses are guided by a professional code of ethics (American Nurses Association, 2011), but they often lack the advanced training to apply ethical decision-making models when faced with ambiguity or contradiction. Instead, nursing staff make intuitive decisions guided by their personal perceptions of what is right, despite ethical premises that moral decisions are socially rather than individually determined (Solum, Slettebo, & Hauge, 2008). Administrative personnel, on the other hand, often respond more to legalities rather than to ethics (Hoffmann & Tarzian, 2005) and those who are part of larger organizations must adhere to policies mandated by the corporate entity.

Ethical dilemmas often result in stress for staff (Bolmsjö, Sandman, & Andersson, 2006) as well as feelings of anger, helplessness, and frustration (Turkoski, 2000). Thus, it is not surprising that staff request more education and time in dealing with ethical decision making (Gjerberg et al., 2010). One proposed model of ethical decision making for nurses working with older residents (Bolmsjö et al., 2006) illustrates some underlying principles generally accepted in long-term care, as well as the related conflicts that arise. In this model, the overarching goal is for residents "to live as good a life as possible" as indicated by living "the kind of life a particular resident wants and desires to live" (p. 252). However, there are ethical constraints to staff supporting the wishes of all residents in a group setting, in that respecting any one individual's self-determination must be balanced by fairness to other residents. Further, care plans should be evidence based, and any interventions must fall within the roles and responsibilities of the given staff member. In addition, structural constraints such as legalities, resources, guidelines, and staff competence influence the extent to which optimal outcomes may be realized. Thus, these realities must be considered when staff follow the four steps to arrive at an ethical decision: (a) identify and describe the normative situation; (b) identify and describe the different alternatives that are possible in view of situational variables; (c) assess each alternative; and (d) decide, implement, and evaluate the selected alternative (Bolmsjö et al., 2006). The use of this model for ethical decision making may help staff recognize what is important from the perspective of the resident and realistic within the constraints of the situation, and so improve the care planning process.

Within a community of residents, the best outcome for one resident could conceivably impinge upon optimal outcomes for other residents or the setting as a whole, and so it might be necessary to modify the environment or care practices to preserve the rights of all. For example, a resident and his or her family might be granted privacy during the end-of-life period by setting aside a room for use in such instances, thereby allowing a roommate the autonomy to continue living his or her life while the dying resident has privacy and dignity.

At all times, staff, family, and medical personnel must balance respect for autonomy and beneficence, while avoiding paternalism, coercion, and conflicts of interest (McClure & Bosek, 2008). However, long-term care settings are a special case in point, in that restricted and varying resources of both the setting (e.g., number of private rooms) and the resident (e.g., residents who are and are not cognitively intact) often create ambiguous ethical situations, especially at the end of life.

CURRENT KNOWLEDGE REGARDING THE END OF LIFE IN LONG-TERM CARE

There is less research on dying in long-term care settings than in dying in acute care hospitals or at home. Many of the studies in long-term care that exist indicate poor care provided by untrained staff resulting in unrelieved pain, family dissatisfaction, and unnecessary hospitalizations in a regulatory environment that does not recognize palliative care (Miller et al., 2004). Furthermore, earlier studies suggest barriers to hospice involvement in long-term care such as communication difficulties between long-term care staff and hospice personnel, misunderstandings by staff regarding hospice goals and values, and insensitivity of hospice personnel to relationships between long-term care staff and residents (Keay & Schonwetter, 2000; Keay et al., 1994).

On the other hand, evidence also indicates that individuals who receive hospice care while dying in long-term care have better outcomes (Hallenbeck, Hickey, Czarnowski, Lehner, & Periyakoil, 2007). Two outcomes consistently associated with hospice use are use of alternative pain treatments and reduced hospitalizations (Munn, Hanson, Zimmerman, Sloane, & Mitchell, 2006). It is possible, although not established, that having support from hospice enables families and residents to refuse hospitalizations that they otherwise would accept.

Other documented advantages of hospice involvement include improved pain and symptom management (Stevenson & Bramsom, 2009); more attention to emotional and spiritual needs; greater family satisfaction (Stevenson, & Bramson, 2009); and reduced Medicare costs (Gozalo, Miller, Intrator, Barber, & Mor, 2008). In addition, there is evidence that hospice does not hasten death (Parker-Oliver, Porock, Zweig, Rantz, & Petrowski, 2003) and that in some cases, hospice recipients actually live longer than terminally ill elders without hospice (Connor, Pyenson, Fitch, Spence, & Iwaski, 2007). Of note, there is some suggestion that it might not be hospice per se that improves outcomes, but rather knowledge that an individual is at the end of life that changes care and so relates to improved outcomes (Munn et al., 2006).

While suggesting that hospice involvement improves the quality of care and quality of life at the end of life, these studies are inconsistent in informing quality standards. For example, some studies measure psychosocial outcomes and some do not (Blevins & Deason-Howell, 2002; Candy, Holman, Laurent, Davis, & Jones, 2010). Furthermore, medical care cost savings achieved by hospice are not universal, as they vary by disease, length of hospice care, and hospice provider (Gozalo et al., 2008), as well as by race, in that minority groups are less likely to use hospice (Kwak, Haley, & Chiriboga, 2008). That said, family satisfaction appears to remain consistently higher when hospice care is received, regardless of these variations (Hallenbeck, Hickey, Czarnowski, Lehner, & Periyakoil, 2007). This latter point is not to suggest that family satisfaction should be considered the gold standard outcome criterion, however. Given the long-recognized incongruence of family perspectives with those of residents, better gold standard outcome criteria might be the resident's quality of life and quality of dying, or absence of depression or anxiety. Admittedly, these outcomes are less often noted in the literature (Candy, Holman, Leurent, Davis, & Jones, 2010). Fortunately, new work is suggesting criteria by which end-of-life care (e.g., decision-making process, counseling, and communication) and outcomes (e.g., quality of life for patient, quality of life for family) might be assessed (van Soest-Poortvliet et al., 2011).

Indeed, hospice use in long-term care has grown significantly over the previous decade, increasing from 6% of nursing home deaths in 1998 (Kapo, Morrison, & Liao, 2007) to 15% in 2000 (Mitchell, Teno, Miller, & Mor, 2005). More recently, a 2005, four-state study of end of life in both nursing homes and assisted living communities found hospice use rates of 27% (Dobbs, Hanson, Zimmerman, Williams, & Munn, 2006), and other data indicate that one-third of nursing home decedents were enrolled in hospice in 2006 (Miller, Lima, Gozalo, & Mor, 2010). Looking at it from the perspective of hospice clients, almost one third (29%) of current hospice recipients are long-term care residents (NHPCO, 2010), again attesting to the notable use of hospice in long-term care. Further, in addition to benefits according to hospice patients, there is evidence that nonhospice residents receive enhanced end-of-life care when hospice is active in the nursing home (Welch, Miller, Martin, & Nanda, 2008).

CHALLENGES RELATED TO HOSPICE IN LONG-TERM CARE

Despite these demonstrated benefits and increased use of hospice in long-term care, there are site-specific challenges to hospice involvement, especially in nursing homes. First, settings must "invite" hospice into the facility, either through a working relationship or formal contract. Second, they must refer eligible residents for hospice enrollment. Then, once a resident is enrolled, hospice and long-term care staff must coordinate care. Finally, the death experience itself must be managed within the context of long-term care.

Each of these critical points will be detailed in the upcoming paragraphs, but first it must be noted that long-term care settings are only partially adapted to respond to each for various reasons. One reason is the variability of long-term care residents themselves; some are actively dying but others are not, meaning that the needs of dying residents must be given attention while attention is simultaneously given to those with lesser needs. Another challenge relates to resources. Dying long-term care residents differ in their functional capacities, and many long-term care settings themselves lack sufficient resources, such as a sufficient number of staff who are trained in hospice or palliative care. A further complication relates to the fact that 75% of long-term care decedents have some form of cognitive impairment (Munn et al., 2007), meaning that family members become centrally involved in end-of-life decision making despite the fact that their perspectives are not always congruent with those of the resident nor in the resident's best interest. Finally, long-term care settings are responsible for caring for their residents when hospice personnel are unavailable at critical times in the dying process. While all of these points present specific ethical dilemmas, they also present an opportunity for long-term care and hospice staff to demonstrate ethical decision making.

Inviting Hospice Into the Care Setting

Long-term care is among the few institutions in which there must be a working agreement or formal contract with a hospice provider in order for residents to receive hospice care while residing there (Miller, Intrator, et al., 2004). The decision to contract with a hospice provider is based upon a number of factors. For one, there are financial disincentives to hospice use. Hospice is funded by the Medicare Hospice Benefit (MHB) (Miller, Teno, & Mor, 2004), and residents who also are eligible for Medicare Part A (which reimburses rehabilitative nursing home care after a hospital stay) must choose between the two Medicare benefits. Reimbursement to the nursing home through Part A is significantly higher than the hospice benefit, and it is paid directly to the nursing home rather than through a third party. On the other hand, the MHB is paid directly to the hospice provider (Stevenson & Bramson, 2009), who then transfers monies to the nursing home, thus delaying nursing home reimbursement. Further, while the MHB covers nursing care, medical social services, physician services, counseling, physical therapy, occupational therapy, and speech-language pathology services, it does not include room and board; therefore, in some instances, the long-term care provider must continue to bill either the resident or Medicaid, creating another complexity to involving hospice (Dobbs, Hanson, Zimmerman, Williams, & Munn, 2006).

One important consideration affecting whether a hospice contract is signed or hospice is used in the setting is the nursing home administrator's attitudes toward hospice (Buchanan, Choi, Wang, & Ju, 2004). While nursing home administrators are generally positive toward hospice, they view hospice as supplementing rather than replacing the care they provide (Dobbs et al., 2006). Administrators face a paradox in that while hospice involvement may improve care for the individual resident who is at the end of life, the MHB provides considerably less financial support than Medicare

Part A. In consideration of this financial disincentive, an administrator must determine whether the value added to individual resident care is substantial enough to outweigh the financial losses and complications associated with care coordination. Over time, the financial loss could negatively impact staffing levels and consequently care to other residents. Indeed, nursing home personnel often cite meeting the needs of other residents as paramount in their inability to meet the intense and focused needs of dying residents.

Another potential disincentive to hospice is the hospice philosophy of treating the family as well as the resident as the unit of care. While nursing homes recognize the importance of the family unit, their client is the resident, and as such they are responsible for ensuring resident rights, including self-determination. However, family wishes are not always congruent with resident wishes for end-of-life care, and determining what roles relatives should have in decision making is sometimes problematic (Dreyer, Forde, & Nortvedt, 2009). Further, family members may not even know a resident's wishes and may disagree among themselves about end-of-life decisions (Gjerberg et al., 2010). There also are instances of families interfering with appropriate care for dying residents, especially when distant family members are absent until the resident is actively dying. Staff describe family as "coming out of the woodwork" and demanding care (such as taking vital signs despite the discomfort it might cause in repositioning the resident) (Munn et al., 2008). In sum, expanding the focus of health care from the resident to the family does not necessarily result in the best interest of the resident (Dreyer et al., 2009).

The following case example illustrates the complex situations that may arise regarding family decision making:

A hospice social worker contacted a nursing home for admission of a patient with advanced cancer. The nursing home personnel agreed to admit the patient with the expectation that death was anticipated within 2–3 weeks. When the patient was admitted, the hospice nurse's admission note indicated that she was actively dying. Despite this critical time, the hospice nurse left the nursing home shortly after the admission, and the resident died within hours, with no support from hospice and under the care of nursing home staff who were unfamiliar with her. When questioned why hospice moved a patient in the last hours before death, the hospice social worker indicated that the family did not want the patient to die in their home. While it is possible that the patient would not have experienced a better death surrounded by her family, it is not at all clear that being transferred to a nursing home to die there is what she would have desired. Further, this incident frustrated the nursing home staff, who were limited in their ability to care for the woman due to their lack of familiarity with her, as well as the administrator, who was responsible for renewing the hospice contract.

This case illustrates a challenge associated with inviting hospice into the setting. Also, it is an extreme yet real indication of poorly coordinated care. The absence of hospice staff at the time of the resident's death speaks to the difficulties associated with such an absence. Indeed, this case reflects, in the extreme, three of the four ethical foci described in this chapter: inviting hospice; coordinating care; and managing the death experience.

The matter of inviting hospice into the long-term care setting is further complicated by the fact that although "hospice" refers to an overarching philosophy of care, providers differ in the quality of care provided. For example, nonprofit hospices tend to provide fewer services than contracted (OIG, 2011). In addition, hospice use itself is variable within long-term care settings. Also, regional variation exists such that settings in the South (especially Florida) and metropolitan areas are more likely to use hospice (Miller et al., 2004). Furthermore, the majority of hospice referrals are received from a small percentage of providers (Miller & Mor, 2002). More specifically, although 87% of nursing homes have hospice agreements, only 30% actually have hospice enrollees (Stevenson & Bramson, 2009). Thus, hospice services in long-term care continue to appear underutilized (Hoffmann & Tarzian, 2005; Winn & Dentivo, 2004). Taken together, these data suggest that while hospice use has increased, use differs across geographic areas, individual hospice providers, and long-term care settings.

Referring Eligible Residents to Hospice

The statistics in the preceding paragraph indicate that while many long-term care settings contract with hospice, many do not refer eligible residents to hospice. This underuse may relate to the fact that for persons of all ages and in varied residential settings, it is difficult to "diagnose dying" (Ellershaw & Ward, 2003). In fact, there are no precise parameters to the period referred to as the end of life (Powers & Watson, 2008). This difficulty is even greater in long-term care where older adults are less likely than younger persons to die of an illness with a predictable trajectory such as cancer (Miller et al., 2004), and more likely to suffer from multiple comorbidities. This ambiguity creates an indeterminate state with no clear point at which chronic illness becomes terminal. Ideally, an interdisciplinary medical team reaches consensus on a resident's terminal status (Ellershaw & Ward, 2003), but even licensed nurses and doctors, when available, often do not recognize the end of life until the resident is actively dying (Munn et al., 2006).

As noted earlier, an undergirding ethical principle in all health care settings is that of self-determination. For cognitively intact long-term care residents, supporting this principle includes keeping resident information confidential (Gropper & Giovinco, 2000), even from family and friends unless the resident grants permission. However, it is more difficult to balance respect for autonomy with beneficence when cognitive impairment is involved. These situations have fostered a model of shared decision making in which the resident (when able), family, and medical personnel discuss medical decisions together, including the option of using hospice (Heyman & Gutheil, 2006). The literature suggests that the situation is not straightforward, however, because in many instances when relatives are involved in the decision-making process, they lack information on end-of-life options and feel burdened by the responsibility (Dreyer et al., 2009). Conversely, there may be a relief to choosing hospice care, as it narrows the continuum of end-of-life medical treatment, which ranges from aggressive resuscitation to active euthanasia (Dumas & Ramadurai, 2009). This paradox reflects the struggles of acknowledging the end of life versus seeking to extend life as long as possible.

Optimally, end-of-life decisions are made early in the long-term care stay and in conjunction with physicians (Casarett et al., 2005). Unfortunately, physicians are not typically present in nursing homes (Shield, Wetle, Teno, Miller, & Welch, 2005) and are generally not expected to be present in assisted living communities. Thus, it falls on other medical personnel (e.g., licensed nurses, social workers) to determine a resident's cognitive status, identify the terminal state, and counsel residents and families regarding medical decision making, including the use of hospice.

Much like the population as a whole, for residents who are cognitively intact, their refusal to discuss dying is singularly significant in failing to make medical decisions regarding the end of life, including a hospice referral (Heyman & Gutheil, 2006). Similarly, because hospice enrollees waive the right to receive reimbursement for curative care (Stevenson & Bramson, 2009) some residents and families see involving hospice as "giving up" (Ford, Nietert, Zapka, Zoller, & Silvestri, 2008), and so they do not consider a hospice referral until it is obvious that death is days or hours away. Residents and families are not the only ones with a proclivity against end-of-life considerations, in that even some long-term staff and doctors are hesitant to discuss death and dying or do not see themselves as providing end-of-life care (Miller et al., 2004). At other times, staff such as nursing home social workers are tasked with conducting these discussions, yet they too are apologetic about raising the possibility of hospice and may hesitate broaching a discussion of dying if they feel incompetent to deal with death (Ellershaw & Ward, 2003).

Finally, staff attitudes and misconceptions regarding the hospice philosophy create barriers to supporting hospice involvement. Long-term care staff often see themselves as knowing the resident best and perceive no added value of involving hospice personnel (Welch, Miller, Martin, & Nanda, 2008), or at minimum, they want to continue their role providing care for these individuals for whom they have cared for many years (Zimmerman, Sloane, Hanson, Mitchell, & Shy, 2003). In other cases, staff believe that hospice hastens death and that essential care will be withheld if a resident enrolls in hospice (Schockett, Teno, Miller, & Stuart, 2005).

These perceptions and misconceptions present barriers to timely hospice referrals in both nursing homes and assisted living communities. However, once the referral is made, there are other challenges that present additional ethical dilemmas, including the need for care coordination.

Coordinating Care With Hospice

The difficulties of coordinating care when long-term care and hospice staff are providing end-of-life care for a resident are well documented. In nursing homes, care plans are required to be developed from scheduled minimum data set (MDS) assessments; when hospice becomes involved, it assumes overall responsibility for developing and managing the plan of care (Miller et al., 2004). However, because hospice staff are not continually present in the long-term care setting, long-term care staff remain involved in carrying out the plan of care, including medication management.

The coordination of care related to medication management is especially important when treating pain. Treating pain at the end of life has different goals than managing pain associated with chronic illness (which might instead require "as needed" as opposed to prescheduled administration), a situation with which long-term care staff may be more familiar. Although the pain protocol is likely to be determined by hospice personnel, some nursing home staff may be reluctant to follow hospice protocols due to misconceptions about the effect of opioids (Dumas & Ramadurai, 2009). Also, the administration of "as-needed" pain medication may be delayed in cases when residents do not reveal the extent of their discomfort to avoid upsetting family or annoying care providers, or in response to ageist attitudes about pain being part of old age (Duncan, Forbes-Thompson, & Bott, 2008).

The administration of pain medications is especially complex when residents with dementia are not able to verbalize their needs, and appropriate care depends on recognizing discomfort based on individualized nonverbal cues. In this case, it is not the nurses as much as it is the certified nursing assistants (CNAs) who administer 90% of direct care to residents who are reported best able to recognize such cues (Duncan et al., 2008). Indeed, one of the most important factors in improving end-of-life care in nursing homes has been identified as increasing nursing assistant time (Miller et al., 2004; Zimmerman, Sloane, et al., 2003). Unfortunately, CNAs are not generally included in the care planning process and voice dissatisfaction at being ignored by hospice personnel (Munn et al., 2008). Nonetheless, hospice involvement does seem to result in improved pain and symptom management for both hospice recipients and other dying residents in the same setting (Duncan et al., 2008)

The matter of care coordination relates to more than medication management, however, and anecdotal evidence suggests that long-term care staff "pull away" from hospice recipients, seeing their role in care as diminished. This pulling away is unfortunate, as hospice staff are not always available at critical times (Parker-Oliver & Bickel, 2002). When hospice staff are not available and long-term care staff perceive a diminished role, there arises the possibility that residents "fall through the cracks" and actually receive less care rather than more. It is also intuitive, although not established through research, that should hospice agencies have limited staff, they would prioritize care for community-dwelling patients for whom there are no other care providers, assuming that long-term care staff would provide care for their residents in their absence. In a recent OIG report, 31% of cases examined indicated hospice services to nursing home residents were not provided with the frequency indicated in the plan of care (OIG, 2011). In the end, care coordination is crucial, as despite hospice involvement, the long-term care setting retains the responsibility for resident care (Stevenson & Bramson, 2009). Here, the salient ethical dilemma is whether the preponderance of end-of-life care is improved when hospice is provided. While data suggest that it is, the issues presented earlier suggest that there may be some aspects of care that are not improved, and may actually be worsened, when hospice is involved.

Recent regulations have sought to clarify the responsibilities of both the long-term care setting and hospice, with the intent of reducing cost while improving care. For example, hospice personnel are required to orient nursing home staff to the hospice philosophy of care, "including hospice policies and procedures regarding methods of comfort, pain control, symptom management, as well as principles about death and dying, individual responses to death, patient rights, appropriate forms, and record keeping requirements" (Code of Federal Regulations, 2010, 42 §418.112(f)). These regulations support communication between hospice personnel and long-term care staff and reinforce the role of hospice as expert in end-of-life care provision. However, they do not overcome the day-to-day challenges of implementing care.

There is also a potential tension of coordination in relation to the overall perspective of care. Over time, long-term care has come to embrace a more social, as opposed to strictly medical, model of care—as illustrated by using the term "residents" as opposed to "patients" for those who receive care. This holistic view continues throughout the dying process. Depending on the particular hospice provider, medicalization embedded in hospice care could impede coordination. Instead, exemplars of hospice-nursing home care coordination that work particularly well focus on a social rather than a regulatory or medical model of care (Hodgson & Lehning, 2008) and are person centered rather than task focused (Miller et al., 2004). In high-performing nursing homes, administrators describe hospice as a partner in care and demonstrate considerable effort in establishing good working relationships. In these cases, positive relationships also existed among hospice personnel and nursing home staff and families of residents. In fact, in high-functioning partnerships, roles between hospice and the nursing home are said to be blurred, a change to the traditional hierarchical structure that is often present (Hodgson & Lehning, 2008).

Managing the Death Experience

A fourth critical point in which ethical dilemmas arise in the use of hospice in long-term care settings is managing the death experience itself. A consistent outcome associated with hospice involvement is the reduction of unnecessary hospitalizations at the end of life and consequent cost savings. Hospitalizations have indeed been reduced in nursing homes, underscoring the agreement of care providers, patients, and their families that palliative care occur in the nursing home rather than the hospital (Dumas & Ramadurai, 2009). The matter is not quite that straightforward, though, as decisions to discharge are also affected by supply factors. When hospital beds are readily available and nursing home occupancy rates are high, residents are more likely to be discharged to hospitals than when the reverse is true (Decker, 2008).

The situation in assisted living communities differs from that in nursing homes, however. In terms of the end-of-life experience, these residential settings more closely approximate life within a community because they are not nearly as medically equipped as are nursing homes; in fact, in light of their limited capacity, some state regulations do not allow medically compromised residents to remain in assisted living. In Florida, for example, a resident must be transferred out of assisted living if he or she is not able to evacuate the setting on his or her own (Polzer, 2011). However, some states—including Florida—will allow residents to remain in assisted living as they decline beyond impairment levels deemed appropriate as long as hospice is involved. Still, it must be recognized that half of assisted living communities do not have licensed nursing staff on-site (Stearns et al., 2007), and even more do not have them on-site during the evening and night shifts. In these settings or at these times, should an emergency arise and hospice personnel are not available, there may be little choice but to send the resident to the hospital for skilled care. Nonetheless, despite exemptions that allow for dying in place, some assisted living communities routinely discharge dying residents to hospitals or nursing homes because other residents are uncomfortable witnessing the end-of-life experience. This situation exemplifies a common ethical dilemma in long-term care that underlies many others: weighing the needs of the individual against the well-being of the community as a whole.

Another important aspect in managing the death experience is the practice of calling hospice first when there is a change in resident status. In fact, a common practice among some hospice providers is to place an adhesive sticker on the front of the resident's chart that states: "Call hospice first." However, existing data indicate that hospice staff are unavailable 25% of the time when requested (Parker-Oliver & Bickel, 2002). Further, contacting hospice first may delay or even override family contact, such as in the case when hospice was called at the time a resident was dying, but family members did not learn of the death until several hours after the resident died, when a nursing assistant answered the telephone in the resident's room. In another instance, hospice personnel did not provide the "comfort kit" needed for a resident who was actively dying. As it was the weekend, no one from hospice was available to deliver the kit to the nursing home. Instead, the nursing home staff obtained a prescription from the medical director and the resident's family purchased the necessary medication from a local pharmacy. When the resident died later that evening, the hospice social worker requested that the family remain at the nursing home until she could arrive, to provide bereavement care. The family, however, felt that hospice had failed in their primary responsibility of providing a comfortable death, and so they were not interested in waiting for hospice personnel to provide other services. Here again, absence at a critical point, when the resident was actively dying, seems to perhaps overcome the advantages associated with hospice involvement and raises ethical questions and areas requiring further attention.

Thus, the matter of hospice availability in long-term care settings may be one that raises the most concern, as it cuts across all four critical points at which ethical dilemmas arise. Before an administrator is willing to contract with hospice, and before residents can be referred, and before care can be coordinated, and before the dying experience can be managed, it is important to understand the capacity of any particular hospice organization to provide care—both overall, and to a given patient at a given time, as the capacity of hospice organizations often varies over time. As in all cases, the promise of care is only as good as the delivery of that care.

HOSPICE ORGANIZATIONS AS CONSULTANTS IN END-OF-LIFE CARE FOR FACILITY RESIDENTS

Nursing homes and assisted living communities are, and will continue to be, sites of death for a significant number of older adults in the United States. As such, high-quality end-of-life care is important and the characteristics of nursing home and assisted living communities need to be taken into account when developing care models. Current research indicates that hospice involvement in the long-term care end-of-life experience leads to positive outcomes such as fewer hospitalizations and enhanced pain management. The literature also supports an acknowledgment of hospice clinicians as experts in end-of-life care. However, there are ethical issues that arise at four points within the process: inviting hospice into the community, referring residents to hospice, coordinating care between hospice and long-term care staff, and managing the death experience. Significant in all of these issues are the tensions of managing the care of many residents while also caring for a smaller number of actively dying residents, as well as the documented absence of hospice personnel at critical times during the dying process.

Recognizing and directly addressing the ethical issues between hospice providers and long-term care administrators, staff, residents, and families may help resolve some of these issues. In cases when they cannot be readily resolved, a partial solution may be to use hospice in a consultant role. Certainly, the dilemma should not be resolved by discounting the benefits of hospice, as a recent qualitative study found that five different stakeholder groups (residents, bereaved family members, licensed nursing staff, paraprofessional staff, and social workers) all believed that hospice staff had advanced expertise in areas of pain and symptom management as well as providing support and education for residents and their families (Munn, 2012). This expertise is characterized as both knowledge of and experience in dealing with the dying process.

Notwithstanding the expertise of hospice, the role of hospice as a consultant is reasonable because in some cases, long-term care settings are able to provide care similar to that of hospice when a resident's death is expected, suggesting that being able to anticipate death is key to providing better care (Munn et al., 2006). Further, despite the expertise of hospice providers, long-term care staff do not want to relinquish the caregiving role they had for years at the time that a resident is dying (Zimmerman, Sloane, et al. 2003).

Thus, considering that it is unrealistic to expect third-party care providers to be available in the same manner as long-term care staff—and that the expectation of ready availability cuts across all four critical points at which ethical dilemmas arise—it may be best for hospice to be considered not only as a care provider but also as a consultant. Such a role maximizes the expertise that hospice brings and mitigates the grave issue of the absence of hospice personnel during critical points in care. Indeed, model programs of hospice consultation have been successful (Miller et al., 2004). Partnering this consultation with training (e.g., recognition of pain in cognitively impaired residents [Hanson et al., 2008]) for long-term care staff (Miller & Han, 2008) and empowering staff to deliver end-of-life care (Ellershaw & Ward, 2003) seems a beneficial mode of care provision for long-term care settings.

If hospice personnel undertake more of a consulting role, however, the revenue to hospice will significantly decline (Huskamp et al., 2010). Ironically, such a dilemma mirrors what long-term care administrators currently experience when faced with a choice between higher Medicare Part A reimbursement and accepting the MHB. It is not clear to what extent hospice entities, which can be for-profit agencies, would relinquish the current model for a less lucrative one that better empowers long-term care staff. The driving force, of course, should be the outcomes for residents who are dying in nursing homes and assisted living settings.

REFERENCES

American Nurses Association. (2011). *Code for nurses with interpretive statement.* Retrieved April 2014, from http://nursingworld.org/MainMenuCategories/ EthicsStandards/CodeofEthicsforNurses/Code-of-Ethics.aspx.

Asch-Goodkin, J. (2000). The virtues of hospice. *Patient Care for the Nurse Practitioner*, 3(11), 6–8, 13–4, 17–20.

Assisted Living Federation of America (ALFA). (2011). *Facts and figures*. Retrieved April 2014, from http://www.alfa.org/alfa/Facts_and_Figures.asp.

Bern-Klug, M., ed. (2010). *Transforming palliative care in nursing homes: The social work role*. New York, NY: Columbia University Press.

Bern-Klug, M., Gessert, C. E., Crenner, C.S., Buenaver, M., & Skirchak, D. (2004). 'Getting everyone on the same page': Nursing home physicians' perspectives on end-of-life care. *Journal of Palliative Medicine*, 7(4), 533–544.

Blevins, D., & Deason-Howell, L. M. (2002). End-of-life care in nursing homes: The interface of policy, research, and practice. *Behavioral Sciences and the Law*, 20, 271–286.

Bolmsjö, I. A., Sandman, L., & Anderson, E. (2006). Everyday ethics in the care of elderly people. *Nursing Ethics*, 13(3), 249–263.

Buchanan, R. J., Choi, M., Wang, S., & Ju, H. (2004). End-of-life care in nursing homes: Residents in hospice compared to other end-stage residents. *Journal of Palliative Medicine*, 7(2), 221–232.

Candy, B., Holman, A., Leurent, B., Davis, S., & Jones, L. (2010). Hospice care delivered at home, in nursing homes and in dedicated hospice facilities: A systematic review of quantitative and qualitative evidence. *International Journal of Nursing Studies*, 48, 121–133.

Casarett, D., Karlawish, J., Morales, K., Crowley, R. Mirsch, T., & Asch, D. A. (2005). Improving the use of hospice in nursing homes: a randomized control trial. *Journal of the American Medical Association*, 295, 211–217.

Centers for Disease Control and Prevention (CDC). (2011). *Faststats*. Retrieved April 2014, from http://www.cdc.gov/nchs/fastats/nursingh.htm.

Centers for Medicare and Medicaid Services (CMS) (n.d.). Nursing Home Quality Initiatives. Retrieved April 2014, from http://www.cms. gov/Medicare/Quality-Initiatives-Patient-Assessment-Instruments/ NursingHomeQualityInits/index.html.

Centers for Medicare and Medicaid Services (CMS). (2010). *Nursing home data compendium 2010 edition*. Retrieved April 2014, from http://www.cms.gov/ CertificationandComplianc/Downloads/nursinghomedatacompendium_508. pdf.

Code of Federal Regulations, 42 § 418.112.D. Retrieved April 2014, from http://www. ecfr.gov/cgi-bin/text-idx?SID=586987110f0d24acfd6b32dfc415fb98&node=4 2:3.0.1.1.5.4.5.7&rgn=div8.

Connor, S. R., Pyenson, B., Fitch, K., Spence, C., & Iwaski, K. (2007). Comparing hospice and non-hospice patient survival among patients who die within a three-year window. *Journal of Pain and Symptom Management*, 33(3), 238–246.

Csikai, E. L., & Bass, K. (2000). Healthcare social workers' views of ethical issues, practice, and policy in end-of-life care. *Social Work in Health Care*, 32(2), 1–22.

Decker, F. H. (2008). Dying in a nursing home: The role of local bed supply in nursing home discharges. *Journal of Aging and Health*, 20(1), 66–88.

Department of Health and Human Services, Health Care Financing Administration. (1989, February 2). *Federal Register/Rules and Regulations*, 54(21). Washington, DC: US Government Printing Office.

Dobbs, D., Hanson, L., Zimmerman, S., Williams, C., & Munn, J. (2006). Hospice attitudes among assisted living and nursing home administrators and the Long-term Care Hospice Attitudes Scale. *Journal of Palliative Medicine*, 9(6), 1388–1400.

Dreyer, A., Forde, R., & Nortvedt, P. (2009). Autonomy at the end of life: Life prolonging treatment in nursing homes—relatives' role in the decision-making process. *Journal of Medical Ethics, 35,* 672–677.

Dumas, L. G., & Ramadurai, M. (2009). Pain management in the nursing home. *Nursing Clinics of North America, 44,* 197–208.

Duncan, J. G., Forbes-Thompson, S., & Bott, M. J. (2008). Unmet symptom management needs of nursing home residents with cancer. *Cancer Nursing, 31*(4), 265–273.

Ellershaw, J., & Ward, C. (2003). Care of the dying patient: The last hours or days of life. *British Medical Journal, 326,* 30–34.

Engle, V. F. (1998). Care of the living, care of the dying: Reconceptualizing nursing home care. *Journal of the American Geriatric Society, 46,* 1172–1174.

Federal Interagency Forum on Aging Related Statistics (FIFARS). (2011). *Older Americans 2010: Key indicators of well being.* Retrieved April 2014, from http://www.agingstats.gov/agingstatsdotnet/Main_Site/Data/2012_Documents/Docs/EntireChartbook.pdf

Fleming, D. A. (2007). Responding to ethical dilemmas in nursing homes: Do we always need an "ethicist." *HEC Forum, 19*(3), 245–259.

Ford, D. W., Nietert, P. J., Zapka, J., Zoller, J. S., & Silvestri, G. A. (2008).Barriers to hospice enrollment among lung cancer patients: A survey of family members and physicians. *Palliative and Supportive Care, 6,* 357–362.

Fowler, F. J., Coppola, K. M., & Teno, J. (1999). Methodological challenges for measuring quality of care at the end of life. *Journal of Pain and Symptom Management, 17*(2), 114–119.

Frytak, J. R., Kane, R. A., Finch, M. D., Kane, R. L., & Maude-Griffin, R. (2001). Outcome trajectories for assisted living and nursing facility residents in Oregon. *Health Services Research, 36,* 91–111.

Gozalo, P., Miller, S. C., Intrator, O., Barber, J. P., & Mor, V. (2008). Hospice effect on government expenditures among nursing home residents. *Health Services Research, 43*(1), 134–153.

Gjerberg, E., Forde, R., Pedersen, R., & Bollig, Georg. (2010). Ethical challenges in the provision of end-of-life care in Norwegian nursing homes. *Social Science and Medicine, 71,* 677–684.

Gropper, R. G., & Giovinco, G. (2000). Confidentiality in home and hospice nursing: Protecting vulnerable populations. *Home Healthcare Nurse, 18*(3), 161–164.

Hallenbeck, J., Hickey, E., Czarnowski, E., Lehner, L., & Periyakoil, V. S. (2007). Quality of care in a veterans affairs' nursing home-based hospice unit. *Journal of Palliative Medicine, 10*(1), 127–135.

Han, B., Tiggle, R. B., & Remsburg, R. E. (2008). Characteristics of patients receiving Hospice care in home versus nursing homes: Results from the National Home and Hospice Care Survey and the National Nursing Home Survey. *American Journal of Hospice and Palliative Medicine, 24*(6), 479–486.

Hanson, L. C., Eckert, K., Dobbs, D., Williams, C. S., Caprio, A. J. Sloane, P. D., & Zimmerman, S. (2008). Symptom experience of dying long-term care residents. *Journal of the American Geriatric Society, 56,* 91–98.

Hanson, L. C., Henderson, M., & Rogman, E. (1999). Where will we die? A national study of nursing home death. *Journal of the American Geriatric Society, 47,* 9.

Hawes, C., Rose, M., & Phillips, C. D. (1999). *A national study of assisted living for the frail elderly.* Beachwood, OH: Meyers Research Institute.

Hawes, C., Phillips, C. D., Rose, M., Holan, S., & Sherman, M. (2003). A national survey of assisted living facilities. *Gerontologist, 43*(6), 875–882.

Heyman, J., & Gutheil, I. A. (2006). Social work involvement in end-of-life planning. *Journal of Gerontological Social Work, 47*(3–4), 47–61.

Hicks, T. (2000). Ethical implications of pain management in a nursing home: A discussion. *Nursing Ethics, 7*(5), 392–398.

Hodgson, N. A., & Lehning, A. J. (2008). Palliative care in nursing homes: A comparison of high- and low-level providers. *International Journal of Palliative Nursing, 14*(1), 39–45.

Hoffmann, D. E., & Tarzian, A. J. (2005). Dying in America-an examination of policies that deter adequate end-of-life care in nursing homes. *Journal of Law, Medicine, and Ethics, 33*(2), 294–309.

Hodlewsky, R. T. (2001). Staffing problems and strategies in assisted living. In S. Zimmerman, P. D. Sloane, & J. K. Eckert (Eds.), *Assisted living: Needs, practices and policies in residential care for the elderly* (pp. 78–91). Baltimore: Johns Hopkins University Press.

Huskamp, H., Stevenson, D. G., Chernew, M., & Newhouse, J. P. (2010). A new Medicare end-of-life benefit for nursing home residents. *Health Affairs, 29*(1), 130–135.

Jones, A. (2002). The National Nursing Home Survey: 1999 summary. *Vital Health Statistics, 13*(152). Retrieved May 20, 2014 from http://www.cdc.gov/nchs/data/series/sr_13/sr13_152.pdf.

Kapo, J., Morrison, L. J., & Liao, S. (2007). Palliative care for the older adult. *Journal of Palliative Medicine, 10*(1), 185–209.

Keay, T. J., Fredman, L., Taler, G. A., Datta, S., & Levenson, S. A. (1994). Indicators of quality medical care for the terminally ill in nursing homes. *Journal of the American Geriatric Society, 42*, 853–860.

Keay, T. J., & Schonwetter, R. S. (2000). The case for hospice care in long-term care environments. *Clinics in Geriatric Medicine, 16*, 211–223.

Kiely, D. K., & Flacker J. M. (2003). The protective effect of social engagement on 1-year mortality in a long-stay nursing home population. *Journal of Clinical Epidemiology, 56*, 472–478.

Kwak, J., Halely, W. E., & Chiriboga, D. A. (2008). Racial differences in hospice use and in-hospital death among Medicare and Medicaid dual-eligible nursing home residents. *Gerontologist, 48*(1), 32–41.

Magaziner, J., German, P., Zimmerman, S. I., Hebel, J. R., Burton, L., Gruber-Baldini, A. L., . . . Kittner, S. (2000). The prevalence of dementia in a statewide sample of new nursing home admissions age 65 and older: diagnosis by expert panel. *Gerontologist, 40*, 663–672.

McClure, M., & Bosek, M. S. (2008). Ethical obligations and concerns when trying to achieve a patient's wishes: Palliative care clinical nurse specialist. *JONA's Health Care Law, Ethics, and Regulation, 10*(3), 77–79.

Mezey, M., Dubler, N. N., Mitty, E., & Brody, A. A. (2000). What impact do setting and transitions have on the quality of life at the end of life and the quality of the dying process? *Gerontologist, 42*(Special Edition III), 54–67.

Miller, S. C., & Han, B. (2008). End-of-life care in U.S. nursing homes: Nursing homes with special programs and trained staff for Hospice or palliative/end-of-life care. *Journal of Palliative Medicine, 11*(6), 866–877.

Miller, S. C., Intrator, O., Gozalo, P., Roy, J., Barber, J., & Mor, V. (2004). Government expenditures at the end of life for short- and long-stay nursing home residents: Differences by hospice enrollment status. *Journal of the American Geriatric Society, 52*, 1284–1292.

Miller, S. C., Lima, J., Gozalo, P. L., & Mor, V. (2010). The growth of hospice care in U.S. nursing homes. *Journal of the American Geriatric Society, 58*, 1481–1488.

Miller, S. C., & Mor, V. (2002). The role of hospice care in the nursing home setting. *Journal of Palliative Medicine, 5*(2), 1–7.

Miller, S. C., Teno, J. M., & Mor, V. (2004). Hospice and palliative care in nursing homes. *Clinics in Geriatric Medicine, 20*(4), 717–734.

Mitchell, S. L., Morris, J. N., Park, P. S., & Fries, B. E. (2004). Terminal care for persons with advanced dementia in the nursing home and home care settings. *Journal of Palliative Medicine, 7*(6), 808–816.

Mitchell, S. L., Teno, J. M., Miller, S. C., & Mor, V. (2005). A national location of death for older persons with dementia. *Journal of the American Geriatric Society, 53*, 299–305.

Mollica, R. (1998). *State assisted living policy, 1998*. Retrieved May 20, 2014 from http://aspe.hhs.gov/daltcp/reports/1998/98state.htm.

Morgan, L. A., Gruber-Baldini, A. L., & Magaziner, J. (2001). Resident characteristics. In S. Zimmerman, P. D. Sloane, & K. Eckert (Eds.), *Assisted living: Needs, practices and policies in residential care for the elderly* (pp. 144–172). Baltimore, MD: Johns Hopkins University Press.

Munn, J. (2012). Telling the story: Perceptions of Hospice in long-term care from five stakeholder groups. *American Journal of Hospice and Palliative Medicine, 29*(3), 201–209.

Munn, J., & Adorno, G. (2008). By invitation only: Social work involvement at the end of life in long-term care. *Journal of Social Work and End of Life and Palliative Care, 4*(4), 333–357.

Munn, J., Dobbs, D., Meier, A., Williams, C., Biola, H., & Zimmerman, S. (2008). The end-of-life experience in long-term care: Five themes identified from focus groups with residents, family members, and staff. *Gerontologist, 48*(4), 485–494.

Munn, J., Hanson, L., Zimmerman, S., Sloane, P. D., & Mitchell, C. M. (2006). Is hospice associated with improved end-of-life care in nursing homes and assisted living facilities? *Journal of the American Geriatric Society, 54*(3), 490–495.

Munn, J. C., Zimmerman, S., Hanson, L. C., Williams, C. S., Sloane, P. D., Clipp, E. C.,...Steinhauser, K. E. (2007). Measuring the quality of dying in long-term care. *Journal of the American Geriatrics Society, 55*(9), 1371–1379.

Murphy, K., Hanrahan, P., & Luchins, D. (1997). A survey of grief and bereavement in nursing homes: The importance of Hospice grief and bereavement for end-stage Alzheimer's disease patient and family. *Journal of the American Geriatric Society, 45*, 1104–1107.

National Center for Assisted Living (NCAL). (n.d.). *Assisted living resident profile*. Retrieved May 20, 2014 from http://www.ahcancal.org/ncal/resources/Pages/ResidentProfile.aspx.

National Hospice and Palliative Care Organization (NHPCO). (2010). *NHPCO Facts and figures: Hospice care in America*. Alexandria, VA: National Hospice and Palliative Care Organization.

Nelson, M. L., Schrader, S. L., & Eidsness, L. (2009). 'South Dakota's dying to know': Personal experiences with end-of-life care. *Journal of Palliative Medicine, 12*(10), 905–913.

Office of the Inspector General (OIG). (2011). *Medicare hospice care for beneficiaries in nursing facilities: Compliance with Medicare coverage requirements*. Retrieved April 2014, from http://www.oig.hhs.gov/oei/reports/oei-02-06-00221.pdf.

Park-Lee, E., Caffrey, C., Sengupta, M., Moss, A. J., Rosenoff, E., & Harris-Kojetin, L. D. (2011). *Residential care facilities: A key sector in the spectrum of long-term care providers in the United States* [NCHS Data Brief, No. 78]. Hyattsville, MD: National Center for Health Statistics.

Parker-Oliver, D., & Bickel, D. (2002). Nursing home experience with hospice. *Journal of the American Medical Directors Association, 3*(2), 46–50.

Parker-Oliver, D., Porock, D., Zweig, S., Rantz, M., & Petroski, G. F. (2003). Hospice and non-hospice nursing home residents. *Journal of Palliative Medicine, 6*(1), 69–75.

Phillips, C. D., Holan, S., Sherman, M., Spector, W., & Hawes, C. (2005). Medicare expenditures for residents in assisted living: Data from a national study. *Health Services Research, 40*(2), 373–388.

Porock, E., Parker-Oliver, D., Zweig, S. C., Rantz, M., & Petroski, G. F. (2003). A profile of residents admitted to long-term care facilities for end-of-life care. *Journal of American Medical Directors Association, 4*, 16–22.

Polzer, K. (2011). *Assisted living: State regulatory review.* Washington, DC: National Center for Assisted Living (NCAL). Retrieved April 2014, from http://www.ahcancal.org/ncal/resources/Pages/AssistedLivingRegulations.aspx.

Powers, B. A., & Watson, N. M. (2008). Meaning and practice of palliative care for nursing home residents at the end of life. *American Journal of Alzheimer's Disease and Other Dementias, 23*(4), 319–325.

Schockett, E. R, Teno, J. M., Miller, S. C., & Stuart, B. (2005). Late referral to hospice and bereaved family member perception of quality of end-of-life care. *Journal of Pain and Symptom Management, 30*(5), 400–407.

Shield, R. R., Wetle, T., Teno, J., Miller, S. C., & Welch, L. (2005). Physicians 'missing in action': Family perspective on physician and staffing problems in end-of-life care in the nursing home. *Journal of the American Geriatric Society, 53*, 1532–1657.

Schockett, E. R., Teno, J. M., Miller, S. C., & Stuart, B. (2005). Late referral to Hospice and bereaved family member perception of quality end-of-life care. *Journal of Pain and Symptom Management, 30*(5), 400–407.

Smith, W. R., Kellerman, A., & Brown, J. S. (1995). The impact of nursing home transfer policies at the end of life on a public acute care hospital. *Journal of the American Geriatrics Society, 43*, 1052–1057.

Solum, E. V., Slettebo, A., & Hauge, S. (2008). Prevention of unethical actions in nursing homes. *Nursing Ethics, 15*(4), 536–548.

Stearns, S. C., Park, J., Zimmerman, S., Gruber-Baldini, A. L., Konrad, T. R., & Sloane, P. D. (2007). Determinants and effects of nurse staffing intensity and skill mix in residential care/assisted living settings. *Gerontologist, 47*(5), 662–671.

Stevenson, E. G., & Bramson, J. S. (2009). Hospice care in the nursing home setting: A review of the literature. *Journal of Pain and Symptom Management, 38*(3), 440–451.

Turkoski, B. B. (2000). Home care and hospice ethics: Code for nurses. *Home Healthcare Nurse, 18*(5), 308–316.

US Census Bureau. *The 2010 statistical abstract: The national data book.* Retrieved April 2014, from http://www.census.gov/compendia/statab/cats/births_deaths_marriages_divorces.html.

van Soest-Poortvliet, M. C., van der Steen, J. T., Zimmerman, S., Cohen, L. W., Munn, J., Achterberg, W.,...de Vet, H. C. W. (2011). Measuring the quality of dying and quality of care when dying in long-term care settings: A qualitative content analysis of available instruments. *Journal of Pain and Symptom Management, 42*(6), 852–863.

Welch, L., Miller, S. C., Martin, E. W., & Nanda, A. (2008). Referral and timing of referral to Hospice care in nursing homes: The significant role of staff members. *Gerontologist*, *48*(4), 477–484.

Winn, P. A. S., & Dentivo, A. N. (2004). Quality palliative care in long-term care settings. *Journal of American Medical Directors Association*, *6*, S89–S98.

Zerzan, J., Stearns, S., & Hanson, L.C. (2000). Access to palliative care and hospice in nursing homes. *Journal of the American Medical Association*, *284*(19), 2489–2494.

Zimmerman, S. I, Gruber-Baldini, A.L., Sloane, P. D., Eckert, J. K., Hebel, J. R., Morgan, L. A....Konrad, T. R. (2003). Assisted living and nursing homes: Apples and oranges? *Gerontologist*, *43*(SI-II), 107–117.

Zimmerman, S., Love, K., Sloane, P. D., Cohen, L. W., Reed, D., Carder, P. C., and the CEAL-UNC Collaborative. (2011). Medication administration errors in assisted living: scope, characteristics, and the importance of staff training. *Journal of the American Geriatrics Society*, *59*, 1060–1068.

Zimmerman, S., Sloane, P. D., & Eckert, J. K. (Eds.) (2001). *Assisted living: Needs, practices and policies in residential care for the elderly*. Baltimore, MD: Johns Hopkins University Press.

Zimmerman, S., Sloane, P. D., Eckert, J. K., Gruber-Baldini, A. L., Morgan, L. A., Hebel, J. R.,...Chen, C. K. (2005). How good is assisted living? Findings and implications from an outcomes study. *Journals of Gerontology: Series B*, *60*(4), S195–204.

Zimmerman, S., Sloane, P. D., Hanson, L., Mitchell, C. M., & Shy, A. (2003). Staff perceptions of end-of-life care in long-term care. *Journal of the American Medical Directors Association*, *4*, 23–26.

Zimmerman, S., Munn, J., & Koenig, T. (2006) Assisted living settings. In B. Berkman (Ed.), *Handbook of social work in health and aging* (pp. 677–684). New York, NY: Oxford University Press.

CHAPTER 10

Cardiopulmonary Resuscitation in Hospice

Ethically Justified or an Oxymoron?

MURIEL R. GILLICK

Few topics have generated more discussion in the bioethics literature than the withdrawal or withholding of medical interventions, and no technology has stimulated more debate than cardiopulmonary resuscitation (CPR). Home hospices might have been expected to be immune to controversies about CPR since hospice care is focused on accepting imminent death and allowing it to occur without sophisticated technological interventions. But, in fact, hospice staff, ethicists, and agencies regulating hospice have all argued about the appropriateness of requiring that dying patients enrolled in hospice choose whether to accept CPR. Given that the philosophy of hospice is to promote comfort and dignity in patients near the end of life, is it ethical to even offer CPR to patients enrolled in hospice?

THE SPECIAL STATUS OF CARDIOPULMONARY RESUSCITATION

To understand why CPR might be considered an option within the hospice framework, it is useful to begin by examining why designating a patient do not resuscitate (DNR) or, to use the preferred term, do not attempt resuscitation (DNAR) continues to generate controversy. Closed chest massage was first reported to be successful in treating ventricular arrhythmias 50 years ago (Kouwenhoven, Jude, & Knickerbocker, 1960). Initially recommended as a means of responding to sudden, unexpected death, typically in the setting of an acute myocardial infarction, it quickly became routine practice for any patient whose heart stopped beating. This, in turn, led to the recognition that occasionally CPR should *not* be attempted, and the first DNR orders were written (Clinical Care Committee of the Massachusetts General Hospital, 1976; Rabkin, Gillerman, & Rice, 1976). But DNR orders were sometimes misused, instituted unilaterally by physicians without the consent or awareness of patients. After a scandal in New York State in which hospital staff surreptitiously labeled medical charts with purple dots to designate patients DNR, states began legislating the process by which patients could acquire a DNR status and hospitals began establishing their own DNR policies (McClung & Kamer, 1990).

Building on both legislative and hospital mandates, professional organizations such as the American Heart Association (AHA) developed advice for when the use of a DNAR order was ethically justified (AHA, 2005). Because of the inability to predict with absolute certainty whether a given patient will survive attempted CPR, the American Heart Association concluded in its most recent guidelines that "all pediatric and adult patients who suffer cardiac arrest in the hospital setting should have resuscitative attempts initiated unless the patient has a valid DNAR order or has objective signs of irreversible death (eg, dependent lividity)" (Morrison et al., 2010, p. S669). In short, attempting CPR for a patient whose heart has stopped is the default response.

The analogous British guidelines, jointly issued by the British Medical Association, the Resuscitation Council (UK), and the Royal College of Nursing, likewise establish CPR as the standard in the event of a cardiac arrest (British Medical Association, Resuscitation Council, & Royal College of Nursing, 2007). They recognize that "when a patient is in the final stages of an incurable illness and death is expected within a few days, CPR is very unlikely to be clinically successful" but stop short of recommending unilateral DNAR orders (British Medical Association et al., 2007, p. 8). Instead, the guidelines indicate that senior clinicians should explain the risks and benefits of CPR "in a sensitive way" (p. 10) but that "if patients still ask that no DNAR decision be made, this should usually be respected" (p. 13). Both case law and spokespersons of the major religious traditions have affirmed the right of competent, terminally ill patients to request a DNAR order (Burns, Edwards, Johnson, Cassem, & Truog, 2003).

Electing to forgo attempted resuscitation in the event of a cardiac arrest is imbued with special significance because an arrest is one of the only truly life-or-death clinical situations. Patients whose hearts have stopped and who are not breathing will die if no attempt is made to resuscitate them (although many will die even if the attempt is made). Patients who appear to be ventilator dependent, by contrast, may turn out to be able to breathe on their own, as was the case with Karen Ann Quinlan, who survived for 9 years after the New Jersey Supreme Court authorized withdrawal of respiratory support in the first widely publicized "right to die" case (Colby, 2006). Similarly, select patients with fever who are presumed to require antibiotics for survival sometimes do just as well (or just as poorly) regardless of whether they receive antibiotics, as was found in one study of individuals with advanced dementia (Fabiszewski, Volicer, & Volicer, 1990).

Some of the controversy surrounding CPR is related to persistent misunderstandings about what it entails and its likelihood of benefit: The lay public—and some physicians (La Puma, Silverstein, Stocking, Roland, & Siegler, 1998)—suffer from the erroneous belief that "DNR" means more than not instituting CPR, that it implies withholding of other potentially beneficial interventions. Physicians and patients also continue to widely overestimate the chance of successful CPR, due in no small measure to television dramas that show two thirds of patients who undergo CPR in the hospital living to be discharged home (Diem, Lantos, & Tulsky, 1996). The reality, however, is that fewer than one fifth of patients over age 65 who sustain an in-hospital cardiac arrest survive to discharge (Ehlenbach et al., 2009) and fewer than 8% survive after out-of-hospital CPR (Sasson, Rogers, Dahl, & Kellermann, 2010), statistics which have remained constant for decades.

IS CARDIOPULMONARY RESUSCITATION IN HOSPICE ANY DIFFERENT FROM CARDIOPULMONARY RESUSCITATION IN THE HOSPITAL?

In the hospice environment, the all-or-nothing character of CPR is just as stark as in the hospital or the nursing home. Despite the acceptance of death that is presumed to undergird a decision to enroll in a hospice program, agreement to a DNAR status entails an explicit acknowledgment that life-prolonging measures will be forgone. Hospice programs rightly emphasize all that they *will* provide (e.g., pain medication, oxygen, psychosocial support) but also need to acknowledge what they will *not* routinely provide (e.g., interventions such as hospitalization, chemotherapy, and CPR). In the hospice setting, where patients typically have a prognosis of 6 months or less, the likely outcome of attempted CPR is considerably lower than in the population as a whole.

While it is understandable that some patients with advanced illness might choose CPR, it is nonetheless somewhat surprising that *hospice* patients would request attempted CPR. After all, patients with advanced illness are not compelled to enroll in a hospice program. They do so because they have chosen comfort as their primary goal and are willing to forgo potentially life-prolonging therapy in the interest of comfort. Some argue that this is an unfair choice: Patients may well accept the inevitability of death, wish to focus on comfort, and embrace the home care services and intensive symptom management offered by hospice without wishing to forgo life-prolonging treatment such as antibiotics for infection or a blood transfusion for anemia. In fact, many patients who might benefit from hospice services decline them because they will have to forgo what they regard as beneficial palliative treatment (Fishman et al., 2009). Increasingly, "open access" hospice is available to patients whose overriding but not exclusive goal of care is comfort. However, open access hospice is intended to ensure that patients do not have to forgo beneficial palliative treatments such as radiation therapy or palliative chemotherapy; it is not intended to permit patients to have access to death-denying treatment as well (Wright & Katz, 2007). But for patients who do choose to enroll in conventional hospice, with both its advantages and its limitations, why is it ethically required for them to be able to choose CPR but not ethically required that they be able to choose surgery, chemotherapy, or hospital care?

AUTONOMY AND JUSTICE: THE CASE FOR THE RIGHT TO CHOOSE CARDIOPULMONARY RESUSCITATION IN HOSPICE

The principal argument for why hospice patients should be able to choose whether to undergo CPR is that it is essential in order to honor their autonomy (Fine & Jennings, 2003). A secondary concern is fairness—the belief that it would be discriminatory to fail to offer such a choice (Watson, Regnard, & Randall, 2009). The autonomy argument is that patients have the right to determine which medically justifiable treatments they will or will not undergo. From this perspective, they should be able to decide whether to have chemotherapy, radiation therapy, intensive care unit (ICU) care—or CPR. The discrimination argument is that offering CPR is part of accepted medical practice and failing to offer it in hospice would "result in confusion" by excluding hospice patients from "good practice," thereby creating poorer and therefore inequitable care.

The claims about autonomy assume that a patient's right to determine what is done to his or her body entails both a *negative* right to be free of

unwarranted intervention and a *positive* right to demand possibly beneficial treatment. The former was established as early as 1914 in the United
States when Justice Benjamin Cardozo ruled that a person "of adult years
and sound mind has a right to determine what should be done with his
own body," defining treatment instituted without a patient's consent as
assault (*Schloendorff v. Society of N.Y. Hospital*, 1914). A positive right, the
right to demand specific therapy (as distinct from the more general right
to medical care), is not generally accepted as having a firm basis in law or
ethics and is viewed by many as inconsistent with professional ethics (Brett
& McCullough, 1986).

Favoring the right to choose CPR based on a patient's right to
self-determination is predicated on CPR representing a meaningful choice.
Offering a patient an ineffective or harmful treatment is a false choice. If
CPR in the setting of the final stage of a terminal illness is not beneficial
(see the discussion of futility later in this chapter), then it should not be
available. Patients near the end of life have numerous choices to make—
about where they wish to die, whether they prefer full pain relief or mental lucidity, and whether they want simple, potentially life-prolonging
measures such as oral antibiotics, for example—without muddying the
decision-making waters by introducing treatment options that cannot
achieve their stated aims.

The autonomy argument for CPR in hospice also implies that the hospice benefit itself is ethically suspect, precisely because it does not "cover"
all possible medical treatments. Indeed, any insurance plan—and in the
United States the hospice *insurance benefit* is, practically speaking, intimately intertwined with all hospice *programs*—would similarly be potentially unethical. After all, every insurance plan places restrictions on what
services it will pay for. While some states have legislated a requirement
that particular types of treatment be covered—for example, chemothera-
peutic drugs that are listed in one of several compendia in some states and
infertility treatments in others—outside these limitations plans have the
freedom to design and market their own mix of services. Many patients
have little choice of health insurance plan—their only option is the plan
offered by their employer—but all insured patients who meet hospice's
clinical criteria have the option of either enrolling in hospice or continuing
with their existing plan. It is difficult to understand why restrictions on
what plans can cover are ethical but exclusion of CPR from hospice is not.

With respect to the claims about discrimination, the argument is that
if patients enrolled in hospice cannot have attempted CPR but similar
patients outside hospice can, then those in hospice programs are unfairly
discriminated against. Their care would be jeopardized, the argument

goes, because failure to include CPR in the package of services provided by hospice would lead to "confusion" among clinicians and substandard care (Watson et al., 2009). There is simply no evidence that the physicians and nurses who care for hospice patients provide poor care because their approach differs from that of mainstream medicine; on the contrary, there is ample evidence that allowing patients to enroll in hospice *and* to remain "full code" engenders confusion among clinicians. Clinicians caring for patients in a hospice understand that the patient has chosen to be treated outside the hospital and to forgo invasive treatments such as those typically provided in an ICU setting. But when they observe a patient's clinical status deteriorating—perhaps he is developing a rapid respiratory rate or his blood pressure is dropping or his heart rate is accelerating—"standard" treatment for someone who is willing to undergo CPR is to transfer the patient to the hospital in anticipation of an imminent cardiac arrest or to institute treatment intended to prevent a cardiac arrest. Caring for patients who simultaneously want attempted CPR but do not wish to be transferred to a hospital or undergo aggressive interventions creates confusion.

Insisting that clinicians provide treatment that they regard as inappropriate can also produce moral distress. In the intensive care setting, requiring experienced nurses to participate in aggressive procedures such as CPR for patients who are not expected to survive has resulted in depression, anxiety, and job dissatisfaction (Robichaux & Clark, 2006). Physicians likewise report that subjecting dying patients to CPR is inconsistent with the maxim to "do no harm" and hence most hospital DNAR policies allow physicians to transfer patients to other clinicians if they cannot resolve disputes about CPR.

REGULATORY REQUIREMENTS AND THE CARDIOPULMONARY RESUSCITATION DECISION

In both the United States and the United Kingdom, regulatory authorities appear to mandate that patients enrolling in hospice be allowed to decide on their code status. The Patient Self-Determination Act (PSDA), part of the Omnibus Budget Reconciliation Act of 1990, which requires all US health care institutions receiving federal funds to offer patients the opportunity to complete an advance directive but which prevents those institutions from requiring patients to complete an advance directive, has been interpreted as implying that hospices cannot require a specific advance directive—such as a DNAR status—as a prerequisite for admission. On April, 20, 2000, a memorandum from the Centers for Medicare and Medicaid Services (CMS), which oversees much of hospice care in the United States, further stated that hospices must provide CPR for enrolled patients who have a cardiac arrest and do not have a DNR order, though many hospices have inferred that calling 911 suffices to meet the CPR requirement. A 2001 response by the Ethics Committee of the National Hospice and Palliative Care Organization to CMS argued that the government's logic was flawed for a variety of reasons: A requirement to perform CPR is inappropriate because the primary function of hospices is to provide symptom management of a terminal illness and the insistence on hospices providing CPR fails to recognize both that CPR may be medically contraindicated and that it is not in fact mandated by the PSDA (Swiger, 2002).

The British guidelines on CPR also assert that all competent patients have a right to choose their code status and do not exempt hospice patients (British Medical Association et al., 2007). However, the guidelines include a proviso that "If the clinical team believes that CPR will not re-start the heart and maintain breathing, it should not be offered or attempted. CPR (which can cause harm in some situations) should not be attempted if it will not be successful" (p. 8). Likewise, the 2010 guidelines of the American Heart Association state that CPR is inappropriate when clinically futile, though the authors limit prospective determination of futility to patients who present with "objective signs of irreversible death (eg, decapitation, rigor mortis, or decomposition)" (Morrison et al., 2010, p. S666). Both sets of guidelines implicitly or explicitly acknowledge that CPR should not be attempted if it is futile to do so. Is CPR futile in hospice patients?

FUTILITY

As much ink has been spilled in the bioethics literature over the concept of futility as over CPR itself. The upshot of the futility debates is that futility is rejected by most ethicists as a basis for the withdrawal or withholding of treatment (Helft, Siegler, & Lantos, 2000). Invoking futility is typically a surrogate for disagreement about the goals of care, not a technical statement about the inherent uselessness of a medical intervention (Truog, Brett, & Frader, 1992). For example, in the paradigmatic case of Helga Wanglie, an elderly woman maintained on a ventilator while in a persistent vegetative state, the ventilator was held by her physicians to be futile because it could not return her to her prior state of independent functioning, whereas it was viewed by her husband as effective since it sustained her, albeit in a vegetative state (Capron, 1991). Despite the concerns expressed by ethicists about the futility label, physicians continue to invoke futility as a justification for refusing to administer a test or procedure and many hospitals have futility policies (Halevy & Brody, 1996). Some states, such as Texas, have a statutory approach to futility disagreements, although this typically entails delineating a process for dispute resolution rather than defining futility (Fine & Mayo, 2003). What is the evidence of efficacy of CPR in hospice patients?

The data on CPR in advanced illness suggest it very rarely works. A recent meta-analysis found that survival after CPR of patients with cancer was 9.5% in patients with local disease, 5.6% in patients with advanced disease, and 2.2% for cancer patients in the ICU, who may be clinically comparable to patients in the last 6 months of life (Reisfield et al., 2006). One study that specifically looked at patients with terminal cancer found no survivors among patients in whom progressive clinical deterioration preceded the cardiac arrest (Ewer, Kish, Martin, Price, & Feeley, 2001). There are similarly virtually no survivors of attempted CPR in nursing home residents, a population with advanced age and multiple comorbidities (Applebaum, King, & Finucane, 1990). But the prognosis is slightly more uncertain in patients with advanced organ failure such as heart or lung disease (Carew, Zhang, & Rea, 2007), where the end-of-life trajectory differs from that of patients with cancer or dementia, and who increasingly enroll in hospice near the end of life (Dy & Lynn, 2007). It is this lingering doubt, this small probability that the outcome of attempted CPR might be different in hospice patients with severe heart or lung disease, that motivates some commentators to suggest that CPR cannot be considered futile for all hospice patients.

As with other futility arguments, the real issue is the goals of care and not the statistics about the results of CPR (Council on Ethical and Judicial Affairs, 1999). Whether the likelihood of survival is less than 1% or less than 5%, it is surely very, very low: Even with automated external defibrillators, the overall success rate of out-of-hospital CPR remains 8% and that includes young people with an arrhythmia associated with an acute myocardial infarction who may be expected to respond well to defibrillation (Eisenberg & Psaty, 2010). Patients enrolled in hospice (or their families) who request CPR are fundamentally rejecting the hospice premise to "accept natural death" and are advocating instead the application of intensive technology in a last-ditch effort to stave off the inevitable.

SYMBOLIC VALUE OF CARDIOPULMONARY RESUSCITATION

CPR in hospice has an extremely low likelihood of preserving life; it is inconsistent with the basic hospice philosophy; and refusing to administer

CPR to hospice patients does not infringe on their autonomy as they can simply decline to enroll in hospice. Is there any role for CPR in hospice patients? Clearly, for some patients, a DNAR status is of great symbolic significance. They wish to accept hospice for the services it offers, but they feel that explicitly agreeing to forgo resuscitation constitutes deprivation. This perception is reinforced when hospice personnel, whom the patient has typically just met at the time of hospice enrollment, appear to be badgering them to accept a DNAR status. The essence of the problem is lack of trust between the clinicians and the patient (Henderson, Fins, & Moskowitz, 1998). While building a trusting relationship with the patient might ultimately lead to acceptance of a DNAR status, it may be best to accept the emotional importance of remaining "full code" initially, provided that it does not signal a more general desire for ongoing life-prolonging treatment (Gillick, 2009). Other medical therapies are also widely administered for symbolic reasons, such as artificial nutrition in patients with advanced Alzheimer's disease, even when there is no scientific evidence that such treatment prolongs life or prevents problems such as aspiration, pneumonia, or pressure ulcers (Gillick & Volandes, 2008).

In some cases, it is the family for whom CPR serves an important symbolic role. Family members may feel that when the end finally comes, they will be their loved one's executioners if they do not authorize one final attempt to intervene. Family members often serve as surrogate decision makers for incompetent patients near the end of life; moreover, hospice, unlike most contemporary Western medical institutions, regards the family as the unit of care. While it may seem to undermine individual patient autonomy to perform CPR for the benefit of the family (Yarborough, 1988), in fact patients not uncommonly take their family's needs and wishes into consideration in their personal decision making. Just as patients frequently reject life-prolonging treatment because they do not wish to be a burden to their families (Singer, Martin, & Keiner, 1999), they may opt for possibly life-prolonging treatment to satisfy their families. In some ethnic groups, patients routinely defer decision making to the family, commonly the eldest son (Blackhall, Murphy, Frank, Michel, & Azen, 1995). As long as a choice to accept symbolic CPR at the end of life does not impose undue suffering on the patient—and while unsuccessful CPR is not a dignified way to die it is typically painless because the patient is unconscious during the procedure—it is an ethically acceptable option.

In other cases, cultural values drive the wish to pursue CPR. There is widespread evidence that African Americans, Latinos, and Chinese Americans tend to favor aggressive care near the end of life to a greater extent than White Americans and are less inclined to accept hospice care

(Greiner, Perera, & Ahluwalia, 2003). Explanations for the observed differences in preference abound. It may be due to distrust of the medical establishment, particularly in the African American community, in the setting of a long history of discrimination and mistreatment (Crawley et al., 2000). It may be due to limited health literacy rather than to race or ethnicity, as was found in one study of the role of video in helping patients determine their preferences for medical care in the event they developed advanced dementia: Significant differences in preferences between Black and White patients were noted when the subjects were presented with a verbal description of dementia, but after watching a video illustrating the characteristics of advanced dementia, racial differences in preferences vanished (Volandes et al., 2008). The wish for aggressive treatment near the end of life in some ethnic groups may be due to a belief that agreeing to forgo an intervention constitutes "giving up" and itself can precipitate death (Kagawa-Singer & Blackhall, 2001). Alternatively, the request for attempted CPR by terminally ill patients may reflect a lack of understanding of the severity of their illness or of the risks and benefits of the proposed treatments. One study of community-dwelling elders, for example, found that the majority said they would want CPR, but almost all changed their minds when they learned the true outcomes of the procedure (Murphy et al., 1994). If the wish for CPR is based on cultural values rather than a misunderstanding of the facts, then it should be respected. If, however, the factors motivating the interest in CPR also lead to a rejection of the hospice philosophy—and there is compelling evidence that the same patients who wish to remain "full code" also reject hospice care at the end of life—then the patient should not enroll in a hospice program.

TRANSLATING ETHICS INTO POLICY

From a policy perspective, how can hospices balance the competing concerns that affect their decision about whether to offer CPR to enrolled patients and, if they do offer it, how should they implement a "full code" status in practice? The first step is to ensure that the enrollment process allows the hospice clinicians to ascertain whether the patient and family buy into the hospice philosophy. Only if they accept the goal of providing management of symptoms and psychosocial support within the home or hospice facility should patients sign onto hospice.

Once patients opt for what hospice offers—nursing care, personal care, medications, and assistive devices needed to care for a person with a hospice diagnosis, as well as social work and chaplaincy assistance—and agree to accept these services in lieu of conventional technological medical care, they should be given a variety of enrollment materials. These typically include a medication "kit," which has emergency supplies of medications often needed for symptom control, and a special telephone number to contact hospice 24/7, as well as informational brochures about advanced illness. To these standard materials should be added an out-of-hospital DNR form, with the explanation that the medications, the contact number, and the form are all *recommended* but none are *required*. This approach conceptually switches the default from assuming that all patients want CPR attempted unless otherwise stated to assuming that hospice patients will not want CPR attempted, but it does require that they complete a DNAR form to verify their choice. Hospices should further clarify that patients who do not sign the out-of-hospital DNAR form should contact emergency personnel in the event of a cardiac arrest and that hospice providers who witness an arrest would likewise call emergency medical technicians rather than initiating CPR themselves.

A limitation of this proposal is that it expects patients to actively agree to a DNAR status. The behavioral psychology literature has repeatedly demonstrated that individuals behave in ways contrary to their own self-interest when they have to take concrete steps to actively accept rather than to reject an option (Thaler & Sunstein, 2008). However, in the event the patient is transferred to another facility, the hospice's DNAR default will not be accepted by that institution unless a standard out-of-hospital DNR form has been completed. Until such time as the surrounding community accepts a "default DNAR" from area hospices, it is probably best to protect patients by asking them to complete the usual form.

The idea of a default DNAR status for terminally ill patients generally, not just those enrolled in hospice, has been around since the creation of the first DNR orders. Ethicists and clinicians have struggled with whether it is appropriate to raise the issue of CPR with terminally ill patients— whether or not they are enrolled in a hospice program. A provocative editorial in the *New England Journal of Medicine* in 1987 posed the question, "Must we always use CPR?" (Blackhall, 1987). The National Council for Hospice and Specialist Palliative Care Services and the Association for Palliative Medicine of Great Britain and Ireland stated in 2002: "We reaffirm that there is no ethical obligation to discuss CPR with those palliative care patients, for whom such treatment, following assessment, is judged to be futile" (National Council for Hospice and Specialist Palliative Care Services & Association for Palliative Medicine, 2002, p. 280). The British have made the additional argument that it is a human right to be free of "inhuman or degrading treatment," which usually refers to torture but which they also apply to CPR instituted in a dying patient (Manisty & Waxman, 2003). Default DNAR has been introduced in some nursing homes (Gordon, 2003) and has been advocated for patients with advanced dementia (Volandes & Ebbo, 2007).

If it becomes acceptable for physicians to make unilateral DNAR decisions for terminally ill patients, and if such decisions are recognized by all medical facilities, then it will no longer be necessary to separately consider the issue of CPR in hospice. Until then, a strategy of recommending but not requiring a DNAR status—and facilitating this approach by providing out-of-hospital DNAR forms for patients on admission to hospice—may be the best way to balance autonomy and beneficence.

REFERENCES

American Heart Association. (2005). Guidelines for cardiopulmonary resuscitation and emergency cardiovascular care. Part 2: Ethical issues. *Circulation, 112*, 6–11.

Applebaum, G. E., King, J. E., & Finucane, T. E. (1990). The outcomes of CPR initiated in nursing homes. *Journal of the American Geriatrics Society, 38*, 197–200.

Blackhall, L. J. (1987). Must we always use CPR? *New England Journal of Medicine, 317*, 1281–1285.

Blackhall, L. J., Murphy, S. T., Frank, G., Michel, V., & Azen S. (1995). Ethnicity and attitudes toward patient autonomy. *Journal of the American Medical Association, 274*, 820–825.

Brett, A. S., & McCullough, L. B. (1986). When patients request specific interventions: defining the limits of the physician's obligation. *New England Journal of Medicine, 315*, 1347–1351.

British Medical Association, Resuscitation Council, & Royal College of Nursing (2007). *Decisions relating to cardiopulmonary resuscitation*. Retrieved April 2014, from http://bma.org.uk/-/media/Files/PDFs/Practical%20advice%20at%20work/Ethics/DecisionsRelatingResusReport.pdf.

Burns, J. P., Edwards, J., Johnson, J., Cassem, N. H., & Truog, R. D. (2003). Do-not-resuscitate order after 25 years. *Critical Care Medicine, 31*, 1543–1550.

Capron, A. (1991). In re Helga Wanglie. *Hastings Center Report, 21*, 26–28.

Carew, H. T., Zhang, W., & Rea, T. D. (2007). Chronic health conditions and survival after out-of-hospital ventricular fibrillatory cardiac arrest. *Heart, 93*, 728–731.

Clinical Care Committee of the Massachusetts General Hospital. (1976). Optimum care for hopelessly ill patients: A report of the Clinical Care Committee of the Massachusetts General Hospital. *New England Journal of Medicine, 295*, 362–364.

Colby, W. (2006). *Unplugged: reclaiming our right to die in America*. New York, NY: AMACOM.

Council on Ethical and Judicial Affairs. (1999). Medical futility in end-of-life care: report of the Council on Ethical and Judicial Affairs. *Journal of the American Medical Association, 281*, 937–941.

Crawley, L., Payne, R., Bolden, J., Payne, T., Washington, P., & William, S. (2000). Palliative and end-of-life care in the African American community. *Journal of the American Medical Association, 284*, 2518–2521.

Diem, S. J., Lantos, J. D., & Tulsky, J.A. (1996). Cardiopulmonary resuscitation on television: Miracles and misinformation. *New England Journal of Medicine, 334,* 1578–1582.

Dy, S., & Lynn, J. (2007). Getting services right for those sick enough to die. *British Medical Journal, 334,* 511–513.

Ehlenbach, W. J., Barnato, A. A., Curtis, J. R., Kreuter, W., Koepsell, T. D., Deyo, R. A., & Stapleton, R. D. (2009). Epidemiologic study of in-hospital cardiopulmonary resuscitation in the elderly. *New England Journal of Medicine, 361,* 22–31.

Eisenberg, M., & Psaty, B. M. (2010). Cardiopulmonary resuscitation: Celebration and challenges. *Journal of the American Medical Association, 304,* 87–88.

Ewer, M. S., Kish, S. K., Martin, C. G., Price, K. J., & Feeley, T. W. (2001). Characteristics of cardiac arrest in cancer patients as a predictor of survival after cardiopulmonary resuscitation. *Cancer, 92,* 1905–1912.

Fabiszewski, K. J., Volicer, B., & Volicer, L. (1990). Effect of antibiotic treatment on outcome of fevers treated in institutionalized Alzheimer patients. *Journal of the American Medical Association, 263,* 3168–3172.

Fine, P. G., & Jennings, B. (2003). CPR in hospice. *Hastings Center Report, 33,* 9–10.

Fine, R. L., & Mayo, T. W. (2003). Resolution of futility by due process: Early experience with the Texas Advance Directives Act. *Annals of Internal Medicine, 138,* 743–746.

Fishman, J., O'Dwyer, P., Lu, H. L., Henderson, H., Asch, D. A., & Casarett, D. J. (2009). Race, treatment preferences, and hospice enrollment: Eligibility criteria may exclude patients with the greatest needs for care. *Cancer, 115,* 689–697.

Gillick, M. R. (2009). Decision making near life's end: A prescription for change. *Journal of Palliative Medicine, 12,* 121–125.

Gillick, M. R., & Volandes, A. E. (2008). The standard of caring: Why do we still use feeding tubes in patients with advanced dementia? *Journal of the American Medical Directors Association, 9,* 364–367.

Gordon, M. (2003). CPR in long-term care: Mythical benefit or necessary ritual? *Annals of Long-Term Care: Clinical Care and Aging, 11,* 41–49.

Greiner, K. A., Perera, S., & Ahluwalia, J. S. (2003). Hospice usage by minorities in the last year of life: Results from the National Mortality Followback Survey. *Journal of the American Geriatrics Society, 51,* 970–978.

Halevy, A., & Brody, B. A. (1996). A multi-institutional collaborative policy on medical futility. *Journal of the American Medical Association, 276,* 571–574.

Helft, P. R., Siegler, M., & Lantos, J. (2000). The rise and fall of the futility movement. *New England Journal of Medicine, 343,* 293–296.

Henderson, S., Fins, J. J., & Moskowitz, E. H. (1998). Resuscitation in hospice. *Hastings Center Report, 28,* 20–22.

Kagawa-Singer, M., & Blackhall, L. J. (2001). Negotiating cross-cultural issues at the end of life. "You got to go where he lives." *Journal of the American Medical Association, 286,* 2993–3001.

Kouwenhoven, W.B., Jude, J. R., & Knickerbocker, G. G. (1960). Closed-chest cardiac massage. *Journal of the American Medical Association, 173,*1064–1067.

La Puma, J., Silverstein, M. D., Stocking, C. B., Roland, D., & Siegler, M. (1998). Life-sustaining treatment: A prospective study of patients with DNR orders in a teaching hospital. *Archives of Internal Medicine, 148,* 2193–2198.

Manisty, C., & Waxman, J. (2003). Doctors should not discuss resuscitation with terminally ill patients. *British Medical Journal, 327,* 614–615.

McClung, J. A., & Kamer, R. S. (1990). Implications of New York's do-not-resuscitate law. *New England Journal of Medicine, 323,* 270–272.

Morrison, L. J., Kierzek, G., Diekema, D. S., Sayre, M. R., Silvers, S. M., Idris, A. H., & Mancini, M. E. (2010). 2010 American Heart Association guidelines for cardiopulmonary resuscitation and emergency cardiovascular care. Part 3: Ethics. *Circulation, 122*, S665–S675.

Murphy, D. J., Burrows, D., Santilli, S., Kemp, A. W., Tenner, J., Kreling, B., & Teno, J. (1994). The influence of the probability of survival on patients' preferences regarding cardiopulmonary resuscitation. *New England Journal of Medicine, 330*, 545–540.

National Council for Hospice and Specialist Palliative Care Services and Association for Palliative Medicine. (2002). Ethical decision making in palliative care: Cardiopulmonary resuscitation for people who are terminally ill. *Journal of the Royal College of Physicians of Edinburgh, 32*, 280.

Omnibus Budget Reconciliation Act of 1990, Public L. No. 101-508, §4751, 104 Stat. 1388–204 (1990).

Rabkin, M. T., Gillerman, G., & Rice, N. R. (1976). Orders not to resuscitate. *New England Journal of Medicine, 295*, 364–366.

Reisfield, G. M., Wallace, S. K., Munsell, M. F., Webb, F. J., Alvarez, E. R., & Wilson, G. R. (2006). Survival in cancer patients undergoing in-hospital cardiopulmonary resuscitation: A meta-analysis. *Resuscitation, 71*, 152–160.

Robichaux, C., & Clark, A. P. (2006). Practice of expert critical care nurses in situations of prognostic conflict at end of life. *American Journal of Critical Care, 15*, 480–491.

Sasson, C., Rogers, M. A., Dahl, J., & Kellermann, A. L. (2010). Predictors of survival from out-of-hospital cardiac arrest. A systematic review and meta-analysis. *Circulation: Cardiovascular Quality and Outcomes, 3*, 63–81.

Schloendorff v. Society of N.Y. Hospital, 211 N.Y. 125, 105 N.E. 92 (1914).

Singer, P. A., Martin, D. K., & Keiner, M (1999). Quality end-of-life care: Patients' perspectives. *Journal of the American Medical Association, 261*, 163–168.

Swiger, H. (2002). *Hospice care and the institutional barriers to its success.* A paper commissioned by the National Hospice and Palliative Care Organization's Public Policy Committee. Alexandria, VA: National Hospice and Palliative Care Organization.

Thaler, R. S., & Sunstein, C. R. (2008). *Nudge: Improving decisions about health, wealth, and happiness.* New Haven, CT: Yale University Press.

Truog, R. D., Brett, A. S., & Frader, J. (1992). The problem with futility. *New England Journal of Medicine, 326*, 1560–1564.

Volandes, A. E., & Ebbo, E. D. (2007). Flipping the default: A novel approach to cardiopulmonary resuscitation in end-stage dementia. *Journal of Clinical Ethics, 18*, 122–139.

Volandes, A. E., Paasche-Orloff, M., Gillick, M. R., Cook, E. F., Shaykevich, S., Abbo, E. D., & Lehmann, L. (2008). Health literacy not race predicts end-of-life care preferences. *Journal of Palliative Medicine, 11*, 754–762.

Watson, M., Regnard, C., & Randall, F. (2009). Should hospices be exempt from following national CPR guidelines? *British Medical Journal, 338*, 1176–1177.

Wright, A. A., & Katz, I. T. (2007). Letting go of the rope: Aggressive treatment, hospice care, and open access. *New England Journal of Medicine, 317*, 324–327.

Yarborough, M. (1988). Continued treatment of the fatally ill for the benefit of others. *Journal of the American Geriatrics Society, 36*, 63–67.

CHAPTER 11

Moral Meanings of Physician-Assisted Death for Hospice Ethics

COURTNEY S. CAMPBELL

The voluminous literature in biomedical ethics on physician-assisted death has presumed there are primarily only two parties with significant interests, the physician and the patient, and has neglected the contexts of end-of-life caregiving, including hospice care. This is a very problematic oversight, since in states such as Oregon and Washington, where physician-assisted death is not a philosophical abstraction but a legalized caregiving reality, the vast majority of terminally ill patients who seek to use the method of physician-assisted death to end their life are hospice patients. According to the Oregon Department of Human Services (ODHS), 90.1% of terminally ill patients who have used the state's precedent-setting "Death With Dignity" law to end their life with a physician's prescription from 1998 through 2013 have been enrolled in hospice care (Oregon Public Health Division, 2014). The statutes in Oregon and Washington are virtually verbatim. The corresponding figure for Washington State for 2009–2012 is 84.6% (Washington State Department of Health, 2012, 2013). The role of hospice in patient decisions about physician-assisted death can present difficult and defining ethical questions for hospice programs and their staff, as illustrated in the following examples.

Vignette 1

A terminally ill patient enrolls in hospice care, and after discussion with her care-givers and attending physician, makes a request for a prescription to end her life in accord with the Oregon Death With Dignity Act. The patient is informed that the hospice respects the patient's legal right to pursue the process to obtain a medication from her physician, and that regardless, the hospice will continue to provide customary hospice care. However, as stipulated by the hospice's policy on involvement with patient requests for a medication to end life, the hospice will not have a staff person or nurse in attendance when the patient takes the medication. The patient understands this, and then informs the hospice team not to inform her family members of her intent to use the Death With Dignity process, as is the patient's right under the law. The patient is divorced from her husband, who has strong religious commitments, and believes that disclosure of her request to family members would generate substantial disruption in an already difficult family situation.

The patient receives a prescription for the medication, obtains it, and takes the medication attended by persons from the patient rights advocacy organization, Compassion & Choices, and dies without any complications. Following customary practice, Compassion & Choices then contacts the hospice program requesting a hospice staff member to provide confirmation of death, and a hospice nurse arrives at the home shortly thereafter to confirm death.

Soon after the hospice nurse arrives, the patient's daughter comes to visit her mother and is aghast to find her mother deceased. The daughter feels betrayed by the hospice and questions the nurse, asking "Why didn't you tell us about this?" The nurse confides to her staff supervisor that she experienced moral distress over this circumstance and felt that she had deceived the family and the daughter.

Vignette 2

A hospice nurse developed a professionally meaningful caring relationship with a cancer patient and his family over 3 months. The nurse is aware that her patient has requested a prescription from his attending physician to end his life as permitted by Oregon's law. As this prospect approaches, the patient asks the nurse whether she will be present when the patient takes the medication (the law requires the patient to self-administer the medication).

The nurse has a professional but deep commitment to this patient, and she has expressed how meaningful it has been to be a "companion on the journey" of her patient. In considering the patient's request for her presence, however, the nurse is cognizant of the written policy of her hospice program, which affirms the right of hospice patients to choose any legal end-of-life option, but prohibits any hospice staff or volunteer from attending the dying of a patient using the Death With Dignity law. This prohibition encompasses not only attending the dying of the patient at the time of self-administration of the medication but also the duration between self-administration and the time of patient death.

The nurse is conscientiously committed to the purposes of hospice care and views hospice nursing as her "calling" or vocation. However, the request of her patient generates moral conflict for her regarding fulfilling responsibilities of devoted patient care, nonabandonment of patients, and fidelity to her hospice program and its policies. The nurse determines she will attend the patient's use of the medication "as a friend, not as a nurse."

The comparatively recent legalization of physician-assisted death (or "death with dignity") statutes in Oregon (Oregon Revised Statute, 1994) and Washington (Revised Code of Washington, 2008) has generated a set of ethical questions and decisions for hospice programs and their staff as to whether they will participate in the physician-assisted death process and to what extent they will incorporate physician-assisted death within the services provided by hospice caregiving (Campbell, Hare, & Matthews, 1995). Hospice programs in Vermont now face similar questions and decisions (Vermont Statutes Annotated, 2013). These questions have also been considered by national organizations such as the National Hospice and Palliative Care Organization (NHPCO, 2005), the Hospice and Palliative Nurses Association (HPNA, 2011), and the American Academy of Hospice and Palliative Medicine (AAHPM, 2007) and anticipated by hospice programs in diverse areas of the country where physician-assisted death is yet to be formally legalized (e.g., Colorado, Montana, Massachusetts).

This chapter seeks to identify and analyze some of the ethical questions inevitably encountered by hospice programs and their staff in the context of the trend toward greater social acceptance of legalized physician-assisted death as an option in end-of-life caregiving. Insofar as these questions are faced by hospice staff as professionals caring for specific patients, as illustrated in the preceding vignettes, as well as by hospice programs and organizations in the formulation of policy or practical caregiving directives, the chapter also seeks to examine alternative positions hospice programs could assume toward legalized physician-assisted death. An important aspect of this discussion is a call for hospice programs to make use of the moral resources embedded in the traditions of the philosophy of hospice care (NHPCO, 2000; Stoddard, 1992). The chapter will use as an initial point of departure a brief overview of a study recently conducted by the author regarding the extent of participation by Oregon hospice programs in that state's existing "Death With Dignity" statute.

The Oregon Death With Dignity Act was passed by a citizen referendum in 1994 and became legally effective in October 1997. In its basic feature, it allows terminally ill patients to request of their attending physician a prescription for "medication for the purpose of ending [the patient's] life in a humane and dignified manner" (Oregon Revised Statute ch. 127.805, §2.01, 1994). The legal statute itself makes no mention of hospice care, other than stating that patients must be informed by their attending physician of hospice as a "feasible alternative" to a request for life-ending medication (ch. 127.815, §3.01). Nonetheless, for a variety of reasons—including the high quality of hospice care, the near statewide access to hospice programs, and the endorsement of influential patient advocacy organizations such as Compassion & Choices of Oregon—hospice care has evolved, at least in states where assisted death is now legal, from being situated as an "alternative" to physician-assisted death to being perceived as a comprehensive program of end-of-life care whose philosophy is fundamentally consistent with the aspirations for dying and death of terminally ill patients who may be contemplating requesting a life-ending medication.

This perspective of compatibility between hospice and physician-assisted death is espoused by the Oregon Hospice Association (OHA), which emphasizes that "dying Oregonians need not choose *between* hospice and physician aid-in-dying" (OHA, 2009); that is, the OHA contends that the idea of hospice as a "feasible alternative" as presented in the statute or public discourse is a false "either-or" choice when the practical reality is "both-and": both quality hospice care and the option for physician-assisted death. The OHA takes an advocacy position in "support of patient choice" and affirms that individual hospice programs "should never deny a person its services because he or she has asked a doctor for a prescription, even when the hospice intends to exercise its right to not be involved."

In 2009–2010, the author and a research assistant conducted a study (Campbell & Cox, 2010) of all in-state member hospices of the Oregon Hospice Association (with the exception of hospices associated with correctional facilities) to assess the involvement of individual hospices in the Oregon statute. They also sought to determine whether the hospice programs represented a concept of hospice care as an alternative to physician-assisted death, a concept of compatibility of hospice with physician-assisted death, or reflected some different perspective or even hybrid approach. The study was assessed as exempt following review by the institutional review board chair. We contacted 65 OHA-affiliated hospice programs and requested policy statements, program guidelines, and staff education materials developed by these programs to address patient inquiries about the Oregon Death With Dignity Act. Documents representing policies or educational materials were received from 56 of the 65 Oregon hospice programs. We supplemented these materials with visits to two hospice programs, whose staff members provided experientially informed critiques of our analyses.

In general, this study disclosed a very rich diversity of positions, policies, and practices on physician-assisted death among Oregon hospice programs. This diversity indicated that portraying hospice care only in terms of an "either-or" alternative to physician-assisted death or a "both-and" complementarity is simply conceptually inadequate. While Oregon hospice programs generally understand themselves to assume a minor role in the decision-making processes of patients who exercise their legal rights under Oregon law, nevertheless, virtually all hospice programs set limits to their participation and the participation of staff members. These boundaries stem from ethical values and commitments that the individual hospices take to be at the core of the hospice philosophy of care. The permissions, restrictions, and value rationales invoked in these policy statements thus provide insight on diverse interpretations of the identity and meaning of "hospice" as a distinctive mode of caregiving. Since these values and commitments provide a context for the approach of Oregon hospices to the ethical questions embedded in hospice participation in physician-assisted death, I wish here to present a compressed overview and commentary on findings in the study relevant to hospice ethics.

Concepts of Participation

It is important to offer at the outset two framing concepts. First, the question of hospice participation in the Oregon law is an *ethical* question for Oregon hospices because the law itself is essentially silent on hospice involvement. Moreover, one provision of the statute (Oregon Revised Statute ch. 127.885, §4.01, 1994) states there is "no legal requirement to participate" in the law on the part of any health care provider or facility. Thus, the decisions of hospice programs about participation, as reflected in their policy statements, can integrate core hospice values and mission, rather than be exclusively driven by concerns with legal compliance.[1]

Secondly, hospice documents invite ambiguity on the question of what is meant by "participation" by a hospice program. On my analysis, for some hospices, participation (or nonparticipation) can refer to *facilitating the process* delineated by the statute for a patient to receive life-ending medication. At a minimum, this could involve hospice programs in such practices as providing information about the law to a patient, distributing brochures about the law prepared by patient rights organizations (Compassion & Choices of Oregon has distributed brochures about their organization to many Oregon hospices requesting they be given to hospice patients who make an inquiry about physician-assisted death), engaging the patient in conversation about his or her interest or desires, and referral or notification of the patient to his or her attending physician or to a patient advocacy organization. These illustrations, as well as other practices, enable hospice programs to encourage informed decision making by patients or collaboration with the medical community. This involvement in the procedural aspects of the law can be considered a *broad* conception of participation.

For other hospice programs, participation may be understood in a *narrow* sense to refer to the *act* in which the patient ingests the prescribed medication. While by law self-administration of the medication by the patient is required, hospice involvement in the action, as distinguished from the process, might encompass staff procurement or preparation of the medication so that it can be consumed, or staff presence or being a witness to the patient's death, or needs for patient care in the event of medical complications from the medication, a contingency not addressed by the law but that has been reported by the state in 5% of Oregon's cases. "Participation" may thus have a broader or narrower meaning, and some of the moral divergence revealed by the study of Oregon hospices reflects these different understandings of participation.

These moral and policy issues are most directly addressed by the documents of Oregon hospice programs in statements of program policy that affirm a position on physician-assisted death or the Oregon law. The study disclosed eight different positions or policy formulations of Oregon hospices on participation in the Oregon Death With Dignity Act, though for purposes of summation, I will compress these eight formulations into three broad categories.

1. A first position, which I designate as a model of "nonparticipation," was illustrated in the policy documents by phrasing that X hospice "would not cooperate" with or was "opposed" to the law, or that quality hospice care made such a law "unnecessary," or simply that X hospice, as permitted by the law, "does not participate." The affirmation of nonparticipation essentially reflects a model that hospice care is not only a "feasible" but a morally preferable alternative to physician-assisted death. These hospices ($n = 20$, or 36%) use the statutory permission to not participate

in facilitating either the process or the act, and generally express confidence that quality hospice caregiving, including palliation and symptom management, will resolve the underlying concerns or fears (i.e., uncontrolled pain, anxiety about dying) that are held to be the rationale for a patient to make a request for life-ending medication. It is also worthy of mention that several nonparticipating hospices, though not a majority, have an affiliation with a religious tradition and thus may rely on specific religious values or moral teachings, in addition to the tradition of hospice values they may invoke.

2. A second broad cluster of hospices reflect what may be designated as "qualified participation," a model identified in the documents by phrasing that X hospice does not "actively" or does not "directly" participate in the Oregon law. These hospices (n = 16, or 29%) tended to reflect the distinction between broad and narrow senses of participation explicated earlier; that is, they understand participation in the educational aspects of the process preceding the act of ingestion to be permissible in hospice care, whereas a boundary is drawn with respect to involvement in those practices pertaining to the patient's action, which comprise "active" or "direct" participation. To be sure, the cluster of hospices in this model of qualified participation manifest differences regarding the extent of process participation as well, but these practices are developed through extensive caregiving guidelines for staff members, rather than being included as part of the policy or position statement itself. There is no claim in the statements of these hospice programs that quality hospice care is the panacea for every patient who expresses interest in life-ending medication or that hospice care is intrinsically incompatible with or a morally preferable alternative to physician-assisted death. Nonetheless, these hospices do place limits to programmatic and staff involvement, including, in almost all cases, restrictions on staff presence when medication is ingested.

3. A third set of hospices, which can be designated as "respectful participation," reflect a model of participation by hospice programs that "follow the provisions of the statute" or law. The concept of "respect" here has two foci: hospices respect and rely on the state to regulate the practice, including oversight of the physician–patient relationship; at the same time, these hospices also affirm support for the regulatory rationale of the law, namely, "respect for patient self-determination," including patient choice about the method of bringing life to an end. This cluster of hospices (n = 19, or 34%) are closest to the perspective reflected by the Oregon Hospice Association that hospice philosophy and care can be compatible with physician-assisted death, although arguments

can be made in the model of respectful participation that a patient's choice for physician-assisted death *ethically* should not be a first resort and may even be a last resort, and not, as implied by the law, one resort among many at the end of life (Quill, 2008). The respectful participatory model draws on hospice values to warrant the broad sense of procedural participation, but it recognizes that the law's stipulation of patient self-administration of the medication sets a limit on hospice assistance with medication distribution and the act of ingestion. Nonetheless, the majority of these hospices do accommodate narrow participation by permitting hospice staff to be present for the patient or the patient's family upon request or invitation and some (though not all) devote attention to staff member's responsibilities for patient care in the event of complications.

Values in Language and Policy

At stake for hospice ethics, of course, is not only the model of hospice participation, that is, the statement of program policy, but also the values that inform the reasoning that leads to these three broad positions. However, prior to a discussion of hospice values, it is important to address a premoral consideration, a consideration that needs some resolution for a moral discussion to occur: The study disclosed that the diversity in policies and practices among the Oregon hospices extends to, and is likely shaped by, differences over what to call the set of actions by which a terminally ill patient enrolled in hospice care makes a request of a physician for life-ending medication that is subsequently self-administered by the patient. As noted earlier, the statutory title for this process is designated as "death with dignity" by state law, and this language is used by 25% (n = 14) of the Oregon hospice programs. However, the most common designation, used by 52% (n = 29) of the hospices, is that of "physician-assisted suicide," which is the phrasing adopted by the National Hospice and Palliative Care Organization. The remaining 23% (n = 13) use the language of "physician-assisted death" adopted by the American Academy of Hospice and Palliative Medicine. Strikingly, no hospice program uses the language of "physician aid-in-dying" adopted by the state hospice association or by the patient rights organization Compassion & Choices.

The implications of this linguistic diversity for hospice ethics are evident. If hospice programs frame their prospective involvement as a form of participation in some fashion in a patient's suicide, then incorporating the practice into hospice care is likely to encounter an exceedingly high bar of justification, because hospice from its modern historical origins has sought to provide the kind of quality end-of-life care that at the very least would diminish prospects of a patient's suicide (Saunders, 1991–92). Participation, even in the broad sense, could seem to make a hospice program morally complicit in an action that hospice has long sought to prevent and that tends to be interpreted in hospice discourse as a "failure" of hospice care. It is perhaps no surprise then that all of the Oregon hospice programs whose policy documents use the language of "physician-assisted suicide" to refer to the legalized actions in question state their policy position in terms of "opposition," "noncooperation," or "nonparticipation." And conversely, the hospice programs whose documents use the languages of "physician-assisted death" or "death with dignity" are more inclined to hold a policy position that reflects qualified or respectful participation and generally affirm respect for patient choices and the relationship of physician and patient.

The diversity of hospice languages clearly mirrors the conceptual diversity within national organizations, biomedical ethics, and in public discourse generally; that is, this phenomenon is not unique to the hospice context. Nevertheless, one central task for hospice ethics is conceptual clarification and movement toward consensus on terminology. It is important for hospice ethics to not have the ethical issue decided in advance through the selected phrasing of important concepts. Physician-assisted "suicide" clearly implies a morally negative evaluation of an action that is understood as discontinuous with the tradition and philosophy of hospice care. Physician "aid-in-dying" suggests there is no moral issue to confront, or at least any moral issue distinctive to the patient's request, and that the act is compatible with hospice philosophy and tradition, whereas language affirming "death with dignity," while consistent with the phrasing of the legal statute and more politically palatable (Jones, 2007), presents a positive moral evaluation, and for some, even entails a moral obligation. The language of "physician-assisted death," by contrast, seems to leave the ethical question open, allowing for discussion and rational argumentation to be presented without linguistic prejudgment. The American Academy of Hospice and Palliative Medicine contends it adopted the language of "physician-assisted death" in its policy statement based on "the belief that it captures the essence of the process in a more accurately descriptive fashion than the more emotionally charged designation physician-assisted suicide" (AAHPM, 2007). While this is not the place to make the argument, it seems that hospice ethics would do better to begin its discourse on this question using the language of "physician-assisted death"; this phrasing will be used throughout this chapter.

The diversity of programmatic positions and conceptual phrasing notwithstanding, the policies of Oregon hospices on physician-assisted death generally manifest fidelity to a core set of values held to represent commitments in the hospice philosophy of care. These commitments include (1) the philosophy that death is a natural continuation of the human life span, (2) that each dying patient manifests a fundamental dignity to be affirmed, (3) that hospice care aims to promote the quality of a patient's remaining life through the highest level of caring practices, (4) that the family is recognized as integral to quality patient care, and (5) that embedded in these practices is a distinctive devotion to symptom and pain management and bereavement care (Byock, 1998). In turn, these core values can provide justification for more specific ethical responsibilities of particular relevance to how hospice programs respond to laws or requests from patients regarding life-ending medication. In descending order of frequency, the Oregon hospice policies make explicit reference to the following ethical responsibilities in at least 50% of the policy documents:

- Respect for the patient's right to self-determination (n = 44 or 79%)
- Hospice care will neither prolong nor hasten death (n = 33 or 59%)
- Hospice programs respect decisions made within a physician–patient relationship (n = 33 or 59%)
- Hospice care is committed to enhancing the quality of life at the end of life (n = 29 or 53%)
- Hospice caring will never abandon patients or their families (n = 28 or 50%)

While not an exhaustive list of hospice values in general or of ethical precepts in the PAD policies of the Oregon hospice programs, these five precepts have reasonably broad appeal and may often be implicit in caregiving practices even if not explicitly identified in a policy. They can provide some common substantive ground or morality to give normative guidance to hospice programs in developing policies and practices regarding physician-assisted death. As is true of broad values or principles in general, these precepts require specification in particular contexts and applications, something that the Oregon hospice policies studied seldom carried out. Furthermore, while these precepts would seem to provide ethical direction for the general array of caregiving issues that hospice programs and staff encounter, they are not, without specification, adequate by themselves for the context of physician-assisted death.

Indeed, were hospice programs to rely exclusively on the preceding commitments in addressing physician-assisted death, the programs would very quickly encounter moral conflicts that lack any clear resolution or means of reconciliation, including the tension between the historical hospice commitment to "not hasten death" and the contemporary commitment to "respect self-determination" when a patient makes a request of a physician for life-ending medication. The method by which most Oregon hospices evade this conflict is, subsequent to the provision of basic information about patient options under the law, to (1) remove themselves from the decision-making process to a significant extent and (2) defer to decisions made by the patient in consultation with his or her attending physician.

On one hand, this strategy succeeds in ensuring that physician-assisted death does not evolve into what might be called "hospice-assisted" death. However, it also means that hospice care assumes instrumental value in a plan of care whose ends have been chosen by the patient and physician outside the hospice context. Although the intrinsic goods of hospice care may be diminished by this approach, for many hospice programs this is an acceptable and legitimate compromise that advances the patient's interests in a dignified death without involving hospice in practices beyond its scope and mission.

Furthermore, the invited presence of a devoted staff member at the medication ingestion seems consistent with the hospice commitment to "nonabandonment of patients," but it is a practice that is not allowed by the majority of the Oregon programs ($n = 31$, 55%) and is permitted by only a small minority ($n = 11$, 20%). In this circumstance, an unarticulated value (at least in the policies) overrides not only the precept of nonabandonment but also respect for the patient request for caregiver presence. In the site visits where the author probed the rationale for this restriction, what was articulated in conversation was language roughly equivalent to a value of "preserving the integrity and image of hospice." As illustrated in vignette 2 earlier, one nurse commented that were she to receive such a request for presence from a patient, "I would go, but as a friend, not as hospice staff on duty." Other hospice staff and program directors expressed concern that staff presence during dying would foster public perceptions that hospice encourages or condones physician-assisted death or assumes responsibility for ensuring that the patient's death occurs without complications.

My point here is not to resolve these conflicts or assess the cogency of the arguments but simply to note that while the five broadly stated precepts in Oregon hospice policies present common ground for hospice ethical discussion of physician-assisted death, they are not in the context of PAD internally consistent nor are they comprehensive. Ultimately, hospice ethics will need to engage in specification of these norms or precepts, or prioritization of a particular norm, as is the case with those hospice programs, as well as the Oregon Hospice Association, which have elevated respect for patient choices to primary significance, or identify a primary norm to which to appeal in cases of value conflict, as the "hospice integrity and image" value appears to function in the restrictions on staff presence.

Moral Ordeal and Moral Opportunity

As illustrated by the study, the emergence of physician-assisted death legislation has raised very difficult questions for Oregon hospices about the adequacy of the hospice philosophy of care, about programmatic mission and integrity, and about staff commitments, including accommodation for conscientious refusal. Jennings (2011) has elegantly articulated why such legislation can present hospice with a moral ordeal. Jennings observes that contemporary hospice manifests "the dynamics of the essential ethical tension between a substantive conception of good dying and a respect for individual autonomy" (p. 4). This tension emerges directly in the context of physician-assisted death legislation as a defining question of identity for hospice: "Legalization [of PAD] would liberate dying people from what hospice had been teaching could be a meaningful and valuable time of life. On the other hand, a major part of the quality of living while dying that hospice champions is autonomy, respect, and dignity. How could hospice stand against that?" (p. 4).

In examining the ethical argumentation regarding hospice participation in physician-assisted death, an important question is where the stronger burden of justification rests. I say "stronger" burden, rather than simply "burden," because each of the three broad positions of nonparticipation, qualified participation, or regulatory participation infringes or overrides an important hospice value. Is the ethical burden greater for those programs that affirm that physician-assisted death is compatible with and expands upon the caregiving services hospice customarily provides? Such a position incorporates the cultural priority of patient self-determination and affirms it as a hospice value. Moreover, it gives expression to the hospice value of nonabandonment of patients. However, it can seem to neglect the commitment to not hasten death as well as the more general hospice philosophical understanding of finding relational fulfillment, an expanded self-awareness, and personal meaning in the dying process.

Is the ethical burden then greater for those programs who see physician death as an alternative essentially outside the parameters of hospice care (and, for some, outside the realm of policy regulation)? This perspective affirms the hospice commitment to never hasten death, as well as the philosophical claim of the hospice tradition that the dying process always has pedagogical significance. These pillars of nonparticipation are typically combined with a normative assumption: Quality hospice care, including pain control and symptom management, makes physician-assisted death unnecessary for hospice patients. This point does not deny the significance of a legal choice for patients of physician-assisted death, but it claims that patients will be less likely to exercise that choice when provided quality hospice care. This aspiration is expressed in the following statement from one policy: "Hospice will always address the needs of the terminally ill with compassion, dignity, and respect, hopefully alleviating their concerns sufficiently that the smallest number of people would choose this new [PAD] option."

However, this perspective does not give full acknowledgment to patient self-determination and the background hospice philosophical commitment to empower patients and families to assume responsibility and control in the dying process. It may also presume a hospice vision of a good dying or good death for patients, or as Jennings (2011) expresses it, "a conception of human flourishing while dying," that is not shared by patients (p. 4). This invokes the specter of paternalism that contemporary bioethics has rejected, even while acknowledging that substantive visions of the good are appropriate within certain communal contexts, such as religious traditions. It may also rely on a noble aspiration about hospice care that may not sufficiently match the responsiveness needed for actual patient needs. Finally, insofar as hospice programs would customarily permit staff to attend the death of a patient upon request, the restrictions set by hospice programs on staff presence at the death of patient who consumes a life-ending medication seem clearly to infringe the precept of nonabandonment. Philosophically, do all hospice patients experience equality of treatment in death, or are some deaths vocationally and morally different?

The burden of justification for the model of qualified participation is generated in part by matters of internal consistency and integrity. The perspective appears to share the understanding that hospice care and physician-assisted death can be compatible and complementary, but a profound ambivalence is signaled by the policy language restricting "active" or "direct" participation by the hospice and its staff. While I have interpreted the intent of such language as signifying a permission to participate in the process, but proscribing any facilitation, either instrumentally or symbolically, in matters pertaining to medication and the act of ingestion, this differentiation requires justification. It can be morally questionable to portray providing information to patients, conversation with patients, collaboration with physicians, and referrals to patient advocacy organizations and other hospice practices as equivalent morally to "passive" participation or "indirect" involvement. Part of the moral burden for qualified participatory hospices is one of transparency, and more broadly, one of more substantive reflection about the boundaries and identity of hospice care. If a hospice program permits some involvement in the process, for example, to further ends of informed patient decision making, what changes ethically when a patient who has received ongoing hospice care from enrollment makes a request for a staff member to be present when he or she consumes life-ending medication?

For each of these alternative approaches, ethical justification ultimately requires discourse regarding the fundamental purposes and mission of hospice. Hospice programs seeking to maintain fidelity to the hospice philosophy of care are presented with a moral ordeal in the context of physician-assisted death. The question then is whether this moral ordeal can be transformed into a moral opportunity. Our visits to hospice programs led to conversations that revealed that, unsurprisingly, hospice programs and staff seek to avoid the difficult questions, intellectual tensions, and moral ordeals generated by physician-assisted death, be they at the philosophical, programmatic, or practice level. Staff members indicated reticence to engage in conversation about the issue as a philosophical or policy matter because of concerns that it could prove disruptive to the team philosophy of care that is no less core to hospice self-identity. Some caregiving staff clearly experience moral distress in physician-assisted death circumstances (Schwarz, 2003). Moreover, a substantive discussion, however respectful, dialogic, and civil, was sometimes viewed as an unproductive diversion from the practical immediacies of caregiving facing hospice staff. However, to avoid the conversation is to recognize only the ordeal and miss the opportunity that physician-assisted death can offer hospice programs to engage meaningfully with its philosophical traditions of care, even when, and especially when, they generate moral tensions. Caring for patients who inquire about physician-assisted death can be a catalyst for hospice programs to identify and specify the constitutive ethical values formative of hospice identity and integrity, and to embody processes of conversation that can generate new insights and consensual approaches to formulating hospice policy on deeply controversial matters.

Based on the Oregon experience of the past 16 years, I think a strong case can be made that quality and comprehensive hospice care, coupled with extensive efforts in physician and public education, and implementation of palliative care measures, substantially diminishes the frequency of patient resort to life-ending medications (Campbell, 2008; Jackson, 2011). The numbers of Oregon terminally ill patients who exercise their legal rights to obtain a prescription to end life are approximately 10% of the projections of proponents of the law prior to its passage (opponents of the law tended to have even higher projections). That hospice programs enroll comparatively few patients who make a request for a life-ending medication is attributable at least partly to the efficacy of quality hospice care; nevertheless, this may often function as a self-serving article of faith for hospice programs, and the claim is in need of empirical substantiation. It is striking, for example, that *How to Die in Oregon*, the 2011 award-winning documentary on the experience of numerous Oregon Death With Dignity patients never once mentions hospice care (Richardson, 2011).[2] Even the best hospice care does not entirely eliminate all patient requests for physician assistance in death.

However, this argument is most compelling in circumstances when hospice care is directed toward the alleviation of patient pain. If the case for legalized physician-assisted death were exclusively based on the relief of pain at the end of life, then the principles of beneficence and caring would seem to warrant policies of hospice nonparticipation. But neither the Oregon or Washington statutes mention alleviation of patient pain as a personal rationale or a medical indication for a terminally ill person to request a life-ending medication. Moreover, a minority of Oregon patients ($n = 177$, or 23.7%) who have actually used the law have informed their physicians that they were concerned about receiving inadequate medication to control their pain. Instead, the legal rationale for the statutes is very explicitly to respect patient self-determination at the end of life, and that rationale affirms a value that, though secular and political in origin, has been integrated into hospice philosophy as a corollary to the commitment to empower patients (and family) to the extent possible with control over the process of dying. This is the value cited with most frequency in the Oregon hospice program documents on physician-assisted death, and it is the concern mentioned most frequently by Oregon patients ($n = 684$, or 91.4%) who receive life-ending medication, far surpassing the number of patients who express concerns about inadequate pain treatment.

This does not bestow on patient self-determination moral priority necessarily, but it also means the value cannot be summarily dismissed. As developed in the biomedical ethics literature generally, a legally recognized right supporting patient self-determination, including self-determination about the method and timing of death through physician assistance, generates a negative right, a right against others, including hospice programs, of noninterference with the patient's exercise of the right. The possession of a negative right does not, however, generate a positive right, or a right against others for assistance in the exercise of that right. Put another way, a negative right cannot impose on others, whether members of the medical community or hospice staff, a positive duty of participation or assistance (Beauchamp & Childress, 2009, pp. 352–353). The Oregon statute recognizes this distinction between negative and positive rights by giving terminally ill patients an entitlement to physician assistance in death, while stipulating there is "no legal duty to participate" on the part of any health care provider or facility. In the context of hospice, the extent of involvement or participation by hospice programs and staff will turn on understandings of the scope and boundaries of hospice care.

To be sure, in some Oregon hospice settings, hospice values are supplemented by religious values and commitments, including values of life's sanctity and responsible stewardship, to justify the restrictions on personal liberty. In practice, in such hospice settings, a patient request for life-ending medication seldom arises because patients self-select another hospice. Nonetheless, nonparticipating hospice programs bear a responsibility to address the following kinds of questions to satisfy their burden of justification: Who ultimately is empowered or authorized to make decisions regarding the kinds of end-of-life care hospice will provide? What are the purposes or objectives for nonparticipation, and are these purposes compatible with the moral traditions of hospice philosophy? What alternatives are available to patients enrolled in a nonparticipating hospice so they can no less experience a dying process with respect, dignity, and integrity? What are the benefits and the burdens of nonparticipation, and upon whom do the benefits and the burdens fall? What expectations are there that these benefits can be achieved, and are these expectations (e.g., complete control of pain) reasonable?

This does not diminish the burden of justification required of hospices who have opted for regulatory or qualified participation in physician-assisted death. Given the hospice tradition that dying can be a meaningful part of living, that death is a natural part of the life process, and the ethical precept that death should not be hastened because it brings a premature end to the meaningful experience of dying, a case needs to be made as to how physician-assisted death can be incorporated within hospice care without substantial compromise to these constitutive commitments. That case is more evaded than made when the hospice rationale is that death is not hastened by hospice care because the primary decision makers are the physician and patient outside the domain of hospice.

Instead, a set of related questions must necessarily be addressed for justification of participation: What are the causes and goals of hospice participation? Relief of patient pain and respect for patient choice are both legitimate aspirations of hospice caregiving, but they do not necessarily lead to the same conclusion about the necessity of physician-assisted death. Further, how are these causes and goals compatible with the moral traditions of hospice philosophy, including the philosophical claims about the meaningfulness of the dying experience? Has the hospice program provided the full array of its quality care and services to the patient, such that physician-assisted death is not one option among many, but is almost always a last resort?

Finally, what degree of assurance is there that hospice participation will succeed in meeting the interests of both the patient in achieving death "in a humane and dignified manner" and in the hospice program retaining its own moral autonomy and integrity? In particular, what provisions are made by participating hospices for patient care in the event of a patient experiencing complications from ingesting the medication? This contingency is addressed by less than 10% of the Oregon hospice policies ($n = 5$), even though complications have occurred in 5% of the cases. Participating hospices need to devote attention to this question and determine what care they will allow attending staff to provide consistent with hospice ethics. Otherwise, such hospices may be too optimistic about reliance on pharmacological agents and neglect caring skills for patients who experience complications.

If hospice programs and associations can engage these questions of justification (Campbell, 1992)—and this engagement necessarily requires other forms of discourse than are possible in compressed policy documents— in sustained and respectful discourse open to diverse perspectives, then the ethical challenges of physician-assisted death for hospice can become a moral opportunity to develop its tradition and philosophy of care. For some organizations and writers, this approach suggests a different policy option, designated as "studied neutrality."

The Limits of Studied Neutrality

Even though the American Academy of Hospice and Palliative Medicine commends "studied neutrality" in its policy statement on physician-assisted death, it is of interest that the language of "neutrality" was entirely absent in the policy documents of the Oregon hospice programs. The concept of "studied neutrality" was initially articulated by physicians Quill and Cassell

(2003), and it bears scrutiny as a possible alternative to the models of nonparticipation, qualified participation, and regulatory participation presented earlier.

Quill and Cassell (2003) directed their argument toward professional organizations (including hospice organizations) who had or were contemplating presenting position statements on physician-assisted suicide (the common professional phraseology at the time of writing). They contend that a position of "studied neutrality" by an organization can "recognize and respect the diversity of personal and religious views and choices of its members and their patients and [can] encourage open discussion" (p. 210). Quill and Cassell present the example of an influential Oregon task force whose adoption of a neutral position permitted physicians and other caregiving members to promote greater implementation of palliative care measures, helped physicians and other caregivers "with diverse values struggle with how to respond to requests" by patients for life-ending medication, and provided experience for caregivers to develop ways of working with patients who make such requests irrespective of their own position. Ultimately, they contend the model of studied neutrality has the advantage of affirming the professional commitment to nonabandonment of patients while expressing "respect for diversity." The question here is whether the concept of studied neutrality is preferable and feasible for hospice programs.

As noted earlier, the Academy of Hospice and Palliative Medicine has endorsed the position of "studied neutrality" regarding physician-assisted death. What is rather striking about the AAHPM analysis is that the context for patient requests for physician-assisted death is framed as "intolerable" or "intractable suffering." The AAHPM seems to presume quality hospice and palliative care will sufficiently alleviate patient pain, ironically sharing the same assumption on efficacy as Oregon hospices who have opted for nonparticipation. As many have argued, however, suffering is a distinct phenomenological entity that cannot be reduced to severe or extreme pain (Campbell, 1997).

It is important to recall that the statutory rationale for physician-assisted death is not severe or unrelieved pain, nor is it the experience of suffering, but rather an expression of commitment to patient self-determination. Although the AAHPM does not provide an account of suffering, its position statement identifies several sources of suffering, some of which seem in the family of concepts implicit in the self-determination argument, particularly in its recognition that "loss of control and dignity" is a source of suffering. On the other hand, some of the other sources of suffering identified, such as depression, "loss of sense of self," or fears of being a burden to others, could undermine the capacity for self-determination, and thus erode the self-determination rationale.

The interpretation of patient requests for physician-assisted death as a response to intolerable suffering is not beyond the scope of hospice care and the skills of interdisciplinary team members, but it is important to note it is a different context than what is presumed in most of the Oregon hospice policies, where the caregiving issue is principally framed as relief of pain and preservation of quality of life. This may have some impact, then, on whether a policy option of "studied neutrality" is a preferable and feasible option for hospice programs. Ultimately, I contend that though the perspective of Quill and Cassell on "studied neutrality" is suggestive, and perhaps even appropriate in some circumstances, it is not sufficiently comprehensive for the purposes of hospice programs in jurisdictions where physician-assisted death is legalized.

Quill and Cassell focus on caregiving practices, such as palliative care measures and caregiver responsiveness to patient requests, but the content of their phrase "studied" remains elusive. Clearly implicit in their account are responsibilities on the part of professional caregivers to engage in self-examination of personal values, and to devote attention to a "best practices" approach to responding to patient requests. That is to be commended and cultivated, but it hardly seems sufficient professionally or programmatically.

For example, while Quill and Cassell focus their discussion primarily on the ethical self-scrutiny of the individual caregiver, this may be inadequate for the context of interdisciplinary team caring integral to hospice. On one hand, a posture of moral neutrality that emphasizes respect for diverse viewpoints can appear compelling if there is concern that affirming a different program position or even engaging in an open discussion may lead to sharp disagreements that can threaten the unity required in the team model of caring. However, it is important that neutrality not signify to staff a matter about which hospice cannot take a principled moral stand. Physician-assisted death presents both challenges and opportunities to core pillars of hospice philosophy and care and requires mediated substantive conversations even if such a procedure risks conflict.

Furthermore, beyond the examination of personal values implied in the studied neutrality position, a realm of study that should be emphasized is that of professional values and their meaning and scope. While Quill and Cassell would concur with the Oregon hospices that nonabandonment is a core responsibility of physicians, nurses, and other professional caregiving staff, as we have seen, that can at times be difficult to fulfill for some hospice staff because of other conflicting values. It would also seem necessary for the open discussion Quill and Cassell say their position is supposed to encourage for professional staff to have engaged in some study of the relevant statute and be reasonably familiar with philosophical and ethical argumentation on the issue. Finally, hospice staff should devote some study to the traditions and philosophy of hospice care. As articulated by the founder of the modern hospice movement, Dame Cicely Saunders, hospice in its modern origins sought to provide quality care to the terminally ill so patients could avoid two kinds of less preferable modes of dying, technological prolongation of biological life and a hastened death through euthanasia. This is the historical and philosophical context for the emergence of the common hospice ethical precept that hospice care seeks "neither to prolong nor to hasten death." This history seems important to learn and to educate the public and professional communities about, as even prominent physician writers like Atul admit that, before carefully researching the topic, he thought that "hospice hastens death" (Gawande, 2010).

This latter point suggests another inadequacy with the concept of studied neutrality delineated by Quill and Cassell. Their recommendation seems to assume on the part of both professional associations and their members a kind of policy position independent of moral tradition and embedded moral practices. Studied neutrality is, in short, an ethic tailored for an era of maximizing autonomy for organizations and professionals (as well as patients), a procedural ethic for moral strangers who have no shared vision of professional or human flourishing. This may be feasible for certain professional organizations that lack a substantive moral tradition and a philosophy of care, but that is not the case with hospice. Indeed, as Jennings has observed, it is precisely this commitment to a substantive philosophy of hospice care that generates the inescapable "dynamic of ethical tension" when situated in the context of physician-assisted death. Hospice, if it is to retain its identity and integrity, needs to manifest fidelity to its philosophical tradition of care. Hospice can be distinctive not only for its commitment not to abandon patients but also to not abandon the moral tradition upon which its caregiving practices rest.

A third assumption embedded in the concept of "neutrality" as Quill and Cassell develop it may be relevant for some hospice programs, but not for programs in the state of Oregon. As is the case with much of contemporary moral language, such as that of "autonomy" or "rights," neutrality also finds its origins within a political context, and thus it seems much more apt when there is a live policy question under discussion. In anticipation of an impending debate over a legislative statute (Vermont), or a citizen referendum process (Massachusetts), it can be appropriate for professional associations, including hospice programs, to affirm a position of "studied neutrality," provided the issue has been studied in a context of open discussion and the sharing of diverse views and is not a method to avoid ethical engagement. It seems far less compelling, however, when the policy issue has been decided, particularly, as in the case of Oregon and Washington, on the side of affirming legalized physician-assisted death. In the context of legalization, hospice care is very integral to patients who may have recourse to the law, and thus neutrality regarding the enabling statute appears to reflect moral evasion.

As noted, in the study of Oregon hospices, no program used the language of "studied neutrality" or "neutrality" regarding the Oregon law. Our conversations at site visits disclosed use of "neutrality" language in a more circumscribed context, however, that of staff providing information about the Oregon law to hospice patients. While not part of the formal policy statement, an embedded expectation of these hospices was that staff would provide information about the statute in a neutral manner, intending neither to persuade nor dissuade a patient in his or her choice. Whether that is an achievable expectation or an admirable ideal is a reasonable question; my point here, however, is that "neutrality" in the provision of information to patients is performed in service of a commitment to the larger hospice objective of facilitating informed decision making by patients. It is not clear what hospice end is served by the espousal of neutrality toward a practice once it has become a legalized policy and practical option for patients, and as hospice programs and staff face concrete choices about their involvement and participation.

CONCLUSION

Our analysis of the policies of Oregon hospices on the Oregon Death With Dignity Act indicates that while there is widespread agreement among Oregon hospices over the responsibilities of hospice to provide customary hospice care to all patients, that agreement dissipates when the question shifts to determining "customary" care in hospice, and more generally, to identifying the distinctive meaning and purposes of *hospice care*, in contrast to other forms of caring. In this respect, physician-assisted death provides a boundary or defining issue about the scope, meaning, and purposes of hospice and customary care, for the responsibilities or restrictions hospice programs assume relative to the Oregon law are substantially influenced by programmatic understandings of hospice care.

At the risk of overgeneralization, the hospice mission as presented in Oregon hospice PAD policies tends to fall into two (very broad) categories: (1) the hospice role in ensuring *quality at the end-of-life experience* for patients and on *the results* of hospice caregiving interventions; (2) *educational* responsibilities for hospice in supporting *patient self-determination* and *informed choices* about end-of-life care options. Both of these commitments are well rooted in hospice philosophy, tradition, and practice. The hospice responsibility for informed choice and the commitment to high-quality end-of-life care are clearly not incompatible, and in most circumstances these commitments complement each other. Yet physician-assisted death can present one circumstance in which they are not easily reconciled.

In this context, procedures embedded in the studied neutrality posture are important for any hospice program as they contemplate an approach to physician-assisted death. These include ethical self-examination, an attitude of respect toward different values or positions, and opportunities for discussion among hospice staff members. These procedures acknowledge that physician-assisted death is an *ethical* issue for hospice programs and present necessary conditions for meaningful dialogue, while not predisposing the outcome of the discussion.

In an ongoing study of Washington hospice policies, I find it important that several refer to a "personal responsibility" of hospice staff to examine their own values, their views on physician-assisted death, and their commitment to hospice care. This element of moral introspection can be supplemented by attentiveness to values of professional vocation, as well as familiarity with legislative statutes, and ethical reasoning. A studied position in hospice care will engage the moral tradition and philosophy of hospice, including its constitutive values, and an analysis of how the individualistic assumptions of both physician-assisted death legislation and the studied neutrality posture can be integrated within the team and communitarian vision of care espoused by hospice. When these procedures of a personally responsible position are in place, then it seems reasonable to proceed to dialogue and policy development. Then the moral questions posed by physician-assisted death for hospice can be transformed into a moral opportunity for illuminating programmatic self-definition and redefinition. And while, for pragmatic reasons, a posture of moral neutrality might be justifiable for hospice programs and associations to adopt prior to or during a political process debating legalization, it seems much less compelling in the wake of legalization when hospice programs must devote themselves to practical choices in patient care, including responses to patient requests for a life-ending medication.

The procedures for practical caregiving hospices adopt regarding patient requests should be directed and constrained by the overarching purposes and vocation of hospice care.

APPENDIX

To facilitate a process of hospice deliberation, I present in conclusion a comprehensive set of 50 questions that seemed to be presupposed in the Oregon and Washington hospice policy documents. Given the program information we received, this compilation involves reflection on *what question had to have*

Table 11.1. FRAMEWORK FOR HOSPICE DELIBERATION

Hospice Procedure	Framing Questions
Hospice philosophy	What is the mission of hospice (or the agency)?
	What makes hospice distinctive?
	What values support this mission or purpose?
	What is the scope of hospice care?
	What actions would fall outside the realm of hospice care?
Hospice policy	What is the policy of a hospice on participation in the Death With Dignity Act?
	What is the purpose and who is the audience for the policy?
	What language will the policy use to describe the event? (e.g., physician-assisted suicide, physician-assisted death, death with dignity, physician aid-in-dying, self-administration of lethal medication)
	How was/will the policy be composed, and who did/will compose it?
	What will be the rationale for the policy (e.g., religious tradition, professional ethic, hospital policy, hospice mission)?
	Will a hospice participate/facilitate the patient decision-making process prior to self-administration?
	Will a hospice leave the process to be worked out between physician and patient?
	Will a hospice allow staff, upon request, to be present when a patient administers the medication?
Patient access	Will patients receive customary hospice services irrespective of their interests in a lethal medication to end life?
	Will the patient be informed by hospice of all their legal rights and options in end-of-life care?
	Will the hospice notify the patient of the hospice policy regarding their participation in the Act? If so, when and how?

(continued)

Table 11.1. (CONTINUED)

Hospice Procedure	Framing Questions
Patient inquiries	What responsibilities does a hospice have to a patient who makes an inquiry?
	If a patient makes an inquiry or request, what will be the tone of response of hospice staff?
	If a patient has questions about the Act, will the patient be referred to his or her primary care physician for information?
	If a patient has questions about legal options, will he or she be given contact information about community or state resources that can answer his or her questions?
	Will a hospice participate/facilitate the patient decision-making process prior to self-administration?
	Will the hospice provide information (written or verbal) about the law?
	Will the hospice provide educational brochures about the law prepared by nonhospice organizations?
Staff–patient conversations	Will members of the hospice staff have a conversation with the patient about his or her inquiry or request?
	How should hospice staff understand their role in such a conversation?
	Will hospice staff seek to identify physical, emotional, social, or religious factors that may contribute to the patient's request?
	Will hospice staff inform the patient about all alternatives in end-of-life care?
	Will patients be informed that their wishes will be communicated to members of the hospice team?
Patient requests	Will hospice staff be permitted to facilitate the process of informed consent or informed request?
	Are hospice staff permitted to act as witnesses of the patient's request?
	What responsibilities, if any, do staff have (or must refrain from) with regards to the prescribed medication?
	Will hospice staff provide information to the patient or caregivers regarding the safe disposal of medications?
	If requested, will hospice staff be permitted to be present when a patient self-administers the medication?
Team interactions	Will staff be encouraged to consider their own perspectives on whether they can provide care to a patient who makes a request?
	Will a patient inquiry or request be communicated to members of the hospice IDG Team?
	Will staff have a conversation about the plan of care in light of a patient inquiry or request?
	Will the hospice include documentation of patient's request and subsequent conversations in a patient's record?
	What responsibilities do staff have if they wish to discontinue caring for a patient who requests use of the Death With Dignity Act?

(continued)

Table 11.1. (CONTINUED)

Hospice Procedure	Framing Questions
	What responsibilities does the hospice program have should a staff member request to transfer patient care because of moral or ethical concerns about the patient's decision?
	Will hospice staff be permitted to be present when a patient self-administers the medication?
	Will hospice staff be permitted to be present post ingestion but prior to death?
	What are staff responsibilities should they make a home visit post ingestion and prior to death?
	What are staff responsibilities post death to the family?
Provider relations	What is the role of the hospice relative to the attending physician?
	Will the hospice notify the attending physician of a patient's interest in a lethal medication?
	Will the hospice provide information about pharmacies that will dispense the prescribed medications?
Community resources	Will the hospice refer a patient with questions about the law to the Washington State Web site?
	Will the hospice refer a patient with questions to patients' rights advocates such as Compassion and Choices?
	Will the hospice refer a patient to other providers in the community?

been asked for a precept or practice to appear in a policy statement. I have organized these questions primarily around the kinds of interactions a hospice program or hospice staff might have with various stakeholders in a patient's decision, including the patient; other members of the hospice team; other health care professionals or institutions; and community resources or organizations beyond the hospice program (see Table 11.1).

NOTES

1. In the wake of passage of the Oregon Death With Dignity Act, President Clinton signed The Assisted Suicide Funding Restriction Act of 1997, which prohibits federal funds from being used for purposes of ending life through "assisted suicide, euthanasia, or mercy killing." The Oregon Act also prohibits these actions; however, a majority of Oregon hospices continue to use the language of "assisted suicide" in their policy statements. See http://uscode.house.gov/download/pls/42C138.txt

2. In private conversations with the filmmaker Peter Richardson, I have indicated that the omission of hospice from the Oregon landscape of physician-assisted death documented in the film is a substantive weakness in an otherwise very dramatic and compelling set of stories.

REFERENCES

American Association of Hospice and Palliative Medicine (AAHPM). (2007). *Physician-assisted death*. Retrieved May 21, 2014 from http://www.aahpm.org/positions/default/suicide.html.

Beauchamp, T. L., & Childress, J. F. (2009). *Principles of biomedical ethics* (6th ed.). New York, NY: Oxford University Press.

Byock, I. C. (1998). *Dying well: Peace and possibilities at the end of life*. New York, NY: Riverhead Trade Books.

Campbell, C. S. (1992). Aid-in-dying and the taking of human life. *Journal of Medical Ethics, 18*(3), 128–134.

Campbell, C. S. (1997). Must patients suffer? In R. A. Carson & C. R. Burns (Eds.), *Philosophy of medicine and bioethics* (pp. 247–263). Dordrecht, The Netherlands: Kluwer Academic.

Campbell, C. S. (2008). Ten years of death with dignity. *New Atlantis, 22*(Fall), 33–46.

Campbell, C. S., & Cox, J. C. (2010). Hospice and physician-assisted death: Collaboration, compliance, and complicity. *Hastings Center Report, 40*(5), 26–35.

Campbell, C. S., Hare, J., & Matthews, P. (1995). Conflicts of conscience: Hospice and assisted suicide. *Hastings Center Report, 25*(3), 36–43.

Cassell, E. J. (2004). *The nature of suffering and the goals of medicine* (2nd ed.). New York, NY: Oxford University Press.

Gawande, A. (2010, August 2). Letting go: What medicine should do when it can't save your life. *The New Yorker*. Retrieved May 21, 2014 from http://www.newyorker.com/reporting/2010/08/02/100802fa_fact_gawande.

Hospice and Palliative Nurses Association (HPNA). (2011). *Role of the nurse when hastened death is requested*. Retrieved April 2014, from http://hpna.org/PicView.aspx?ID=1528.

Jackson, A. (2011). Unreconcilable differences? *Hastings Center Report, 41*(4), 6–7.

Jennings, B. (2011). Unreconcilable differences? *Hastings Center Report, 41*(4), 4–5.

Jones, R. P. (2007). *Liberalism's troubled search for equality: Religion and cultural bias in the Oregon physician-assisted suicide debates*, Notre Dame, IN: University of Notre Dame Press.

National Hospice and Palliative Care Organization (NHPCO). (2000). *Hospice philosophy statement*. Retrieved April 2014, from http://www.nhpco.org/i4a/pages/Index.cfm?pageID=5308#2.

National Hospice and Palliative Care Organization (NHPCO). (2005). *Commentary and resolution on physician assisted suicide*. Retrieved May 21, 2014 from http://www.nhpco.org/publications-press-room/nhpco-position-statements.

Oregon Hospice Association (OHA). (2009). *Choosing among Oregon's legal end-of-life options*. Retrieved April 2014, from http://www.oregonhospice.org/endoflifecare_legal.htm.

Oregon Public Health Division. (2014). *Death with Dignity Act annual report: 2013*. Retrieved April 2014, from http://public.health.oregon.gov/ProviderPartnerResources/EvaluationResearch/DeathwithDignityAct/Pages/ar-index.aspx.

Oregon Revised Statute 127.800–127.995 (1994).

Quill, T. E. (2008). Physician-assisted death in the United States: Are the existing 'last resorts' enough? *Hastings Center Report, 38*(5), 17–22.

Quill, T. E., & Cassell, C. K. (2003). Professional organizations' position statements on physician-assisted suicide: A case for studied neutrality. *Annals of Internal Medicine, 138*(3), 208–211.

Richardson, P. D. (Producer & Director). (2011). *How to die in Oregon.* [Motion picture]. United States: Clear Cut Films, New York, NY.

Revised Code of Washington 70.245 (2008).

Saunders, C. (1991-92). The evolution of the hospices. *Free Inquiry, 12*(Winter), 19–23.

Schwarz, J. K. (2003). Understanding and responding to patients' requests for assisted dying. *Journal of Nursing Scholarship, 35*(4), 377–384.

Stoddard, S. (1992). *The hospice movement: A better way of caring for the dying*, New York, NY: Random House.

Vermont Statutes Annotated Title 18, Ch. 113 (2013).

Washington State Department of Health. (2012). *2011 Death with Dignity Act Report.* Retrieved April 2014, from http://www.doh.wa.gov/YouandYourFamily/ IllnessandDisease/DeathwithDignityAct.aspx.

Washington State Department of Health. (2013). *2012 Death with Dignity Act Report.* Retrieved April 2014, from http://www.doh.wa.gov/YouandYourFamily/ IllnessandDisease/DeathwithDignityAct.aspx.

CHAPTER 12

Ethics Committees for Hospice

Moving Beyond the Acute Care Model

JENNIFER BALLENTINE AND PAMELA DALINIS

Health care ethics committees (HCECs) were constituted beginning in the late 1970s to address treatment decisions for incapacitated patients in the acute care setting. Stimuli for creation of HCECs came both from external sources (court decisions, government-level studies, accreditation organizations) and from within health care facilities as practitioners, administrators, and patients grappled with conflicts at the intersection of what could be done, technically and medically, and what should be done, morally and humanely. By the end of the 20th century, HCECs were well established in hospitals and standards of practice had begun to be described in studies and prescribed by authoritative theorists and professional organizations.

The prevalence of ethics committees in hospice organizations, however, can only be estimated. To date, no comprehensive formal study of mechanisms for resolving ethical dilemmas or the presence or operation of dedicated ethics committees in hospice organizations has been undertaken. The limited relevant literature suggests committees may be present in about a third of agencies. Otherwise, hospice organizations appear to access other-facility ethics committees, rely on informal review by administrators and senior clinical staff, or include ethical issues in clinical discussions by the interdisciplinary team. None of these methods is optimal for conducting ethical deliberation rooted in hospice philosophy or achieving best outcomes for patients and organizations. When establishing an ethics committee in a hospice organization, a simple transfer of the paradigmatic model from acute care may not be the best approach. The goals of hospice care, with an emphasis on patient autonomy, comfort, and quality of life, as well as the largely home-based delivery of care by a team of peers, demand that care be organized and delivered much differently than is the case in acute care organizations. This chapter proposes that the difference between care models should inform parallel differences in the structure and function of health care ethics committees in hospital organizations.

Dedicated hospice ethics committees (HoECs) constituted with the necessary adaptations provide a more appropriate context in which to resolve conflicts that arise at the bedside. Additionally, commitment of resources and attention by a hospice organization to an internal ethics committee opens up opportunities for a more expansive exercise of ethical action within the agency as a whole and the community it serves. Following a brief recap of the development of ethics committees in general and a look at what is known about the structure, function, and operations of acute care and hospice ethics committees, this chapter will offer a model for the formation and operation of ethics committees in hospice organizations that is consistent with the hospice philosophy of care and responsive to the unique goals, care delivery model, and care environment of hospice.

A BRIEF LOOK BACK AT HEALTH CARE ETHICS COMMITTEES

Health care ethics committees evolved in response to new ethical dilemmas emerging from rapidly developing medical technologies in the second half of the 20th century. In 1900, death tended to be swift and unequivocal. Medical breakthroughs accelerating through the last century such as antibiotics, insulin, reliable surgery, vaccinations, hemodialysis, cardiopulmonary resuscitation (CPR), organ transplantation, and mechanically assisted respiration and circulation had stunning success as lifesaving and life-prolonging measures. They had equal "success" in prolonging dying and introducing an unprecedented degree of iatrogenic suffering to the experience of illness. By the mid-1990s, the American Hospital Association estimated that 70% of deaths were "managed"—only coming about as a result of a decision to stop a treatment or not start a treatment (Webb, 1997, p. 189). What was once at the hand of fate became a matter of choice with profound legal and ethical implications for all involved.

Concurrent with the development of life-prolonging technologies and treatments, determinations of who would have access to those limited and very expensive resources was a major ethical preoccupation. For example, with the invention of the arteriovenous (AV) shunt in the late 1950s, long-term outpatient dialysis became feasible. However, demand far outweighed the capacity of the handful of dialysis machines available in the early years. The inventor of the AV shunt and founder of the first outpatient dialysis center, Dr. Belding Scribner, "wanted to ensure that decisions were made by the community," and in 1961 turned to the King County (Washington) Medical Society to convene a "Life and Death Committee" with responsibility of deciding who should receive dialysis and who would be denied (Lenzer, 2003, p. 167). Physicians on the committee reviewed the clinical circumstances of the candidates; those who met criteria were passed on to a group of nonmedical community members, who made the final decisions (Altman, 2003). This process generated much controversy at the time but is generally credited with "giving birth" to health care ethics committees as currently understood (Lenzer, p. 167).

Another quickly emerging challenge was that the new technologies and treatments often rendered patients incapable of communicating, either temporarily or permanently, and thus unable to consent to or refuse a proposed course of medical action. Determination of capacity to make health care decisions demanded ongoing clarification of the rights, duties, and liabilities of patients, families, medical professionals, and institutions of care (Presidents Commission, 1983). Increasingly, such clarifications involved the courts and legislative bodies at state and national levels as private tragedies at the crux of the decision-making dilemma played out on the public stage.

Notably the cases of Karen Ann Quinlan in the 1970s (*In re Quinlan*, 1976) and Nancy Beth Cruzan in the 1980s (*Cruzan v. Director, Missouri Department of Health*, 1990) accelerated national awareness of the issues and the need for criteria and procedures for establishing surrogate decision-making authority. In both cases, the patients were young, permanently unconscious, and dependent on technology for life: Karen on a respirator and feeding tube, Nancy on a feeding tube. Neither had written or explicitly stated preferences for treatment under such circumstances. In both cases, after years of caring and hoping, their families had to fight legal as well as medical authorities to achieve what they believed would have been their daughter's preference to discontinue life-sustaining interventions.

The details of the court decisions in these cases are beyond the scope of this chapter and have been well documented elsewhere (Colby, 2002, 2006; Pulrich, 1999; Uhlmann, 1998; Webb, 1997; Zucker, 1999). Suffice it to say that they established fundamental principles underpinning medical decision making, especially by surrogates, and processes for establishing and documenting patient treatment preferences in advance directives. Additionally, the New Jersey Supreme Court decision in the Quinlan case included a provision that if Karen's physicians considered that she had no reasonable hope of recovery, "they shall consult with the hospital 'Ethics Committee' or like body of the institution" and, if the committee agreed, her life support could be withdrawn (Zucker, 1999, p. 163). The Court indicated that such committees could be used to decide similar cases without recourse to the courts. At the time, ethics committees, as distinct from research-focused institutional review boards, hardly existed, but the Court's recommendation quickly motivated hospitals to establish them as a way of avoiding judicial review of each and every fraught case involving end-of-life treatment decisions.

In an early review of the development of hospital-based ethics committees, Rosner (1985) charts a zigzagging path of institutions trying on various models of committee with various purposes: prognosis committees (the type the New Jersey Supreme Court had in mind) to consider appropriateness of withdrawal of life-sustaining treatment; critical care committees to consider criteria for continuing treatment of irreversibly ill patients; bodies primarily charged with education and policy setting; and those whose role was primarily to offer counsel and support to providers in the midst of moral distress.

Taking its cue from the Quinlan decision and these early efforts, the President's Commission for the Study of Ethical Problems in Medicine and Biomedical and Behavioral Research produced one of the first authoritative public documents defining and describing the "institutional ethics committee." Published in the early 1980s, the report recommended an amalgam of the prototypes into one entity that would have as its primary function to undertake systematic discussions designed to protect the interests and rights of incapacitated patients "particularly for decisions that have life-or-death consequences" in order to "ensure their well-being and self-determination" (President's Commission, 1983, p. 5), while also fulfilling educational, policy-setting, and supportive roles.

The Commission set the stage for the development of ethics committees as the preferred venue for consideration of complex ethical dilemmas in the delivery of health care as well as the clarification of related patients' rights regarding treatment preferences and professional responsibilities in a context of proliferating medical advances and breathless social change. This consideration required a style of deliberation beyond the traditionally paternalistic decision making of medicine and the state's interest in preserving life.

A study informing the Commission's work had found that ethics committees then existed in about 4% of hospitals (President's Commission, 1983); by 1984, following adoption by the American Medical Association of a resolution supporting "bioethics committees" in hospitals, over 50% had developed them (Fost & Cranford, 1985; Rosner, 1985). Two significant developments in the early 1990s further accelerated the establishment of institutional ethics committees. The Patient Self Determination Act (PSDA), part of the Omnibus Budget Reconciliation act of 1990, among a great deal else, stated that decision making regarding all complex cases should generally be considered in the health care setting without judicial review (Pulrich, 1999). In 1992 the Joint Commission, the major accreditation organization for hospital facilities, added a standard that hospitals must have "a defined process for handling ethical issues" (McGee, Caplan, Spanogle, & Asch, 2001, p. 61). By the late 1990s, two studies (Fox, Myers, & Pearlman, 2007; McGee et al., 2001) found ethics committees in 93% of responding hospitals and ethics consultation services (by committees, small teams, or individuals) in 100% of facilities with more than 400 beds.

PRESCRIPTION AND DESCRIPTION—ETHICS COMMITTEES IN ACUTE CARE AND HOSPICE

Ethics Committees in the Acute Care Setting

Standards for HCECs developed through the early years as much from descriptions of what the committees were already doing as from prescriptions of what they ought to be doing. Descriptions were offered by studies of ethics committees and consultation services (e.g., Fost & Cranford, 1985; Fox et al., 2007; McGee et al., 2001; President's Commission, 1983; Rosner, 1985) informing prescriptions offered by professional associations (e.g., AMA, 1985; ASBH, 1998), seminal journals (e.g., *The Hastings Center Report, HEC Forum*), major health systems (e.g., the Veterans Health Administration), and expert theorists (e.g., Beauchamp & Childress, 2001; Jonsen, Siegler, & Winslade, 2006), which in turn shaped the composition and activities of the committees and services.

A landmark description/prescription for acute care HCECs was offered in the aforementioned President's Commission for the Study of Ethical Problems in Medicine's 1983 report. The report included model legislation developed by the American Society of Law and Medicine for states wishing to establish ethics committees and grant them appropriate immunities from civil and criminal prosecution. The legislation (prescription) was in large part based on a study (description) undertaken by the Commission of the few extant ethics committees and testimony by members of these pioneering bodies (Presidents Commission, 1983).

The Commission's report and accompanying model legislation established several of the foundational features of ethics committees. Membership should be "diverse"—including clinical disciplines, administration, and lay representatives—in order to ensure varying viewpoints. The committees' primary functions are to review medical treatment decisions with ethical implications, establish guidelines regarding treatment or other medical decisions, and engage in self-education and education of the facility staff on ethical issues (President's Commission, 1983).

In 1998, a taskforce was convened by the Society for Health and Human Values—Society for Bioethics Consultation comprising scholars from medical, legal, nursing, philosophical, and pastoral professions, and representatives from national associations and health systems to develop guidelines for the practice of health care ethics consultation. Published as *Core Competencies for Health Care Ethics Consultation*, by the American Society for Bioethics and Humanities, this booklet has been recently updated (ASBH, 2010) and remains the authoritative prescriptive guide for HCECs. It covers the process of ethics consultation; core competencies, skills, knowledge, and traits for consultation; touches on organizational ethics; and emphasizes the importance of evaluation of consultation outcomes.

In 1999, two groups of researchers conducted studies of ethics activity in the acute care setting: McGee, Caplan, Spanogle, and Asch (2001) focused on ethics committees, looking at prevalence, membership, activities, issues, and outcomes. Fox, Myers, and Pearlman (2007) looked more broadly at ethics consultation services—whether conducted by committees, small teams, or individuals. These two studies, although conducted more than 10 years ago, provide real data on what ethics committees in acute care actually do. Details of the results from the McGee and Fox studies are presented in Table 12.1.

A few key features are most relevant to our discussion: Ethics committees in the acute care setting generally comprise volunteer members, dominated by physicians and nurses but including a smattering of other clinical roles, administrators, attorneys, and rarely community members. Activities span, about evenly in commitment of time, the prescribed triumvirate of education, case consultation, and policy review. Education appeared to be primarily of the committee, rather than of the facility or community by the committee. The median number of annual active case consultations, in a range from 0 to 300, was only 3, and focal issues were topped by patient autonomy/capacity, communication, and conflicts in

Table 12.1. COMPARISON OF FINDINGS IN TWO STUDIES OF HOSPITAL ETHICS COMMITTEES/CONSULTATION SERVICES

Feature	McGee et al., 2001	Fox et al., 2007
Data collected	1999	1999–2000
Data source	National: Random sample of 1,000 hospitals from AHA 1995 membership	National: Random sample of 600 hospitals from AHA 1998 membership
Response rate	36% ($N = 346$)	87.4% ($N = 519$)
Method	100%: Written questionnaire mailed to a random sample (1,000) of US hospital directors	Questionnaire completed with "best informant" 86%: via telephone interview 14%: in writing
Focus of study	Features and activities of HCEC	Features and activities ECS
Type of responding facilities/agencies (majority categories)	81%: No religious affiliation 74%: Not for profit	82%: No church affiliation 52%: Nonacademic 52%: Not for profit
Bed size/ADC	Not reported	45%: <100 38%: 100–299 12%: 300–499 6%: ≥500
Presence of committee or consultation service	93%	81%: present (100% in hospitals with >400 beds) 14%: developing
Time since inception	Median 7 years	47%: 5–10 years 27%: <5 years 26%: >10 years
No. of members	Median 14	n/a
Disciplines (major categories)	Physicians, nurses	Individuals performing ECS: physicians (34%), nurses (31%)
Disciplines (all other)	Equally prevalent: administrators, clergy, attorneys/risk managers, social workers/psychologists, other	11%: Social work 10%: Chaplain 9%: Administrator
Activities (mean % time)	30%: HCEC self-education 28%: Formulating/evaluating policy 20%: Case consultation 15%: Retrospective review of cases	n/a
Supported by facility/ agency budget	Not reported	16% hospitals provided salary support for ECSs
Policy issues addressed by committee (multiple responses possible)	94%: DNR/withdrawal of care 68%: Brain death 68%: Organ donation 25%: Anencephalic infants	Not reported

(*continued*)

Table 12.1. (CONTINUED)

Feature	McGee et al., 2001	Fox et al., 2007
Access to committee or service for consultation	Not reported	95%: "Anyone" may request consultation
Ethics-specific training for HCEC/ECS members	Not reported	45%: Independent learning with no formal training or supervision 41%: Training by formal supervision by experienced ECS member 5%: Fellowship, graduate degree program in ethics
Median no. of consults/year	4 "formal"; 2 "informal"	3 (range 0–300; generally larger the hospital, more the consultations with most in academic facilities)
No. of person-hours devoted to consult	Not reported	Median 6 (range 1–120)
Model for consultation	Not reported	68%: Small team 23%: Full committee 9%: Individual
Method for deliberation	Not reported	87% claimed to use consistent model for deliberation almost none able to describe method. 15 respondents cited Jonsen's 4-box model.
Outcome of deliberation	*As end result of % of consultations across HCECs:* 95%: Recommendations to physicians/staff 73%: Communication with patient/family 39%: Consultation with risk management 5%: Binding decisions	*As end result in % of cases across all ECSs:* 46%: Recommend best single course of action 41%: Recommend range of acceptable options 13%: No recommendation
Method for reaching conclusions	Not reported	51%: Never used voting 8%: Always by voting
Major core issues of consultations (top three)	38%: Patient autonomy/competency 35%: Improving communications 7%: End-of-life issues	Not reported

(continued)

Table 12.1. (CONTINUED)

Feature	McGee et al., 2001	Fox et al., 2007
Explicit goals of consultations (top three)	Not reported	94%: Intervening to protect patient rights
		77%: Resolving real or imagined conflicts
		75%: Causing a change in patient care to improve quality
Documentation	Not reported	93%: In committee records
		72%: In the patient medical record
Reporting of results	Not reported	73%: To chair/committee members
		26%: To authority external to ECS (e.g., administration, IRB, etc.)
		64%: Never reported in writing to patient/family
Evaluation of consultation's effect	Not reported	28%: Formal process:
		13%: by internal review
		7%: by survey or follow-up with participants
		4%: by evaluators external to ECS

ECS, hospital-based ethics consultation service; HCEC, hospital-based health care ethics committee.

goals of care. McGee et al. (2001) found that while "end-of-life issues" per se comprised only 7% of case consultations, "end-of-life situations provided a context for consultation about basic issues framed as patient autonomy or the improvement of 'communication'" (p. 63). Focal issues for policy evaluation/formulation were, however, predominantly in the "end-of-life" domain (brain death, do not resuscitate [DNR]/withdrawal of care, organ donation). Methods for case deliberation varied. Notably, while 87% of respondents reported using a single method consistently for deliberation, almost none were able to describe it. Conclusions were overwhelmingly framed as recommendations, with only a tiny percentage of committees making binding decisions. A minority of consultation services conducted any sort of follow-up or evaluation of their recommendations, and reporting of results was primarily internal to committee chairs and members. The committees received little financial support, even in paid time for members to attend meetings and consultations. Education and qualification of members varied: A small minority held graduate degrees in ethics, whereas most received training either from experienced mentors or via independent study.

Ethics Committees in the Hospice Setting

As noted previously, the prevalence and activities of hospice ethics committees are not well documented. There are indications that hospice organizations have been slower to develop internal ethics committees than have their acute care counterparts. A study of hospice ethics committees in five states, conducted about the same time as the McGee and Fox studies, found that while 73% of hospice agencies had access to an ethics committee, only 23% had committees "within their agency location and 8 percent had regional corporation committees serving more than one location" (Csikai, 2002, p. 267). An informal survey of Colorado hospices, conducted by the Colorado Center for Hospice & Palliative Care in 2008 (CCHPC, unpublished data), found internal committees in only 30% of responding hospices. Additionally, 35% of hospices are currently accredited by the various private accrediting bodies, each of which includes a standard requiring a process or group of qualified professionals to review and resolve ethical issues (http://www.hospiceanalytics.com).[1] These data points suggest that some 50 years into the development of the hospice field and nearly 40 years after *In re Quinlan*, somewhere between 20% and 30% of hospices likely have internal ethics committees.

Hospice's apparent tardiness in fostering internal ethics committees may be explained by a lack of universal regulatory or legislative requirements for clinical ethics resolution, hospice's traditional "outsider" status in the health care field, or even by an assumption that once a patient reaches hospice care, all the hard decisions have been made. Issues of patient autonomy and capacity, surrogate decision making, treatment choices, and withdrawal are hardly absent at the end stage of illness, however. Furthermore, particular features of the hospice approach to care, model of care delivery and environment, not to mention new pressures on hospice, including reimbursement and resource reductions, open access enrollment policies, and market competition, are ripe for the occurrence of ethical conflicts and complexities. Some of these unique issues are touched on in the next section; others are more fully explored throughout this text.

There is some evidence that ethical issues are capturing an increasing degree of attention and conversation in the field. In 2005, the Hospice

Foundation of America dedicated its annual teleconference, usually focused on grief and bereavement, to ethical issues at the end of life, and returned to this topic in 2012. Also in 2005, another tragic case involving withdrawal of the feeding tube from a young woman who was being cared for in hospice (Terri Schiavo) fanned a national firestorm. Fueling, or perhaps responding to, this accelerating interest, two authoritative prescriptions for ethics processes in hospice have appeared in recent years.

First, the National Quality Forum's *National Framework for Preferred Practices in Palliative and Hospice Care Quality* (NQF, 2006) devotes one of eight domains of care to "ethical and legal aspects" and identifies five preferred practices, mainly involving advance care planning and surrogate decision making for incompetent or minor patients. Preferred Practice 37 recommends that palliative and hospice care organizations "establish or have access to ethics committees or ethics consultation across care settings to address ethical conflicts at the end of life" (p. 45).

Second, the National Hospice Organization (now the National Hospice & Palliative Care Organization) issued guidelines for the development of hospice ethics committees as early as 1998. This document was extensively updated in 2007 as part of the organization's initiative to promote consistent hospice quality standards. The booklet *Starting an Ethics Committee: Guidelines for Hospice and Palliative Care Organizations* (NHPCO, 2007) and its companion *Ethical Principles: Guidelines for Hospice and Palliative Care Clinical and Organizational Conduct* (NHPCO, 2006) are excellent resources for hospice-specific ethics committees.

Both the five-state study (Csikai, 2002) and the Colorado survey (CCHPC, unpublished data) turned up extremely small samples and are thus not reliable for making conclusions about the state and operations of ethics committees in hospice organizations. However, along with Fife's (1997) description of VITAS's establishment of regional ethics committees in the 1990s, they do offer some interesting hints at similarities and differences in the role and function of ethics committees in hospice versus acute care. Table 12.2 presents a comparison of the five-state study and the Colorado survey findings.

While only 23% to 30% of responding hospices had internal hospice ethics committees (HoECs), another 40% to 50% of those without HoECs participated on or utilized the services of a committee in another facility, typically a hospital. Those without any ethics committee handled cases by review/discussion between administrator and medical director or palliative care team, or within interdisciplinary team meetings with input from administration. HoECs, where they existed, appeared more broadly interdisciplinary than their hospital cognates, with better representation from

Table 12.2. COMPARISON OF FINDINGS IN TWO STUDIES OF HOSPICE
ETHICS COMMITTEES/CONSULTATION SERVICES

Feature	Csikai, 2002	CCHPC, unpublished data
Data collected	Prior to 2002 (exact time not stated in article)	December 2007
Data source	Five states selected by systematic random stratified sampling from alphabetical list of states (plus one chosen at random): Arizona, Georgia, Maryland, New Jersey, South Carolina, Wyoming	Colorado only: 2008 hospice provider members of the Colorado Center for Hospice & Palliative Care
Response rate	68% (*N* = 182)	73% (*N* = 30)
Method	Phone survey of each hospice in each state; follow-up surveys to social workers/chairs serving on dedicated hospice ethics committees: 25 committees	E-mailed questionnaire
Focus of study	Role of social workers on ethics committees	Features and activities of hospice-based ethics committees (HoEC) or consultation services (ECS)
Type of responding facilities/agencies (majority categories)	75%: Nonprofit	100%: Nonacademic 96%: No religious affiliation 72%: Not for profit
Bed size/ADC	Mean ADC: 136 (range 7–575)	Mean ADC: 94 (range 2–399)
Presence of committee or consultation service	42%: HCEC 23%: HoEC 8%: Regional corporation committees	67%: ECS (HoEC, individual consultant, or other-facility HCEC) 30%: HoEC (all but one in hospices with >100 ADC) 24%: Developing
Time since inception	*HoECs only:* 3.5 years	*HoECs only:* 33%: 1–5 years 33%: 6–10 years 33%: >10 years
No. of members	*HoECs only:* Mean 10 members	*HoECs only:* 33%: 11–15 33%: 16–20 22%: 1–10 11%: >20
Disciplines (major categories in order of prevalence in membership)	*HoECs only:* Nurses, physicians, administrators, lay persons	*HoECs only:* Chaplains, management, nurses, physicians, social workers

(continued)

Table 12.2. (CONTINUED)

Feature	Csikai, 2002	CCHPC, unpublished data
Disciplines (all other, in order of prevalence in membership)	*HoECs only:* Social workers, attorneys, ethicists, psychologists	*HoECs only:* Administrators, community members, attorneys, ethicists, nurse practitioners, CNAs, other
Activities (mean % time)	*HoECs only (in order of frequency):* Policy development and review Case consultation and review Education (seminars, staff in-services)	*HoECs only:* 32%: Retrospective review of cases 31%: HoEC self-education 19%: Active case consultation 19%: Education of agency employees/ volunteers 14%: Formulating/evaluating policy (Sum of percentages more than 100 because not every respondent allocated time to all activities)
Supported by facility/ agency budget	n/a	*HoECs only:* 25% committees had budget or paid staff time for attendance
Policy issues addressed by committee (multiple responses possible)	n/a	*HoECs only:* 25% each for: Advance directives Nutrition/hydration Palliative sedation Refusal of tx Withdrawal of tx Request for nonpalliative tx Safety issues
Access to committee or service for consultation	n/a	*HoECs only:* 100%: Patient, family member, attending MD 94%: IDT member, volunteer 83%: Patient rep, external professional (e.g., SNF staff, clergy, attending MD)
Ethics-specific training for HoEC/ECS members	n/a	*HoECs and ECSs:* 82%: Receive some training
Median no. of consults/ year	n/a	*HoECs & ECSs:* 2.9 (range 0–10)
No. of person-hours devoted to consult	n/a	*HoECs & ECSs:* Mean 4.9 (range 2–30)

(*continued*)

Table 12.2. (CONTINUED)

Feature	Csikai, 2002	CCIIPC, unpublished data
Model for consultation	n/a	*HoECs & ECSs:* 47%: Full committee 47%: Small team 3%: Individual
Method for deliberation	n/a	*HoECs & ECSs:* 50%: By "structured group process" 38%: By "unstructured group discussion" 12%: By structured or unstructured individual analysis/process
Outcome of deliberation	n/a	*As typical end result for % HoECs/ ECSs:* 28%: Recommend best single course of action 44%: Recommend range of acceptable options 11%: No recommendation 1%: Binding decisions
Method for reaching conclusions	n/a	*HoECs & ECSs:* 89%: By consensus, discussion 11%: By voting
Major core issues of consultations (top three)	n/a	*HoECs & ECSs:* 72%: Patient autonomy/competency 56%: Conflict in goals of care 50%: Barriers to delivering care/ treatment choices (tied)
Explicit goals of consultations (top three)	n/a	*HoECs & ECSs:* 83%: Causing a change in patient care that improves quality 77%: Diffusing real or imagined conflicts 77%: Intervening to protect patient rights
Documentation	n/a	*HoECs & ECSs:* 44%: Not recorded in medical record 39%: In the patient medical record 11%: In committee records

(continued)

Table 12.2. (CONTINUED)

Feature	Csikai, 2002	CCHPC, unpublished data
Reporting of results	n/a	To HoEC/ECS leadership:
		44%: Verbal (V); 33%: Written (W)
		To HoEC/ECS members:
		77%: V; 11%: W
		To party requesting consultation:
		61%: V; W: 27%
		To professionals or patient/families
		involved in conflict:
		72%: V; 19%:W
		To authority external to HoEC/
		ECS: 88%: V; 77%: W
Evaluation of consultation's effect	n/a	12%: Formal process

ECS, hospital-based ethics consultation service; HCEC, hospital-based health care ethics committee.

social work, chaplaincy, and management. Laypersons comprised fully a quarter of the committee membership in the VITAS model, and three quarters of the five-state study committees included community members. Financial resources were slightly more abundant in HoECs than in HCECs, with 25% of the former in Colorado receiving budget or paid staff time. HoECs, compared to HCECs, spent twice the time on retrospective case reviews and half the time on policy formulation. In the five-state study, policy was the dominant activity for HoECs. Policy issues tended to focus on advance directives and treatment decisions, notably requests for nonpalliative treatments and safety issues. In Colorado and for VITAS, education was a major activity, including education of the committee and by the committee of the agency and its volunteers, as well as out into the community via conferences and other-facility in-services. VITAS provided extensive training for committee members by professional consultants. The median number of cases and focal issues for case consultations did not differ significantly between HoECs and HCECs, although this may be in part due to the high utilization of hospital committees by hospice agencies. Methods of deliberation in HoECs were evenly split between "structured group process" and "unstructured group discussion." Outcomes typically were recommendations. HoECs were slightly better than HCECs in reporting their recommendations, communicating to parties who requested the consultation, patients and families, those involved in the conflict, as well as committee members and external authorities. Reporting, however, was predominantly verbal rather than written, documentation of cases light, and evaluation lighter still.

Recognizing the limitations of the data from these small sample impressions, it appears that hospice ethics committees are not significantly different in formation or operation from their acute care counterparts, perhaps because hospices have only had the acute care model on which to draw for guidance and because many appear to be utilizing hospital-based committees. In practice, dedicated HoECs do seem to be truly multidisciplinary and more inclusive of community members. Training is not much more rigorous than in hospital settings, but HoECs engage in more external education. Reporting and communication of conclusions is more democratic in hospice than in the hospital setting. These hints point in the direction of some of the important adaptations that are necessary for optimal operation of hospice ethics committees, but none of these studies really grapples with the inherent and unique features of the hospice approach and environment of care and the special promise of ethics committees in hospice.

SPECIAL FEATURES OF ETHICS AND ETHICAL DILEMMAS IN HOSPICE

In developing an internal ethics committee (HoEC), hospice agencies can readily adopt some features from acute care counterparts; other features must be adapted to the hospice environment and or created or transformed to meet the unique needs and challenges of a model of care focused on comfort rather than cure, delivered to patients in the context of families by a team of peers with distributed and discrete responsibilities.

Ethical dilemmas in hospice are rarely "simple" matters of treatment provision or withdrawal to be determined within the confines of a health care facility and the patient–provider dyad. In the acute care setting, the objective of many ethics consultations is to uphold the interests and wishes of the disempowered, overwhelmed patient. Hospice care, particularly when delivered in the patient's home, radically disperses the loci of power, not only between patient and provider but also among members of the team and members of the patient-and-family unit. As more parties are included in the care unit and plan, more perspectives and objectives are likely to come into conflict. When dilemmas occur, robust discussions are likely to ensue in interdisciplinary team meetings, but consultation with an ethics committee can frame the issues in an entirely different structure and allow broader, more objective consideration outside of the self-reinforcing context of the interdisciplinary team (IDT). Let's look at a case:

> Harold, a 62-year-old man with end-stage lung disease, lives with his adult son, Jerrod, in a mobile home park. Harold has been on home hospice for more than 9 months and has declined to the point that he is minimally able to perform activities of daily living. Jerrod has never held a job due to a borderline mental illness. Their diet consists of take-out pizza and canned beans, and the trailer is filled with garbage. All of the IDT members agree that this situation is suboptimal, even dangerous, and will only become more so as Harold deteriorates. Anna, his nurse case manager, believes the hospice should require Harold to move to a nursing home for his own safety and to remain on hospice care. She notes that Jerrod's interaction with his father is not only neglectful but verbally abusive. She believes their bad diet will accelerate Harold's decline. The chaplain and social worker on the team assert that Harold has decisional capacity and has expressed no desire to move. Anna insists that it is unethical for the hospice to allow the situation to continue and believes it is her responsibility to advocate for what is best for Harold as her patient. She is extremely frustrated with her team and what she sees as their failure to provide optimal care for Harold. The team manager suggests a consultation with the hospice ethics committee to seek some objective guidance and recommendation for Harold's plan of care.
>
> The committee hears Anna's many concerns about Harold's situation, her growing distress, her conflict with her IDT, and her personal belief in the ethical imperative for the hospice to take active steps to remove Harold from the situation for his safety. They also hear from other members of the team. The committee discussion focuses on Anna's understanding of professional integrity and the ethical framework of respect for autonomy as expressed in self-determination, as well as the meaning of beneficence and nonmaleficence within the context of hospice care. The ethical framing of the issues leads Anna to reconcile her sense of responsibility for her patient with the patient's expressed wishes and preferences. Further, she is able to see the environment of care as Harold's choice, even though the environment is not ideal. The committee supports Harold's decision to remain in his home, but it also recommends that the hospice team make their concerns clear to Harold and Jerrod, and to offer additional support to Jerrod to assist his understanding of his father's care needs and ability to access helpful resources.

This case illustrates particular challenges and features of ethics committees in hospice. Fundamental tenets of hospice care include supporting the patient's autonomy and independence and providing care in the patient's home whenever and for however long possible. The hospice team is obligated to attend to the patient's assertions of autonomy, even while decision-making capacity diminishes. Thus, Harold's decision to remain in his home was supported. Furthermore, the patient-and-family is the hospice "unit of care," so the hospice team may encounter competing obligations to consider the needs and concerns of the patient's family members, which may diverge from or even clash with those of the patient. Justice demands family members' burdens of caregiving be given as much weight and receive as much attention as the patient's burden of illness. Jerrod, as a family member and potential caregiver, needed additional care and attention from the team.

In evaluating ethical dilemmas in hospice, the balance of beneficence and nonmaleficence is subject to considerable "tipping" depending on whose definition of "good" and "harm" is taken. Anna's definition of "good"— removing Harold from his home—was likely to match Harold's definition of "harm." As Anna's situation illustrates, the hospice team members, too, can experience a degree of moral distress if their duty and desire to provide optimal care is frustrated or their perspectives on best solutions conflict. The egalitarian team model in which all members have an equal voice and are intimately invested in the patient care plan means that the IDT meeting cannot provide the best venue for resolving these intractable dilemmas, as Harold's team discovered. Where the IDT meeting can devolve into an unhelpful echo chamber, an ethics committee consultation best functions as a true sounding board. Here is how.

A NEW PRESCRIPTION FOR ETHICS COMMITTEES IN HOSPICE

For starters, we consider that the ethics committee model, as opposed to ad hoc groups or individual consultants, is the most appropriate for ethics consultations in hospice, as it is a better fit with the team-based, interdisciplinary hospice ethos in general. That said, the ethics function of a hospice organization ought not to be confined to the ethics committee. On the contrary, we see the ethics committee as the ethical hearth of the agency home: the gathering place for focused conversation on ethical matters, foremost, but also the source of moral light and heat for the organization, its patient/family care services, its provider referral sources and partners, and even its geographical and professional community.

Committee Structure, Composition, and Training

Committee Size

HoECs, following the NHPCO guidelines (2007), "must be interdisciplinary, broad based, and consist of members whose backgrounds bring different perspectives to the committee" (p. 10). Specifically, this should include a true representation of clinical disciplines—physician, nurses, social workers, chaplains, certified nursing assistants (CNAs), and volunteers at minimum—as well as members of management/administration and finance, attorneys and/or regulatory experts, and the community. This is likely to make for a large group (77% of the HoECs in the Colorado survey reported more than 10 members, 44% more than 15; in the five-state study, the average membership was 10, and in the VITAS model, 20 [CCHPC, unpublished data; Csikai, 2002; Fife, 1997]).

Interdisciplinary and Interdepartmental Representation

From the descriptions of hospice ethics committees, it appears that HoECs are doing a pretty good job at including core clinical disciplines, except that CNAs and volunteers are underrepresented or even absent. Proportionally, these team members spend far more time with patients and family members than do other members of the clinical team. They are more likely to receive confidences that might betray distress and are more likely to observe interactions that indicate ethical problems. Volunteers, in particular, may be subject to boundary blurring either by patients and family members or the volunteers themselves, which can lead to competing fidelities, questions of professional integrity, or simply mixed messages about the care plan or patient goals. CNAs and volunteers should be included on ethics committees and receive targeted ethics education addressing these issues.

Bereavement counselors can bring a perspective stemming from the after-effects of hospice care. They may hear about interactions with the care team that have left a residue of unresolved distress that complicates grief and delays healing. Other clinical practitioners such as dieticians, physical/occupational therapists, and complimentary therapists should not be overlooked.

Management/administration and legal representatives should be lightly represented. Unfortunately, ethics committees can be perceived as punitive bodies rather than advisory or supportive. Similarly, consultations may be viewed with suspicion by patients and family members as a purely "CYA" ("cover your ass") exercise rather than a process focused on improving quality of care. A committee dominated by administrators, attorneys, and compliance and regulatory personnel is both more likely to be viewed negatively and to function more legalistically.

In addition to being interdisciplinary, HoECs should be interdepartmental in that all service lines of the agency are represented: home-based care and SNF-based care, transitional/palliative care, hospice inpatient facility, and other such distinctions within the organization. Members should be selected not just because of their role-based perspective, however, but also for their personal qualities of reflection, reasoning, and empathy.

Socially Diverse Composition

To the extent practicable, HoECs should include a mix of ethnicities, religions, races, genders, and other demographic characteristics in a way that appropriately reflects the organization's staff and the community it serves. This can be a challenge for hospice agencies, whose workers are predominantly White and overwhelmingly female. While it is true that the hospice patient population is 74.5% non-Hispanic White/Caucasian, many hospice agencies are actively reaching out to non-White communities and diversifying their workforces. Cultural, religious, ethnic, and linguistic diversity are frequent sources of ethical conflicts even within a largely White population (NHPCO, 2013).[2] Having a socially diverse ethics committee will ensure a variety of viewpoints and assist in culturally fraught cases.

Extrainstitutional Perspectives

As Fife (1997) emphasizes, HoECs can benefit from inviting participation from community members (past-patient families, civic or pastoral leaders, patient advocacy groups or disease organizations, business leaders, etc.) or other facilities and services along the continuum of care. The community can be an excellent source from which to fill in social diversity gaps, as well as ensuring against the "CYA" trap. Community members can play another important role—representing community values uncomplicated by specialized medical knowledge. They are good at asking commonsense questions and challenging unconscious assumptions.

Members of health care ethics committees collectively need to possess the skills, knowledge, and capacities required to rigorously address the mission and function of the committee. As such, committee members should be educated in ethical principles and deliberation. Just how educated has been a matter of vigorous debate within the health care ethics community almost as long as there have been ethics committees (Dubler & Blustein, 2007; Fletcher & Hoffman, 1994; Smith, Sharp, Weise, & Kodish, 2010; Williamson, 2007). Advocates for expertise—evidenced by specific academic course work, degrees, or professional certifications—argue that the practice of ethics is no less complex and demanding than the practice of medicine itself: Just as we would not allow a self-taught surgeon to so much as stitch up a gash, we should not allow untrained dilettantes to perform ethics consults, especially in life-and-death matters. As long ago as 1994, the lack of standards and mandatory expertise among ethics committee members and consultants prompted some theorists to "worry that an 'ethics disaster' is waiting to happen" (Fletcher & Hoffman, 1994, p. 336). Lack of training and sophistication in some clinical areas—notably psychology/psychiatry and philosophical/religious questions—was cited even earlier as a likely and troubling weakness in hospice ethics specifically (Klagsbrun, 1982).

On the flipside is the pragmatic "jury model" of ethics consults: Reasonable people with a modicum of specialized training, instruction in the process of ethics consults, and comprehension of the facts of the case can make sound moral judgments—and indeed may do a better job of representing community and societal values than would highly trained specialists. As an early reflection on ethics committees put it, "Making better ethical decisions does not necessarily depend on ethical expertise" (Fost & Cranford, 1985, p. 2688). Even ASBH acknowledges that it is unrealistic to expect that highly trained clinicians volunteering their time could also be expected to undertake advanced study in ethics; furthermore, uniform accredited educational programs for credentialing ethics committee members "could promote the dominance of a particular moral view or technical approach, have an adverse effect on disciplinary diversity, and imply a degree of professionalization that is...premature at best" (ASBH, 1998, p. 32). ASBH does recommend that committees seek to attract persons with varying expertise so that "collectively [the committee members] have the full range of core competencies for ethics consultation" (ASBH, 1998, p.12). This debate is unlikely to be resolved any time soon, so ultimately it is a matter to be decided by each facility or organization. Minimum competencies are desirable in either model, and ASBH's *Core Competencies* (2010) booklet offers detailed guidance.

Constitution of the Committee

The accreditation standards motivating formation of HoECs require some formal structure, such as "organizational policy and procedure [that] outlines the responsibilities of the group and delineates the process for submitting ethical concerns and issues for action" (CHAP, 2004, p. 10). Administrators will likely have to appoint members to nascent committees. Once the committee is established, an application process can be instituted.

Terms of membership and staggered rotation of retiring and new members will keep the committee from becoming too complacent or dominated by a small group or even an argumentative individual (a potential pitfall especially noted by Fife [1997]). We recommend a minimum 2-year term—preferably 3 years—for members, understanding that personal or professional changes might require early resignation and replacement. It takes time to "gel" as a group, as well as to learn and apply the relevant skills. With only about three consults coming to the HoEC in a given year, shorter terms allow fewer opportunities to participate in the core function of the group. The committee chair position, however, can rotate more frequently than every 3 years, but never less often to avoid any overidentification of the committee with a single individual or inadvertent suppression of new perspectives by an entrenched personality.

Because it takes time to "gel," we (and the NHPCO guidelines) recommend monthly or at least bimonthly meetings. The guidelines suggest that active case consultations "should be conducted outside of regular committee meetings" (NHPCO, 2007, p. 10). While this is certainly likely, given the time sensitivity that most cases in hospice are likely to entail, we do not view it as a requirement.

It should be noted that agency leadership must support—but not actively manage—the activities of an ethics committee. Financially, at minimum, the agency should pay for staff time to attend committee meetings and consults. Administrative support can take the form of an assigned record-keeper as well as space and refreshments for meetings. Less tangibly, but perhaps most important, leaders must recognize and uphold the importance of ethical clinical care, organizational behavior, and community relations; a dedicated, agency-based ethics committee can play a key role in all three domains, but only if the leadership grants it importance and authority.

Scope and Mission of Committee Activities

The primary purpose of an ethics committee in any health care setting is "to improve the provision of health care and its outcome through the identification, analysis and resolution of ethical issues as they emerge in clinical cases" (ASBH, 1998, p. 8). The core activities of ethics committees in general—policy review, consultation, and education—are just as appropriate in hospice as in the acute care setting. This discussion will look at each of these activities in the hospice setting, identify their special permutations, and suggest a widening of the ethical lens beyond a tight focus on active, clinical cases.

Policy Review and Development

Policy review and development is an example of the contribution ethics committees can make to the larger organization. Clinical case consultations might prompt development of policies in order to avoid repeating ethical conflicts, generalize conclusions from specific cases, or clarify philosophical positions. The Colorado survey (CCHPC, unpublished data) indicated that hospice ethics committees are spending less than half the amount of time as their acute care counterparts on policy review and development, whereas the five-state study (Csikai, 2002) found policy development to be the dominant activity. Policy review by the ethics committee need not be limited to issues of patient care but could also refer to organizational practices and operations.

Case Review and Consultation

As a core function of HoECs, case review and consultation should be a consistent and frequent activity. If no cases are active, the committee can perform retrospective or practice consultations. There are many models for case consultation, three of which are outlined in detail in the NHPCO guidelines (2007). Whatever model is selected, HoEC deliberations and consultation should have the following four characteristics: (1) HoEC deliberation should be consistent, systematic, and rigorous; (2) it should be focused on ethical principles and issues; (3) it should be evaluated; and (4) it should be faithful to hospice philosophy and goals of care.

Consistent, Systematic, and Rigorous

Recall the finding in Fox et al. (2007) that 87% of hospital consultation services claimed to use a consistent method for each consultation, but almost none were able to describe it. This means that either the method was not consistently used, or it was not much of a method. Consistent, systematic, and rigorous methods have discrete steps, each leading in to the next and culminating in an ethically defensible conclusion. This degree of rigor has two benefits: It keeps the committee focused, and it provides substance and authority to the process should anyone question the conclusions. Without rigor, ethics consultations quickly devolve into the proverbial "frank exchange of views," and conclusions are nothing more than persuasive opinions.

Focused on Ethical Principles and Issues

Another risk in unstructured consultations is that they can become indistinguishable from IDT meetings or care conferences. While some hospices use IDT meetings to discuss and resolve ethical issues (CCHPC, unpublished data), the tenor and goals of discussions in IDT meetings and ethics consultations are significantly different. IDT meetings are focused on clinical interventions and procedures for care. Questions or conflicts may come to the ethics committee as procedural questions: "What are we going to do about Mr. X?" This may be the question that is ultimately answered in the ethics committee recommendations, but the process for getting to the answer in an ethics consultation is entirely different from an IDT discussion.

Let's say Mr. X refuses pain medication due to a religious belief about the redemptive value of suffering, but he insists that hospice staff not tell his adult children of his decision. As his pain increases, his children are naturally upset at the hospice's apparent inability to make him comfortable. The procedural question here is "Should the hospice staff tell the children that their father instructed them to withhold analgesics?" That's the "What should we do?" question, which would appropriately be addressed in an IDT meeting. Ethics consultations back up from the "what" questions and ask the "why" questions, exploring the moral implications of and justifications for choices and consequences. Answers to the ethical questions arrived at

Table 12.3. PROMPTING QUESTIONS FOR ETHICS CASE
CONSULTATION FACT GATHERING IN HOSPICE CARE

Medical Indications

At what stage is the patient in the progression of his/her terminal condition?

How are symptoms being managed? How effectively?

What are patient's goals of care?

How achievable are these goals? How will the care team pursue them?

What are plans if goals cannot be achieved? What are alternatives if symptoms cannot be managed?

Patient Preferences

If competent, what are patient's preferences for care and symptom management?

Does the patient understand the goals of hospice care and are his/her goals in alignment?

Quality of Life

How does patient express/define quality of life? Will interventions support it?

What emotional/psychosocial/spiritual issues are prominent for the patient now and how are they being accounted for in care plan?

How are treatment/care goals supporting and maximizing the patient's definition of quality of life now?

Are there risks, "downsides," or side effects associated with care plans that might undermine the patient's quality of life?

Are patient's expressed preferences for treatment/nontreatment/care consistent with stated goals?

Contextual Factors

Are there family issues affecting patient's preferences for/attitude toward care? How are patient's decisions likely to affect family?

through structured deliberation will likely point directly to a solution to the procedural question, but ethics committees must keep a disciplined focus on the ethical conflicts and questions, temporarily setting aside the procedural concern.

Ethical deliberation begins with gathering the relevant facts of a case in order to have as much information and context as possible and to identify the ethical principles in conflict. In their seminal book on clinical ethics, Jonsen, Siegler, and Winslade (2006) offered the "four-box model," including prompting questions to ensure thorough data gathering from four domains: medical indications, patient preferences, quality of life, and contextual features. While this tool is very helpful, hospice ethics committees may struggle with the acute care assumptions reflected in some of the prompting questions. Table 12.3 offers hospice-oriented prompting questions in each of the four categories identified by Jonsen, Siegler, and Winslade.

This information gathering is only the first step in the process and is intended to assist with the second step, identifying the ethical principles in conflict, including autonomy, justice, beneficence, nonmaleficence, fidelity, honesty, professional integrity, and others.[3] In the case of Mr. X, hospice staff are caught between honoring the patient's wishes (autonomy) and soothing the family's distress (justice), between being faithful to the patient (fidelity) and upholding their obligations to care for both the patient and the family (professional integrity).

With the ethical principles identified, the committee can frame the core ethical question. Ethical questions are couched in ethical language: "Does Mr. X have a right to insist on confidentiality regarding his treatment choices?"; "Does our respect for Mr. X's autonomy overrule consideration of the rights and concerns of his family or the hospice staff?"; "Do hospice staff have a stronger obligation to maintain fidelity with the patient or to professional integrity?"; "Will breaking or maintaining confidentiality achieve a greater good?"

Structured discussions of ethical questions entail in-depth consideration of the ethical principles at issue and the moral implications of choices and outcomes. Not getting sidetracked by care management practicalities or leap-frogging to procedural recommendations prematurely requires a strong facilitator and a respectful committee. As noted earlier, answering the ethical question will likely point directly to a procedural recommendation. For instance, if the committee decides that respect for Mr. X's autonomy trumps alleviating the distress of his family or the hospice staff, the recommendation would be to keep his confidentiality. If the committee were to decide that breaking confidentiality, however upsetting to the patient, would achieve a greater good by calming the concerns of the family and healing the breaches of professional integrity felt by the staff, then the family should be told of the patient's directive.

From both the acute care and hospice ethics committee literature, typical conclusions for case consultations involve one or more (procedural) recommendations arrived at by consensus. Consensus does not mean or require absolute unanimity, and dissenting voices should be heard and recorded. Written documentation of the case should be kept in the records of the ethics committee and/or medical record, and recommendations communicated, preferably in person but also in writing, to all parties involved with an opportunity for questions about the process that led to the recommendation.

Evaluated

Ethics consultations should also have some manner of follow-up to determine the value of the process and efficacy of the recommendations, a step that is often left out. There is considerable discussion in the ethics literature about the importance—and difficulty—of consultation evaluation (ASBH, 2010; Fletcher & Siegler, 1996; Fox & Arnold, 1996). However, evaluation is essential to improve processes and prove the worth of the resources devoted to the committee. Evaluation is complicated by the idiosyncratic nature of the process (each case is different) and competing perspectives of results. In addition, before one can evaluate results, one must determine goals, and "the range of appropriate outcomes for ethics consultations has never been enumerated, and validated measurement tools have not been developed" (Fox & Arnold, 1996, p. 127). Still, on a case-by-case basis, ethics committees can identify goals (e.g., improve patient care, facilitate communication, resolve conflicts, establish guidelines, etc.) and determine success or failure accordingly. Suggestions for evaluation methods are provided in the NHPCO booklet (2007).

Faithful to Hospice Philosophy and Goals of Care

Resolution of ethical dilemmas entails finding the best path toward the ultimate goal of care. In the acute care setting, the goal is to restore a person to good health and function via accurate diagnosis and restorative treatment—in a word, cure. Quality of life is, of course, a consideration, but it is sometimes (perhaps often) subordinated to beating back disease and overcoming injury.

The hospice goal of care is fundamentally and profoundly different: to achieve relief of suffering and support for patients and families in their pursuit of a peaceful and dignified end of life—in a word, comfort. In the hospice approach to care, quality of life for patients and families is paramount. Thus, not only is the nature of the ethical dilemmas likely to be somewhat different in hospice versus acute care settings, the consideration and resolution of those dilemmas should be meaningfully distinct. Applying consultation methods, goals, or evaluations created for the acute care setting to the hospice world is likely to resemble the proverbial pounding of the square peg into the round hole.

Case consultations need not be limited to clinical topics; indeed, the ethics committee can and should serve as a forum for examining organizational issues as well. Marketing and fundraising methods, personnel policies, and business practices are appropriate subjects of ethical scrutiny and analysis. In this way, the hospice ethics committee can inform and ensure ethical behavior and orientations throughout the organization.

Some hospice ethics committees serve as the source of education and consultation for other hospices; equally, they can provide assistance to long-term care facilities, assisted living, home health, and other nonhospital services. Before opening its doors to external organizations, the hospice must assess the burden on resources such services might entail and issues of confidentiality and privacy protections.

Education

Education tends to be the predominant activity of ethics committees in between consults. It is not just a pastime, however; as noted previously, it is critical to the proper functioning of the committee that its members be educated in ethical concepts, methods, and theories and the clinical realities with which they are asked to deal.

The broader educational function of an ethics committee is to expand the knowledge and awareness of ethical issues and processes throughout the organization. Inviting any staff member or volunteer to attend the educational segment of ethics committee meetings is one approach; delivering in-service seminars or participating in new-employee orientation is another. Ethics committee members can act as "ethics ambassadors" always on the lookout for opportunities to introduce the ethical dimension to conversations in all domains of the organization.

As Fife (1997) and Csikai (2002) noted, some hospice ethics committees offer educational programs for the professional or lay community at large. This provides an excellent forum for exploring challenging ideas, debating opposing viewpoints, and promulgating accurate information about emotionally charged or even politicized issues attracting public attention. As the wider societal movement to improve care, ensure comfort, and honor patient's wishes at the end of life gains momentum, as it surely will with the aging of the baby boomer generation, the ethical dimension of health care provision will be increasingly debated in public forums. Hospice organizations have an obligation to engage with these conversations and offer up well-reasoned and morally justified analyses of issues such as right to refuse treatment, distinctions between passive and active euthanasia or between euthanasia and companioned dying, appropriate withdrawal of artificial nutrition and hydration, advance care planning, and access to quality end-of-life care, among others. Hospices especially have an obligation to counter the "death panel" fearmongering that continues to obscure the fundamental good of providing patients and families with the best care possible at a sacred time of life. Examining these issues through an ethical and educational lens can offer a significant service to the community.

A CHALLENGE TO HOSPICE: BRINGING ETHICS TO THE BEDSIDE, BOARDROOM, AND BOULEVARD

The practice of hospice care is steeped in ethical intent: honoring patient's wishes, supporting independence and choice, caring for families as well as patients, and relieving suffering in all its forms are fundamental to hospice philosophy and essential ethical actions. However, inherent does not mean automatic. Ethics, as an orientation and activity, must be maintained—fed and fanned like the fire in the hearth. An internal, dedicated hospice ethics committee provides a mechanism for resolving conflict, a source of education and discussion, a forum for consideration and articulation of moral positions. Furthermore, each of these activities can take place across three distinct but related domains:

At the "bedside"—where the ethical problems concern the specific care of individual patients, and outcomes are recommendations affecting the quality of care for that individual/family

In the "boardroom"—where the problems are more general to entire patient populations or consist in contraventions of the values of the agency as a whole in business and management practices, and outcomes are policies, procedures, and budgetary allocations

On the "boulevard"—where ethical problems that manifest in the agency are either the result of or have significant implications for how health care in general and hospice in particular are practiced and perceived within the community they serve.

In each domain, hospice ethics committees have an opportunity—even duty—to articulate ideals of behavior and moral orientation and provide guidance and inspiration on how best to express those ideals. At the "bedside" means striving for impeccably ethical care of patients and families and resolving conflicts with rigor and compassion. In the "boardroom" means infusing the organization with knowledge of ethics through education and policy review as well as attending to ethical action in marketing and fundraising, management and governance, and employee–supervisor and employee–employee interactions. On the "boulevard" means raising a voice in the public and political debates about health care and end-of-life care, to articulate and uphold ethical positions on issues such as providing care to the indigent, neither hastening nor impeding death, supporting patient autonomy while preserving justice, and focusing always on minimizing suffering and maximizing quality of life for the dying and their families.

A well-educated, active, and supported ethics committee can infuse the entire organization with a "culture of ethics" with profound impact on patient care, organizational strength, and public perception. For those with an eye on the bottom line, a robust ethics committee can foster an active moral community within and beyond the agency in ways that create a significant market differentiator, establish the agency as a "go-to" organization for accurate and rich information, and raise its profile in an increasingly competitive environment.

NOTES

1. At this writing, 947 hospices nationally are accredited by The Joint Commission, 662 by the Community Health Accreditation Program, and 164 by the Accreditation Commission for Health Care (http://www.hospiceanalytics.com).
2. This 2012 figure, while still high, represents a significant drop from 80.5% in 2009. Outreach efforts appear to be diversifying the hospice population—all the more reason for diversity on ethics committees.
3. For more information on these ethical principles and their implications for ethical deliberation, see NHPCO (2006) or Beauchamp and Childress (2001).

REFERENCES

Altman, L. K. (2003, June 22). Dr. Belding H. Scribner, medical pioneer, is dead at 82. *The New York Times*. Retrieved April 2014, from http://www.nytimes.com/2003/06/22/us/dr-belding-h-scribner-medical-pioneer-is-dead-at-82.html?pagewanted=all&src=pm.

American Medical Association (AMA). (1985). Guidelines for ethics committees in health care institutions. *Journal of the American Medical Association, 253*(18), 2698–2699.

American Society for Bioethics and Humanities (ASBH). (1998). *Core competencies for health care ethics consultation*. Glenview, IL: American Society for Bioethics and Humanities.

American Society for Bioethics and Humanities (ASBH). (2010). *Core competencies for health care ethics consultation* (2nd ed.). Glenview, IL: American Society for Bioethics and Humanities.

Beauchamp, T. L., & Childress, J. F. (2001). *Principles of biomedical ethics* (5th ed.). New York, NY: Oxford University Press.

Csikai, E. L. (2002). The state of hospice ethics committees and the social work role. *Omega, 45*(3), 261–275.

Community Health Accreditation Program (CHAP). (2004). *Community Health Accreditation Program core standards of excellence*. Washington, DC: Community Health Accreditation Program.

Colby, W. H. (2002). *Long goodbye: The deaths of Nancy Cruzan*. Carlsbad, CA: Hay House.

Colby, W. H. (2006). *Unplugged: Reclaiming our right to die in America*. New York, NY: Amacom.

Cruzan v. Director, Missouri Department of Health, 497 US 261 (1990).

Dubler, N. N., & Blustein, J. (2007). Credentialing ethics consultants: An invitation to collaboration. *American Journal of Bioethics, 7*(2), 35–39.

Fife, R. B. (1997). The role of ethics committees in hospice programs. *Hospice Journal, 12*(2), 57–63.

Fletcher, J. C., & Hoffman, D. E. (1994). Ethics committees: Time to experiment with standards. *Annals of Internal Medicine, 120*(4), 335–338.

Fletcher, J. C., & Siegler, M. (1996). What are the goals of ethics committees? A consensus statement. *Journal of Clinical Ethics, 7*(2), 122–126.

Fost, N., & Cranford, R. E. (1985). Hospital ethics committees: Administrative aspects. *Journal of the American Medical Association, 253*(18), 2687–2692.

Fox, E., & Arnold, R. M. (1996). Evaluating outcomes in ethics consultation research. *Journal of Clinical Ethics, 7*(2), 127–138.

Fox, E., Myers, S., & Pearlman, R. A. (2007). Ethics consultation in United States hospitals: A national survey. *American Journal of Bioethics, 7*(2), 13–25.

In re Quinlan, 70 NJ 10, 355 A.2d 647 (1976).

Jonsen, A. R., Siegler M., & Winslade, W. J. (2006). *Clinical ethics: A practical approach to ethical decisions in clinical medicine*. (6th ed.). New York, NY: McGraw-Hill.

Klagsbrun, S. C. (1982). Ethics in hospice care. *American Psychologist, 37*(11), 1263–1265.

Lenzer, J. (2003). Belding Scribner. *British Medical Journal, 327*(7407), 167.

McGee, G., Caplan, A. L., Spanogle, J. P., & Asch, D. A. (2001). A national study of ethics committees. *American Journal of Bioethics, 1*(4), 60–64.

National Hospice and Palliative Care Organization (NHPCO). (2006). *Ethical principles: Guidelines for hospice and palliative care clinical and organizational conduct*. Alexandria, VA: National Hospice and Palliative Care Organization.

National Hospice and Palliative Care Organization (NHPCO). (2007). *Starting an ethics committee: Guidelines for hospice and palliative care organizations*. Alexandria, VA: National Hospice and Palliative Care Organization.

National Hospice and Palliative Care Organization (NHPCO). (2013). Hospice facts and figures: Hospice care in America (2012 ed.). Retrieved April 2014, from http://www.nhpco.org/sites/default/files/public/Statistics_Research/2013_Facts_Figures.pdf.

National Quality Forum. (2006). *A national framework for preferred practices for palliative and hospice care quality*. Retrieved April 2014, from http://www.qualityforum.org/Publications/2006/12/A_National_Framework_and_Preferred_Practices_for_Palliative_and_Hospice_Care_Quality.aspx.

Omnibus Budget Reconciliation Act of 1990, Public L. No. 101-508, §4751, 104 Stat. 1388-204 (1990).

Presidents Commission for the Study of Ethical Problems in Medicine. (1983). *Deciding to forego life-sustaining treatment: Ethical, medical, and legal issues in treatment decisions*. Retrieved April 2014, from http://bioethics.georgetown.edu/pcbe/reports/past_commissions/deciding_to_forego_tx.pdf.

Rosner, F. (1985). Hospital medical ethics committees: A review of their development. *Journal of the American Medical Association, 253*(18), 2693–2697.

Pulrich, L. P. (1999). *The Patient Self-Determination Act: Meeting the challenges in patient care*. Washington, DC: Georgetown University Press.

Smith, M. L., Sharp, R. R., Weise, K., & Kodish, E. (2010). Toward a competency-based certification of clinical ethics consultants: A four-step process. *Journal of Clinical Ethics, 21*(1), 14–22.

Uhlmann, M. (Ed.) (1998). *Last rights: Assisted suicide and euthanasia debated*. Grand Rapids, MI: William B. Eerdmanns.

Webb, M. (1997). *The good death: The new American search to reshape the end of life*. New York, NY: Bantam Books.

Williamson, L. (2007). The quality of bioethics debate: Implications for clinical ethics committees. *Journal of Medical Ethics, 24*, 357–360.

Zucker, M. B. (1999). *The right to die debate: A documentary history*. Westport, CT: Greenwood Press.

Ethics and the Future of Hospice

CHAPTER 13

Design for Dying

New Directions for Hospice and End-of-Life Care

BRUCE JENNINGS

There is a growing recognition of the suffering and cost, as well as the benefits, that high-technology medicine has created for critically and terminally ill persons. And there is a dawning—actually by now a high noon—recognition of the staggering social problems that loom in the graying of the baby boomer generation. The population of seniors in the United States is projected to more than double over the next 40 years, rising from 35 million in 2000 to over 88 million by 2050. At that time, one in five Americans will be age 65 years or older. Those 80 years and above will be the most populous age group in the country—32.5 million or 7.4% of the population (Shrestha & Heisler, 2011). America's chronic care, long-term care, and end-of-life care systems are fragmented and patchwork, barely able to cope now, and nowhere near ready to face the human demands within the next generation that these demographic trends will create (Lynn, 2005). The challenge now is to design a more adequate health care system and infrastructure (Gostin, Boufford, & Martinez, 2004; Schoen, Osborn, How, Doty, & Peugh, 2009). This is necessary across the entire life span, of course, but is especially important during the last decade or so of life. This a time marked by incurable, progressive, chronic disease that erodes quality of life and that culminates in a dying process during which technological intervention to prolong life may become both futile and harmful (Lynn, 2004).

Beginning in the mid-1970s, America embarked on a quest to reform and improve medical care and decision making near the end of life. Reform efforts ran along two simultaneous and parallel tracks. One was an individual empowerment (patient rights) strategy aimed at making life-sustaining treatment decisions responsive to the dying patient's personal preferences and values. The second track was an alternative system or model of care (holistic, person-centered, and palliative) that aimed to support meaning, relationality, and dignity for the dying person in the context of surrounding family and friends. The first of these was in place by the end of the 1980s, with the affirmation by the US Supreme Court of the constitutional right of an individual to forgo life-sustaining medical treatment (*Cruzan v. Director*, 1990). The key to its success has been judicial recognition and legislative change. The second track, the hospice and palliative care alternative, was well established by the end of the 1990s. The key to its success has been public financing through the Medicare health insurance system and cultural acceptance.

This chapter will present a discussion of policy issues in end-of-life care that falls into four sections. The first section will review the two reform tracts mentioned earlier in more detail. The second section will examine the attempt to make individual autonomy the design principle of end-of-life care and consider some of its remaining unresolved problems and unanticipated blind spots. The third section discusses the current "relational turn" in end-of-life care and relates it to the system design approach of hospice and palliative care. In the fourth section I sketch a conception for future reforms and improvements in end-of-life care. The conception I propose consists of respect for relational autonomy within the context of an expanded hospice, or neo-hospice, system of evolving medical treatments and caregiving services that are appropriately managed, adjusted, and seamlessly continuous across the trajectory of incurable, progressive chronic illness, especially during the last year or two of life.

Ethics by its very nature offers a design for living; a hospice ethical vision also provides a design for dying that affirms human dignity and the human good. That design is a dynamic, not static, form—a fountain, not a statue. Despite the manifold impediments and challenges present in contemporary health care and society, an ethically robust and practical new design for dying in America is within our reach.

REDESIGNING DYING: TWO STRATEGIES OF IMPROVING END-OF-LIFE CARE

There was a time when a physician was on solid ethical ground in doing "everything possible" to stave off death. The understanding of medical care and the physician–patient relationship were characterized by what might be called the "rescue orientation." The rescue orientation perceives the person confronted with a life-limiting illness as the victim of an attack; this model enlists medicine as the defender and rescuer of the endangered victim. Here the patient's role is largely passive and obedient. His or her benefit derives from the physician's skill and power, which in turn are based on the power of medical science and technology to preserve and prolong life.

Paradoxically, it was medicine's success, rather than its failure, that called the rescue model and patients' passivity into serious question. Advances in critical and intensive care medicine beginning roughly in the 1960s were coming on line to prolong the biological functions of seriously ill patients—mechanical ventilators, intensive care units, kidney dialysis, and the like. These were, for the most part, what Lewis Thomas called "halfway" technologies because they could stave off death and prolong biological functions of life, but they could not necessarily restore the patient to a meaningful mode of being alive (Thomas, 1974).

In the wake of this technological transformation of end-of-life treatment, two things were recognized. First, it became evident that, for perhaps the majority of patients at the end of life, the exact timing and circumstances of one's death were not beyond anyone's control but were in fact the result of specific decisions and choices made by those caring for (physicians) and speaking for (usually family) the patient. Second, thoughtful leaders in medicine, and many family members who had observed the new end-of-life care firsthand, gradually became aware that the experience of dying (for the individual, for the family, and also at times for health care providers) was often a horror. Too many Americans were dying unnecessarily bad deaths—deaths with inadequate palliative support, inadequate compassion, inadequate human presence and witness; deaths preceded by a dying marked by fear, anxiety, loneliness, and isolation; and deaths that effaced dignity and denied individual self-control and choice.

It was not surprising, therefore, that various movements for reform arose to improve end-of-life care. Reform efforts were based on the belief that bad dying was avoidable because it does not reside in dying or death per se, but rather in a dying process that is poorly designed and managed. Our powerful new technology was not being used wisely and judiciously but had succumbed to a kind of technological imperative. Aggressive interventions were not being adequately informed or guided by the patient's own wishes and values. Reductionist medical perspectives, which were the flip side of the new technology and the medical training that went along with it, were displacing more holistic perspectives, and this made it more difficult to see "the patient as person," as one leading bioethicist aptly put it

(Ramsey, 1970). Palliative care was not a priority of mainstream medicine, and the hospice model was only beginning to develop for a limited number of people, such as cancer patients who had "failed chemotherapy."

Thus it was that medicine, ethics, and law came to face a novel and very disturbing question. Should life-extending medical technology be deliberately withheld or withdrawn when the patient refuses to consent to those treatments or when they offer no benefit but only serve to prolong the patient's dying? The answer given—not in one moment, to be sure, but gradually in the accumulating authority and logic of many judicial and professional deliberations—was yes.

Now, if it is ethically and legally acceptable to forgo life-sustaining medical treatments under certain circumstances, then the technological imperative will no longer function as the de facto design principle of end-of-life care. New system design principles will be needed. Two such principles in fact emerged. The first was to allow the dying patient to design his or her own end-of-life care, in accordance with the person's autonomous choices and values, and with the assistance of a surrogate decision maker, if necessary. The second was to have experts in palliative medicine and in holistic psychosocial models of care design an alternative system—often, but not necessarily, physically removed from the hospital setting where the life-sustaining technologies reside—in which relationality (as distinct from individualistic autonomy) and the use of palliative treatments and supports replaces the technological imperative of life-sustaining medical treatment as the design principle and the system default.

Centering the end-of-life care design principle in the autonomy of the dying person entailed a patient empowerment strategy. Working mainly through the medium of the law, but also through ethical persuasion and education within medicine, new norms and decision making standards were put in place to empower and enable individuals to set the terms of their own medical care at the end of life. The law and ethics embraced the right of an individual to consent to or forgo all forms of medical care, and they embraced the use of advance directives to keep the wishes of the individual at the center of the decision-making process if and when the patient lost the capacity to make medical decisions for himself or herself.

The alternative system strategy—in essence the hospice model—located the design principle in palliative techniques, quality of life, and psycho-social-spiritual goals, each of which aims to preserve or restore the relational connections that are meaningful to the dying person so as to mitigate the sense of loss, the isolation, and the final loneliness of the experience of dying. However, it could not rely solely on the empowerment of patients as the planners and generals of their own care. Instead, it required a new kind of end-of-life care system and new kinds of delivery programs or agencies. Working mainly through the medium of health care policy and medical/nursing education, the task of improving end-of-life care was approached by institutionalizing a model and a philosophy or ethic based on the humane values of caring presence, quality of life, dignity, and the relief of suffering; values articulated early on by Saunders and others in the hospice movement, as discussed in Chapter 2 (Cassel & Foley, 1999; Field & Cassel, 1997).

The goal of the system strategy was to orient end-of-life care toward dignity, comfort, symptom management, and meaningful life closure rather than technological intervention to prolong the duration of life. It did so by structuring care planning, treatment pathways, and the decision-making process so that most patients received the most appropriate care for them most of the time, without having to struggle against the prevailing current of automatically aggressive medical interventions. If a given individual wished to have aggressive life-prolonging treatment, then he or she could opt into that decision-making pathway, subject to side constraints of equity and resource availability as well as medical appropriateness. But while opting into disease-modifying or life-extending treatment was available, it was not to be the default presumption of this system. The hospice model would put the rigors and responsibilities of autonomy and empowerment into the background—put them on automatic pilot, so to speak. Forgoing the use of life-sustaining medical technology would not require the effort, determination, or struggle necessary in the hospital environment. Hospice would provide the space or setting designed to facilitate—through symptom control, family involvement and support, counseling—the hard "work" of dying: the achievement of meaningful life closure.

These two strategies were virtually contemporaneous in their origins. And they each were not only expert-driven, top-down reform strategies but also bottom-up social movements—the hospice movement and the so-called right to die movement—that arose out of widespread grassroots dissatisfaction with mainstream medicine. (It should be noted that they also arose in the context of the broader women's health and patients' rights movements.)

In 1975, the family of Karen Ann Quinlan in New Jersey turned to the courts in search of a solution to what they considered a denial of dignity for their daughter by the power of a new life-sustaining technology, mechanical ventilation. The New Jersey Supreme Court ruled that Karen, who was permanently unconscious after sustaining catastrophic anoxic brain injury, had a right to refuse (or have her guardian refuse on her behalf) life-sustaining medical treatment under the circumstances (*In re Quinlan*,

1976). The Quinlan case constituted the first milestone in the patient empowerment strategy.

Two years earlier in 1974, Florence Wald helped frame the alternative care system strategy by founding the Connecticut Hospice. Wald had been the Dean of the Yale School of Nursing, and she had worked and studied with Cicely Saunders at St. Christopher's Hospice in London. Wald and other hospice pioneers perceived that mainstream oncology was manifestly failing to provide adequate support and continuity of care to incurable cancer patients in the terminal phase of their illness. Hospice was designed to remedy that systemic defect; it was created to provide symptom control, palliative relief from suffering, and meaningful presence and human refuge to dying patients and their families (Corless & Foster, 1999).

AUTONOMY BY DESIGN

The patient empowerment strategy was born in the landmark Quinlan case and has evolved in over 100 appellate-level court rulings, culminating in the US Supreme Court decision in the Cruzan case (*Cruzan v. Director*, 1990), in statutes in all 50 states, and in scores of documents from medicine, nursing, the allied health professions, churches, government commissions, and academic experts in biomedical ethics. As noted earlier, from these sources something like an ethical, legal, and professional consensus has taken shape (Berlinger, Jennings, & Wolf, 2013; Meisel, 1993; Meisel & Cerminara, 2004; National Center for State Courts, 1993). It is centered on the right of the individual patient to refuse any and all forms of medical treatment, including life-sustaining treatment. It is an individualistic and autonomy-respecting consensus. Since it places such a strong emphasis on the voice of the patient in the decision-making process, one of its main goals is to continue to be guided by that voice as much as possible, even when the patient has lost decision-making capacity and can no longer speak or decide for himself or herself—hence the emphasis that has been placed on educating patients to fill out advance directives (living wills and durable powers of attorney for health care).

The central premise of this approach to redesigning and reforming end-of-life care has been that appropriate, quality care requires shifting power from the physician and the "clinic"—the institutional space of knowledge and control (Foucault, 1973)—to the critically ill patient. This is done in the service of respect for autonomy, patient rights, and giving voice, influence, and power to the personal values, beliefs, and choices of the patient. If physician control and benevolent paternalism are reinforced by the rescue orientation, this new approach is one of patient consumer sovereignty and is reinforced by what might be called the "individualistic interests orientation." It does not wish to submit to medical control; it wants to direct medical services. It sees the physician as a technical expert working for the patient in the medical treatment process—a partner and advisor, not the general, the master, or the shepherd. This orientation also sees the dying person, not as a passive "patient" or victim, but as a self-reliant and unencumbered self, still planning and directing his or her life right up to the end. In the final analysis, it sees the patient as a consumer, enlisting medicine in the quest to control the dying process in accordance with his or her preferences and values (Annas & Healey, 1974).

Of course, large numbers of critically and terminally ill persons have lost the capacity to express preferences and to make decisions about their own medical care by the time key end-of-life choices have to be made. The *Quinlan* court in New Jersey had asked, What would Karen have wanted done? One obvious solution to this problem is an advanced declaration by the patient regarding medical treatment. Beginning in California, such an approach, quickly dubbed a "living will," was recognized explicitly in state law in the 1970s (California Natural Death Act, 1991). More recently another approach, centered on a designated person rather than a treatment directive, has been followed using the durable power of attorney for health care. Taken together, these two approaches have come to be called "advance directives," and the naming of another person as a proxy decision maker has an advantage over a living will or treatment directive because most people find it too difficult to compose detailed advance treatment instructions. In any case, to sustain the patient empowerment design principle in cases where the individual has lost decision-making capacity, the advance directive has become the point of emphasis (McCarrick, 1991).

Although well established in law and public policy, and significantly institutionalized in bodies such as hospital ethics committees, professional guidelines, regulations, accreditation standards for health care organizations, and the like, the design principle of autonomy has failed to achieve the desired response and outcomes in a number of areas. Individuals have not responded favorably to the advance directive concept and what it requires of them and their families. Physicians have not changed their behavior as expected, either. Advance directives seem to have little effect on the aggressive norm of end-of life treatment and on the power of the technological imperative. Principled grounds for differentiating the right to refuse treatment from the right to demand treatment (also known as rationing) have been very controversial when proposed, so autonomy has opened the door to sometimes unreasonable and costly expectations.

Ironically, the individual empowerment strategy has been criticized as biased against those with disabilities, particularly cognitive disabilities. And it has been seen as imposing a culturally, racially, and class-biased perspective onto groups holding different values and attitudes toward end-of-life care and death, dying, and decision making. Finally, the logic of the individual empowerment approach seems to lead in the direction of legally recognizing a right to medical assistance with suicide or physician aid in dying (PAD), as it has come to be called. PAD is much more controversial in society at large than is the notion of the right to refuse invasive, life-prolonging medical treatment. Nonetheless, advocacy efforts to accept PAD continue, and to date it has been legally authorized (with many preconditions and procedural safeguards) in Oregon, Washington, Montana, and Vermont, and abroad in the Netherlands and Switzerland.

In short, the individual empowerment strategy suffers from unresolved conceptual dilemmas and tenacious pockets of public misunderstanding and cultural resistance. It is rationalistic, individualistic, and consumeristic in ways that, however well they may work in everyday life in a consumer society, seem strangely dissonant and inappropriate near the end of life. To frame end-of-life care as first and foremost an issue of individualistic interests and empowerment is to misconstrue the cultural meaning of care and to slice thin the moral responsibilities of family members as caretakers for the dying. The end stage of a progressive, incurable illness is not the best time to micro-manage one's own medical care and to wage battles on behalf of autonomous selfhood (Hawkins, Ditto, Danks, & Smucker, 2005). Caring, family solidarity, mutual respect, love, and attentiveness to the dying person are the qualities most needed then. The empowerment paradigm has been rather suspicious of families, and it embraces the legal fiction that they are and should be empty conduits of the patient's wishes (Nelson, 1992: Nelson & Nelson, 1995). Mothers and fathers, brothers and sisters, and companions all lose their thick, long-lived ties with the dying person and become "surrogates" or "proxies," cold, artificial terms to denote an impersonal role.

Moreover, rights are undermined in practice unless they are exercised in the context of dialogue and relationships of shared experience and meaning. The individualistic interests orientation sees dying patients' rights as claims of noninterference by others; the relational orientation sees rights as bonds of interpersonal respect and support. Empowerment backfires when it isolates people rather than bringing them together in communion and communication.

Most intriguing of all, the individual empowerment strategy may rest on a fundamental misdiagnosis of the true problem in the first place. The problem may not be so much the allocation of power and the individuation of care at the end of life, as it is a problem of creating a high-quality system to ensure psychosocially appropriate care for all near the end of life, without undue burden on the dying person and the family.

RELATIONALITY BY DESIGN

The hospice movement developed an alternative model of cancer care to better meet the needs of patients who were unresponsive to mainstream treatments and their families. It created community-based, nonprofit agencies to deliver this care. During its first decade hospice was supported by out-of-pocket patient and family payment and by charitable funding. Hospice was then changed significantly by the creation of the Medicare Hospice Benefit in 1983 and the concomitant development of private insurance coverage (Hoyer, 1998; Mahoney, 1998). Since then, enrollment has grown (very rapidly since 2000) and hospice has undergone increasing professionalization and quality improvement. It has also assumed a business orientation as larger for-profit organizations have entered the hospice marketplace. In the 1990s a parallel palliative care initiative, not specifically funded but also not constrained by Medicare eligibility and reimbursement policies, arose and has been growing significantly, especially in hospital settings (Field & Cassel, 1997; Morrison & Meier, 2011).

Hospice and palliative care today offer a well-proven, effective therapeutic model that prevents and manages suffering, maintains quality of life, and reduces illness burden in populations with serious or life-threatening illnesses. This model takes a multidimensional, multidisciplinary approach and is grounded in a holistic bio-psycho-social-spiritual conception of care. In principle, it is beneficial to anyone living with virtually all forms of chronic, progressive life-limiting illness (not only cancer) and is relevant throughout the entire course of the disease (not just in the final 6 months of life). Both the individual patient and the family are considered the unit of care. This model aims to promote ongoing communication to support shared decision making and advance care planning that is sensitive to culture, religion, and other value concerns. It provides comfort and relief from suffering through expert symptom control and management of psychosocial and spiritual needs. It provides practical help in the home and expert management of active dying and its aftermath. It also offers support for family while they are engaged in caregiving and experiencing grief and bereavement. Access to this therapeutic model has grown substantially in the past decade, but it is still limited by policy rules and economic and cultural factors.

What is needed today (and indeed what has been quietly developing since the 1990s at least) is another complex shift in orientation—a movement of tectonic plates in our moral imagination and caring practices, so to speak—to produce a new conceptual foundation for end-of-life decisions. I would call this the "relational turn" in end-of-life care. It is the shift from individualistic interests to a relational and communicative perspective and orientation. In certain respects, this kind of perspectival shift has already begun (Browning & Solomon, 2006; Dubler & Liebman, 1994; Jennings, 2008, 2012; Mackenzie & Stoljar, 2000; Meier, Isaacs, & Hughes, 2010; Morrissey, 2011; Morrissey & Jennings, 2006; Nedelsky, 2013; Sabatino, 1999, 2010; Schneider, 1998). This perspective sees the situation of the critically ill or dying person in relational terms; that is, dying is a process that takes place within a system of interrelationships and a network of shared meanings. The relational orientation combines respect for developmental personhood with recognition of the inherent dignity of all human beings and their need for care, presence, and relief of suffering. It is based on the insight that human beings are not self-sufficient or self-sovereign individuals but are relational and interdependent selves. To live well while dying is to navigate those relationships and meanings intact through the shoals of crisis; to die well is to preserve, and perhaps repair, those relationships right up until the end, and even beyond in the memory of those who survive.

To be sure, the relational orientation is not altogether new; it has been there all along in the alternative care system strategy that has run parallel to the individual empowerment strategy in end-of-life care reform. Throughout its own brief history, hospice has been one of the forces preparing the way for this shift. The future of hospice lies with the development of this relational turn in end-of-life care and with the capacity of the hospice movement and care model to contribute high-quality standards of care and a depth of moral imagination to it. Indeed, the distinctive disposition of the hospice movement has always had a strong affinity with the relational orientation toward the dying person and the nature of his or her existential situation. The relational orientation, as it is expressed and embodied in hospice care at its best, brings to the foreground the complex nexus of social and cultural relations among human beings, with their extraordinarily diverse and powerful cognitive, affective, and communicative capacities.

The fact that this relational orientation is particularly apt with regard to the human experience of dying and death should come as no surprise.

The confrontation with one's own mortality in the context of a progressive and incurable condition that will almost certainly prove fatal in the near future is one of the most intense and fragile moments in human life. For the past 50 years or so, life near the end of life has been invaded and colonized by hard medical technologies. Their benefit in prolonging life can be great, but their destructive potential is alarming. They can destroy the delicate, vulnerable social fabric of families and the tissue of meaning that dying patients and families need in order to get a grip on the terrible thing that has befallen them. When it was technologically impotent, medicine (together with religion) presided over social rituals and cultural meaning during the dying process. Relationships and identities were repaired and renewed—with family and friends at hand, with an opportunity to reconcile with those estranged, to forgive and to ask forgiveness. Today, medicine and medical treatment decisions set up a dynamic that makes that social ecology unstable at best, impossible at worst (Kaufman, 2005).

As it has developed so far, the hospice movement in America has maintained an ambivalent posture toward the individualistic interests orientation's assumptions. It began with a different understanding of the problem to be solved at the end of life. Instead of empowerment, the hospice movement was primarily motivated to bring an alternative model of end-of-life care to dying people and their families. This model was rather limited in scope and was thought of as pertaining mainly to end-stage cancer patients who wished to die at home. By the early 1980s a demonstration study of the hospice model had proven its feasibility and effectiveness. A major policy development was the creation of a public insurance benefit for hospice for the elderly and the poor, the Medicare Hospice Benefit (MHB). Enacted by Congress in 1982 and implemented in 1983, the MHB created a large source of new funding for hospice programs and expanded access to these services. But this expansion did not bring about a broader application of the hospice model of care because the hospice philosophy became equated— mistakenly in my view—with the peculiar eligibility requirements of the MHB. So hospice came to be regarded, not as a model for end-of-life care generally, but rather as a kind of last resort alternative, after life-extending medical treatments had become futile or unduly burdensome and after a decision had been made to forgo them. This was assumed to be appropriate only during the last 6 months of life, even though at roughly the same time many courts were explicitly rejecting the idea that such a short duration of life expectancy should be a precondition for the legal and ethical right to refuse life-sustaining treatment (Meisel, 1993). This hiving off of a more relational and holistic approach to end-of-life care until after the rest of medical care had run its course, as it were, was a key factor in making the individualistic, empowerment orientation the sole focus for end-of-life care ethics in mainstream medical settings. It has also resulted in hospice care being stigmatized as a death warrant, a dead end, an abandonment, and a loss of hope.

The future of hospice lies in making its services more comprehensive and flexible and in placing it more seamlessly within the continuum of chronic and end-of-life care. This is a system issue and thus converges with the parallel need for a systemic approach to decision making about the use of life-sustaining technology near the end of life (Connor, 2007-2008).

A NEW HOSPICE VISION FOR CARE OF THE CHRONICALLY DYING

Let's pause at this point and take stock of where we are. I believe that the history of end-of-life care reform in the last 35 years can best be understood as a shift from the rescue orientation to the individualistic interest orientation—from doctor knows best to doctor as partner, collaborator, and consultant; from the ill body as an object of intervention and manipulation to the ill person as a subject of interests and preferences who inhabits an ill body; from the passive sick role to the active role of a consumer. That shift was monumental, and there is no question of going backward to re-embrace medical control as the ethical paradigm. Nonetheless, in practice if not in theory, the force of the technological imperative and the appeal of the rule of rescue are still very often determinative, especially in cases involving surrogate decision making. So the cultural and ethical struggle between technology and autonomy as end-of-life care design principles continues. Viewed as a cultural struggle to win hearts and minds, I do not think patient empowerment will prevail, in part because that contest (not in courts, but in individual cases at the bedside in hospitals) is played out in a system and in a setting where the deck is stacked against autonomy.

To fulfill the original vision of the patient empowerment strategy will paradoxically require giving up the notion that each patient can build his or her own uniquely personalized system and menu of end-of-life care. A new system, not uniquely personalized but made up of generic pathways and presumptions, must be built to bolster the patient empowerment strategy. Those presumptions are rebuttable and those pathways have exit options, but this generic system, drawing on our knowledge of incurable, progressively degenerative and debilitating chronic disease, will be designed to meet the needs and values of most dying patients and their loved ones, most of the time.[1]

Indeed, the new system I envision will synthesize the two design principles of autonomy and relationality, and that will be a key to its success. Separately the design principle of autonomy and the design principle of relationality have now reached the limits of their viability. A reformed system of care provision, delivery, and financing must span the trajectory of the most common and eventually fatal illnesses (cardiovascular disease, solid tumor cancers, pulmonary disease, dementia, and progressive frailty and debility). If it is based on the design principles of both relationality and autonomy, it can realize the ideal of treating the patient as a subject or a person and tailoring the care plan to the needs and values of the individual more effectively than the patient empowerment approach does (Fins, 2006; Morrison & Meier, 2004).

My reasons for thinking this about autonomy as a design principle have already been mentioned. In terms of how the design principle of relationality operates in practice, hospice as it has developed provides an instructive example, which indicates, I think, that hospice also has reached the end of its tether, and the time has come to expand and build on that experience and to broaden its design elements. Hospice enrollment has grown significantly in the last decade, but as an end-of-life care system it is too narrow and too late. Hospice today is hemmed in by regulatory and financial structures that limit its capacity to realize the full potential of its philosophy to improve end-of-life care. It has been ghettoized in the overall health care system so that very late referrals limit both the duration and the depth of its ability to meet the relational needs of dying persons.

To be sure, quality control and professional standards in hospice have improved and it has matured as a professional field. This has been essential ethically and necessary in order to justify the social support and expenditure of billions of dollars that hospice has received. But as a field thrives, in the competitive market economy of health care in the United States, it also attracts investments and business enterprises that are not always mission driven or consistent with the core values of hospice as a caring practice. It is crucial to maintain a critical scrutiny of these developments, from the point of view of the hospice vision I have in mind here, for they could subvert that vision.

So, where do we go from here? A commitment to what justice requires in caring for the needs of the dying must be translated into tangible institutional structures and policy mandates. It must come to inform those things that motivate behavior in the health care system—from social marketing to professional education and from the provision of funding for services to the cultivation of a professional calling. Making it tangible requires a new vision of hospice and palliative care, one that holds firm to many of the traditions and values of the hospice movement but finds new and more flexible organizational forms through which to express those values, a vision that my colleagues and I have elsewhere called "value-based hospice." This conception and the reasons why it is vital are summarized as follows:

> The nature and goals of [hospice] need to be redefined. We must envision hospice as a potentially new paradigm of social health care for an aging society. If we can learn how to define, organize, finance, and deliver hospice care properly, then we may have found the key to coping with the major problem of caring for staggering numbers of persons with chronic, degenerative disease—the number one problem of the health care systems of the developed world for the next fifty years. Chronic, degenerative disease requires patients and families to make difficult adjustments and transitions in their lives as they pass through various stages and phases of their disease. The experience of chronic disease blends gradually into the experience of dying. The flow and rhythms of hospice, as well as its goals and care plans, must be allowed to match the rhythms of chronic illness, as chronic illness becomes an increasingly widespread social condition. Of all the existing structures and specialties in health care today, hospice has the best chance of successfully transforming itself into this chronic care social medicine of the future. (Jennings, Ryndes, D'Onofrio, & Baily, 2003, p. S4)

This vision and organizational approach are based on three characteristics of the original hospice philosophy of care: (1) Hospice provides expert assistance with the management of the "condition" of the dying person and her family. (2) Hospice is flexible and dynamic in developing new expertise and services to meet changing community needs. (3) In managing a patient's condition, hospice provides continuity of caregiving and care planning, across a broad continuum of settings and services, as the person moves along a trajectory of chronic, debilitating, and life-limiting illness. These characteristics reflect goals that hospice has sought to adhere to; but their implications extend well beyond what we currently designate as "hospice" alone. They also provide elements for a restructuring of the entire system of care in the final chapter of life.

Condition Management

At the heart of this new vision and a system that could embody its practice is the notion of "condition management." Hospice has been successful because it has therapeutically responded to the consequences of the patient's illness—his or her total condition or situation. That is to say, hospice and palliative care should respond to the patient's embodied and relationally embedded personhood, not just his or her disease, symptoms, or isolated body and self. This stands in contrast to a focus on the biomedical aspects of a pathological process, without much regard for the psychological and social aspects of the patient's lived experience of the disease or the implications of the disease state for family members or others. The notion of "managing" a total human situation or condition implies a respect for the integrity and participation of both patient and family members and betokens an active process of controlling symptoms and handling aspects of everyday life so that they do not undermine the kinds of relationships, reminiscences, communication, feelings, and activities that the patient finds meaningful and that give remaining life its positive quality.

The emotional and social meaning of "condition"—the consequences of disease on the lives of patients and those around them—may be at least as important to patients as the physical impairment itself (Helman, 1990; Kleinman, Eisenberg, & Good, 1978). Historically, a keystone of hospice philosophy has been the dictum that "the patient and family are the unit of care." Attention to the needs of caregiving family members has been found to improve consumer satisfaction levels and result in lower health care utilization among family caregivers, many of whom subsequently suffer from significant physical illness or emotional stress, especially if they are not adequately supported by professional services.

Organizational Flexibility

Amid the wide variety of programs and services that make up the hospice world today, there are signs of an expansive movement toward earlier intervention in the disease trajectory, more continuity of care across a greater number of settings, and more responsiveness to community needs and functions beyond those associated with end-of-life care for individual patients and families. Some hospices are not only clinical care delivery agencies but are also becoming public health agencies and institutions of health education and health promotion.

This is one reason that it is a significant mistake to equate hospice care as such with the range of services and eligibility requirements contained in the MHB or to define hospice agencies as entities that solely or predominantly serve patients who qualify under the MHB. In reality, existing hospice programs are quite diverse, and it is useful to distinguish among three basic types of agencies, each of which is certified under the Medicare program but only one of which is primarily focused on MHB patients. These three types can be called Medicare hospices, community hospices, and comprehensive hospice centers (von Gunten & Ryndes, 2005). Medicare hospices, as the name implies, primarily serve patients eligible for the MHB and receive a very high proportion of their income from Medicare. Most of these programs are small, and many of them are independent. They have limited ability to tolerate financial risk or to innovate in their services. Community hospices also rely on Medicare reimbursement but go beyond the Medicare population to offer services to patients who are not medically or emotionally ready for traditional hospice care, as well as to the community at large. Comprehensive hospice centers are community hospices with a dedicated academic mission. They are committed to improving care through professional education and research, and they are often of exceptional size, community position, and philanthropic fundraising capacity. Some are attached to medical and nursing education programs and serve as teaching hospices.

In its early days, hospice was attractive to many patients and families because the alternative was dying in pain or becoming dependent on providers who saw them as failures. Today, as life-extending treatments are increasingly available, patients and families are understandably leery of being compelled to choose between receiving care to extend life, on the one hand, and care directed toward their comfort, on the other. Difficulty in making this decision delays access to hospice for many dying patients— often until they have only days or hours to live.

Requiring that MHB enrollees forgo restorative therapies also has become an impediment enhancing the quality hospice care, because it has created a ghetto structure that often excludes hospices from initiatives to integrate different kinds of care. For many years, hospice pioneers, palliative care specialists, and some consumer advocates have viewed curative and palliative care as complementary approaches that should be provided in a changing mix over the course of an illness to meet patient needs. Some hospices are now adopting and implementing "open access" policies that permit patients the option of accessing certain potentially disease-modifying treatments, such as radiation and chemotherapy for more than simply palliative purposes, while remaining on the hospice program. This is especially applicable to pediatric hospice, but it has yet to become a widespread practice. For those in the last months or weeks of life, the intention to avail oneself of a range of medical treatments may not be widespread. But as one sees the hospice model changing and moving upstream into earlier stages of a progressive chronic illness, this kind of open-access approach will be crucial. As an early response to this problem, the Patient Protection and Affordable Care Act (2010, §3140) mandates demonstration projects in multiple sites that will test the effect of allowing concurrent hospice and conventional care on both quality and cost (Medicare Payment Advisory Commission, 2011).

Continuity of Care Across a Continuum of Services

In its conceptual meaning, hospice is best understood as a form of care, not an institutional venue or a physical facility, like a hospital or a nursing home. Some hospices do have inpatient facilities, but those remain the exception rather than the rule in the United States. Hospice providers are peripatetic: They travel from setting to setting and patients rarely come to them. Consequently, hospice professionals often find themselves in a dual-provider role with home care agencies, nursing homes, and hospitals. This experience has taught hospice how to negotiate the fissures and crevices of the American health care system. Even when hospice is called in very shortly before the patient's death, as happens in about one out of three cases, patients and families often establish relationships with hospice providers and rely on them to orchestrate dealings with pharmacies, community physicians, other health care providers, sometimes clergy, and even neighbors and friends. In the future aging society and in the emerging health care system, more universal access to insurance coverage will come on the condition of greater accountability and cost containment. Hospice, which was in fact the pioneering prospective payment and managed care form of health care delivery, should be in a good position to build on its experience base and provide enhanced continuity across institutional settings. This will be of benefit for patients and families unfamiliar with the complexities of health system, as well as those wrestling with complex clinical and personal decisions.

Having someone serving as a broker or "case manager" in a bewildering system can often be just as important to patients and families as the provision of medical and nursing care and symptom management. And for those who qualify, the MHB is literally the only program in the entire American health care system that allows patients and families to forget about financial worries and to concentrate instead on the hard work of grieving and living in the face of dying. To complement this blessing, families need to be assured that the right type of services, medicine, and equipment will be available to the patient as he or she moves through the trajectory and changing needs of illness. Hospice at its best is *condition management for continuity of care across a continuum of services*. This formulation is a mouthful, but every term is important in it. It is one of the principal contributions that hospice is in the best position to provide, structurally and historically, for end-of-life care.

Hospice must develop new organizational forms if it is to provide these three components to its patients and families and to the communities it serves. The development of such new forms of hospice financing and delivery will tax the creativity and management skills of hospice leaders. It will also require that policymakers leave behind their former emphasis on an individual's categorical eligibility and focus instead on hospice's ability to assume the responsibility and liability for the care of a diverse population. In particular, hospices should be encouraged to implement their continuity of care expertise within a continuum of palliative services, facilitating case management and care planning based on the appropriateness of services given the changes in the patient's and the family's needs over time.

One straightforward reform aimed at increasing access to hospice would be to modify the current MHB by expanding the eligibility criterion of life expectancy from 6 months to 1 year. Yet this would only address the policy and regulatory barriers associated with the 6-month life expectancy rule. It would do little to address the other structural and attitudinal barriers (Casarett, 2007). To address and to overcome the barriers to hospice access in a more comprehensive way, hospice must be reinvented and re-envisioned along the lines shown in Figure 13.1.[2]

Figure 13.1 represents hospice as a provider whose purview ranges across the trajectory of a life-limiting disease. It models a situation in which the traditional hospice as a specialized service and an independent agency with a limited mission has been transformed into a more comprehensive model of hospice care in which hospice becomes the coordinating center for a range of palliative services that can be accessed by patients in

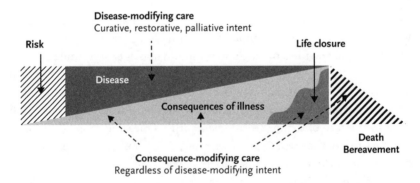

Figure 13.1
Hospice as a continuum of care. (Reprinted from Jennings, Ryndes, D'Onfrio, and Baily, 2003, p. S50, by permission of The Hastings Center.)

various ways as the patient's underlying condition evolves from diagnosis to death. Finally, this image moves away from the distinction between disease-modifying and palliative care to indicate that the benefits of palliative care come not so much from a focus on a biological disease as a focus on the overall situation or condition of a relational self who is navigating the dying process or, for that matter, living (as indeed all of us do) toward and until death.

Many current and narrowly defined hospice policies and regulations, including otherwise laudable efforts to prevent Medicare fraud, are out of step with what is most innovative and creative in the hospice community today. In addition to focusing on the care of those facing a terminal illness, many hospices are active in the delivery or development of philanthropically supported programs for individuals who want symptom management and adaptive counseling even as they pursue active treatment directed toward prolongation of life. These hospices also serve those facing the debilitating effects of aging or the consequences of sudden and catastrophic death. In short, it is clear that these programs have expanded the expression of core interdisciplinary competencies to individuals other than those imminently dying. While the first expression of hospice competencies has been care of the dying, this is not the core hospice competency. The core hospice competency is the interdisciplinary response to the human consequences of chronic disease, disability, and aging—their potential to undermine both autonomy and relationality.

With this in mind, we should begin to think of hospice as offering something of value to many different groups of patients, or to a given patient and family at many points along a spectrum of symptoms and services and across stages of chronic illness. To provide the impetus for policy and practice changes that will increase access to hospice care, we need first to re-envision hospice as a concept of health care—a new way of thinking about the nature and goals of health care itself—rather than an end-stage form of care.

CONCLUSION

How should we view the person who is dying? As a consumer who is purchasing either life-sustaining medical services or palliative and hospice services to stave off pain and suffering at the end? Or as a self embedded in—and flourishing to the extent available through—relationships of shared family, memory, and meaning? Hospice is not entirely alien to the first conception. Indeed, much of our current terminology for organizing and financing hospice and palliative care reinforces, whether deliberately or inadvertently, this first perspective. The consumer perspective does counteract the paternalism of the medical control orientation. But to more fully improve end-of-life care, it is far from sufficient. Law, ethics, and policy must also come to grips with fundamentally interpersonal issues of mortality and meaning. We sometimes seem to talk and act as though dying were solely the concern of the dying person. This is a narrow and short-sighted view.

In making autonomy central to our understanding of the ethics of medical care for the dying and in interpreting the notion of the person in a strongly individualistic way, we create some blind spots that are particularly instructive. One blind spot is the gap between the regulative ideals of ethics and the law and the lived moral experience of the actual persons— physicians, family members, and patients themselves—who make decisions near the end of life. This gap is a warning sign of something amiss in our moral thinking and imagination. The quotidian moral experience of our familial and relational lives as selves—our social embeddedness as persons—serves as an essential corrective to the aspiration for power and the dignity of isolated independence; the will to power and the will to self-affirmation and self-expression.

The challenge facing us is to rebuild, reinforce, and reinterpret our laws, institutions, and practices around the acknowledgment that dying is interpersonal, not strictly individualistic. Hospice at its ethical best has long done this, creating space for families and intimate friends to be close to the dying person. Hospice also recognizes the emotional needs of those same people. Surrogate decision makers and guardians can and should take into account the dying person's concerns for those whose lives will be affected by his or her death. Note that when we understand selfhood from a relational perspective, as embedded and embodied, for dying persons to have concerns of this kind is not an aberrant but a normal response. As challenging, even scandalous as it is to address explicitly, we cannot ultimately dodge the question of what counts as a good death and what counts as good care near the end of life (DelVecchio Good et al., 2004).

The fundamental problem with end-of-life care is structural and institutional in nature. In the modern acute care hospital virtually everything is oriented toward the use of life-sustaining equipment and techniques, not to forgoing them. The informal culture of specialty medicine, the reward system, the institutional pressures faced by family members, the range of choices people in extremis are being asked to make—each of these factors and more make up a system that is remarkably resistant to change when confronted with an ideal, countercultural decision-making model, even one that is to some extent backed up by the force of law and professional ethics.

A countervailing system needs to emerge for end-of-life care, a system centered on care of the person, not simply treatment of the body, and bringing all forms of medical care, disease-modifying and life-extending as well as palliative and quality of life oriented, together in a seamless continuum of services that are case managed and planned in a candid process informed by both solid medical knowledge and inclusive, respectful communication. Until then we will continue to urge the individual to prepare for death in advance, and we will continue to require him or her to make a series of agonizing micro-decisions in order to stay on the right pathway toward death.

I believe that the principal task of the next few years in the end-of-life care domain will be to build out this new system worthy of a palliative vision and an ethical conception of good living while dying (Fins, 2006). We need to continue to refine the decision-making processes and tools that are already in place and to devise new and more culturally sensitive, family systems–oriented strategies of communication and care planning. And we shall need to continue a robust discussion in quest of ethical and conceptual clarity to guide this shift and also to protect against the undue erosion of important patient-centered rights and values. Patient's rights should be reconstrued, but they should not be rejected. It is important to insist on this distinction, for it is not a mere semantic quibble at a time of concerted, often less than careful or discerning, financial cost-containment policy measures targeted at end-of-life care.

I close with the thought that dying is not the worst thing; dying badly is. And while dying is an inevitable part of the human condition, dying badly is not; it is a correctable ethical and system failure.

NOTES

1. Between 2000 and 2003, I codirected a study of access to Hospice Care undertaken by The Hastings Center and the National Hospice Work Group, in collaboration with the National Hospice and Palliative Care Organization and funded by the Arthur Vining Davis Foundations and the Nathan Cummings Foundation. The final report of this study was published as *Access to Hospice Care: Expanding Boundaries, Overcoming Barriers* (Jennings, Ryndes, D'Onofrio, & Baily, 2003). In the remainder of this chapter I draw freely on and paraphrase some of the central findings and arguments of that study, and I highlight aspects of the problem that still remain to be solved today. I am pleased to acknowledge the contribution of my coauthors to this work: True Ryndes, Carol D'Onofrio, and Mary Ann Baily.

2. This conceptual representation is taken from Jennings, Ryndes, D'Onfrio, and Baily (2003). It was developed originally by Dr. Frank Ferris and was used with his permission.

REFERENCES

Annas, G., & Healey, J. (1974). The patient rights advocate. *Journal of Nursing Administration, 4*(3), 25–31.

Berlinger, N., Jennings, B., & Wolf, S. M. (2013). *The Hastings Center guidelines for decisions on life-sustaining treatment and care near the end of life*. (2nd ed. Text rev.). New York, NY: Oxford University Press.

Browning, D., & Solomon, M. Z. (2006). Relational learning in pediatric palliative care: Transformative education and the culture of medicine. *Child and Adolescent Psychiatric Clinics of North America, 15*(3), 795–815.

California Natural Death Act, California Health and Safety Code §§ 7185 to 7194.5 (1991).

Casarett, D. J. (2007). *Is it time to redesign hospice? End-of-life care at the user interface*. [Center for Policy Research, Paper 8]. Retrieved April 2014, from http://surface.syr.edu/cpr/8.

Cassel, C. K., & Foley, K. (1999). *Principles for care of patients at the end of life: An emerging consensus among the specialties of medicine*. New York, NY: Milbank Memorial Fund.

Connor, S. R. (2007–2008). Development of hospice and palliative care in the United States. *Omega (Westport), 56*(1), 89–99.

Corless, I. B., & Foster, Z. (Eds.). (1999). *The hospice heritage: Celebrating our future*. Binghamton, NY: Haworth Press.

Cruzan v. Director, Missouri Department of Health, 497 US 261 (1990).

DelVecchio Good, M. J., Gadmer, N. M., Ruopp, P., Lakoma, M. Sullivan, A. M., Redinbaugh, E.,...Block, S. D. (2004). Narrative nuances on good and bad deaths: Internists' tales from high-technology work places. *Social Science and Medicine, 58*(5), 939–953.

Dubler, N. N., & Liebman, C. B. (1994). *Bioethics mediation: A guide to shaping shared solutions*. New York, NY: United Hospital Fund.

Field M. J., & Cassel, C. K. (Eds.). (1997). *Approaching death: Improving care at the end of life*. Washington, DC: National Academy Press.

Fins, J. J. (2006). *A palliative ethic of care: Clinical wisdom at life's end*. Sudbury, MA: Jones and Bartlett.

Foucault, M. (1973). *The birth of the clinic: An archaeology of medical perception*. New York, NY: Pantheon Books.

Gostin, L. O., Boufford, J. I., & Martinez, R. M. (2004). The future of the public's health: Vision, values and strategies. *Health Affairs, 23*(4), 96–107.

Hawkins, N. A., Ditto, P. H., Danks, J. H., & Smucker, W. D. (2005). Micromanaging Death: Process preferences, values, and goals in end-of-life medical decision making. *Gerontologist, 45*(1), 107–117.

Helman, C. G. (1990). *Culture, health and illness* (2nd ed.). London, UK: Butterworth.

Hoyer, T. (1998). A history of the Medicare hospice benefit. In J. K. Harrold & J. Lynn (Eds.), *A good dying: Shaping health care for the last months of life* (pp. 61–69). Binghamton, NY: Haworth Press.

In re Quinlan, 70 NJ 10, 355 A.2d 647 (1976).

Jennings, B. (2008). Dying at an early age: Ethical issues in palliative pediatric care. In K. Doka & A. Tucci (Eds.), *Living with grief: Children and adolescents* (pp. 99–119). Washington, DC: The Hospice Foundation of America.

Jennings, B. (2012). From rights to relationships: The ecological turn in ethics near the end of life. In K. Doka, C. Corr, & B. Jennings (Eds.), *End-of-life ethics: A case approach* (pp. 3–22). Washington, DC: Hospice Foundation of America.

Jennings, B., Ryndes, T., D'Onofrio, C., & Baily, M. A. (2003). Access to hospice care: Expanding boundaries, overcoming barriers. *Hastings Center Report, 33*(2, Suppl.), S3–S60. Available at http://www.thehastingscenter.org/uploadedFiles/Publications/Special_Reports/access_hospice_care.pdf.

Kaufman, S. R. (2005). *And a time to die: How American hospitals shape the end of life.* New York, NY: Scribner.

Kleinman, A., Eisenberg, L., & Good, B. (1978). Culture, illness and care: Clinical lessons from anthropologic and cross-cultural research. *Annals of Internal Medicine, 88*(2), 251–258.

Lynn, J. (2004). *Sick to death and not going to take it anymore! Reforming health care for the last years of life.* Berkeley: University of California Press.

Lynn, J. (2005). Living long in fragile health: New demographics shape end-of-life care. *Hastings Center Special Report, 356,* S14–S18.

Mackenzie, C., & Stoljar, N. (Eds.). (2000). *Relational autonomy: Feminist perspectives on autonomy, agency, and the social self.* New York, NY: Oxford University Press.

Mahoney, J. J. (1998). Medicare hospice benefit—15 years of success. *Journal of Palliative Medicine, 1*(2), 139–146.

McCarrick, P. M. (1991). *Living wills and durable power of attorney: Advance directive legislation and issues.* National Reference Center for Bioethics Literature, Georgetown University. Retrieved April 2014, from http://bioethics.georgetown.edu/publications/scopenotes/sn2.pdf.

Medicare Payment Advisory Commission (MedPAC). (2011, March). *Report to Congress: Medicare payment policy.* Washington, DC: MedPAC. Retrieved April 2014, from http://medpac.gov/documents/Mar11_EntireReport.pdf.

Meier, D. E., Isaacs, S. L., & Hughes, R. G. (Eds.). (2010). *Palliative care: Transforming the care of serious illness.* San Francisco, CA: Jossey Bass.

Meisel, A. (1993). The legal consensus about forgoing life-sustaining treatment: Its status and its prospects. *Kennedy Institute of Ethics Journal, 2*(4), 309–345.

Meisel, A., & Cerminara, K. L. (2004). *The right to die: The law of end-of life decision making* (3rd ed.). New York, NY: Aspen Law and Business.

Morrison, R. S., & Meier, D. E. (2004). Palliative care. *New England Journal of Medicine, 350*(25), 2582–2591.

Morrison, R. S., & Meier, D. E. (2011). *America's care of serious illness: A state-by-state report card on access to palliative care in our nation's hospitals.* New York, NY: Center to Advance Palliative Care.

Morrissey, M. B. (2011). Phenomenology of pain and suffering: A humanistic perspective in gerontological health and social work. *Journal of Social Work in End-of-Life and Palliative Care, 7*(1), 14–38.

Morrissey, M. B., & Jennings, B. (2006). A social ecology of health model in end of life decision making: Is the law therapeutic? *New York State Bar Association Health Law Journal, 11*(1), 51–60.

National Center for State Courts, Coordinating Council on Life-Sustaining Medical Treatment Decision Making by the Courts. (1993). *Guidelines for state court* decision making in life-sustaining medical treatment cases (2nd ed., Text rev.). St. Paul. MN: West Publishing Co.

Nedelsky, J. (2013). *Law's relations: A relational theory of self, autonomy, and law.* New York, NY: Oxford University Press.

Nelson, J. L. (1992). Taking families seriously. *Hastings Center Report, 22*(4), 6–12.

Nelson, J. L., & Nelson, H. L. (1995). *The patient in the family: An ethics of medicine and the family.* New York, NY: Routledge.

Patient Protection and Affordable Care Act of 2010. Pub. L. No. 111–148, 124 Stat. 119; Pub L. No. 111–152, 124 Stat. 1029 (2010).

Ramsey, P. (1970). *The patient as person.* New Haven, CT: Yale University Press.

Sabatino, C. P. (1999). The legal and functional status of the medical proxy: Suggestions for statutory reform. *Journal of Law, Medicine and Ethics, 27*(1), 52–68.

Schneider, C. (1998). *The practice of autonomy: Patients, doctors, and medical decisions.* New York, NY: Oxford University Press.

Sabatino, C. P. (2010). The evolution of health care advance planning law and policy. *Milbank Quarterly, 88*(2), 211–239.

Schoen, C., Osborn, R., How, S. K. H., Doty, M. M., & Peugh, J. (2009). In chronic condition: Experiences of patients with complex health care needs, in eight countries, 2008. *Health Affairs, 28*(1), w1–w16.

Shrestha, L. B., & Heisler, E. J. (2011). *The changing demographic profile of the United States.* [Congressional Research Service, 7-5700]. Retrieved April 2014, from http://www.fas.org/sgp/crs/misc/RL32701.pdf.

Thomas, L. (1974). *The lives of a cell.* New York, NY: Bantam Books.

von Gunten, C., & Ryndes, T. (2005). The academic hospice. *Annals of Internal Medicine, 143*(9), 655–658.

INDEX

Fife, R. B., 260, 269, 277
Five state hospice ethics study, 259, 260, 261–64t
Florida, 127, 131, 134, 200
Foley, K. M., 47
Food and Drug Administration Modernization Act of 1997 (FDAMA), 123
Forbes Hospice, 25
Fowler, K., 129
Fox, E., 255, 256–58t, 273
Friedman, T., 5–6
Functional assessment staging (FAST) scores, 69
Futile drug therapy, 71
Futility in giving CPR, 215–16

Gabapentin, 68
Gaetz, Don, 23
General Principles of Hospice Care, 42–43
Gillick, M., 6
Grief, 86, 177–79, 260, 268, 293
Griswold, C, L., 151

Hardwig, J., 150, 151
Harrold, J., 4
Health care ethics committees. *see* ethics committees
Health Care Finance Administration (HCFA), 24
Heinz, John, 25
Hermsen, M. A., 104, 105
HIV/AIDS, 157
Hope, role of, 125–27
Hospice, Inc., 20–24, 290
Hospice and Palliative Nurses Association (HPNA), 225
Hospice care
  condition management, 298–99
  continuity of care, 112–13, 301–3, 302f
  definitions, 49
  live discharges, 15
  models generally, 1–2, 23–24, 52–53, 52f
  organizational flexibility, 299–301
  as paradigm shift, 51–53, 52f
  practice of, 53–54
  statistics, 1, 15, 30

value-based hospice model, 296–303, 305n1
Hospice eligibility. *see under* Medicare
Hospice ethics committees (HoECs). *see* ethics committees
Hospice Foundation of America, 259–60
Hospice movement. *see also* Medicare hospice benefit
  cancer treatment, 17–18
  certification, 29, 99–100, 133
  challenges, 14–15
  Connecticut, 20–24
  deinstitutionalization, 25, 26
  euthanasia movement, 19–20
  evolution of generally, 13–14, 295
  Federal funding, legislation, 17, 22–26
  GAO study, 24
  institutionalization, 18–19
  integration, 30–31
  length of stay, 30
  licensure, 22, 24, 29
  managed home care, 27
  models, 23–24
  National Hospice Study (NHS), 24–25
  patients, living *vs.* dying components of, 27, 31
  proprietary hospices, 27, 30
  reimbursement, 22, 25, 27, 30
  religion/spirituality role, 21
  sociopolitical factors, 15–16
  visiting nurses associations (VNAs), 22
Hospice Nurses Association (HNA), 27–30
Hospice philosophy. *see* philosophy of care
How to Die in Oregon, 237, 247n2
Hydromorphone, 61, 64–66
Hyperalgesia, 78

Ibuprofen, 67–68
IDT. *see* interdisciplinary team
Impression management, 115
Individualized health care plan (IHCP), 137
Informed consent, 79, 127–29
Inpatient care
  access, 165–66
  autonomy, 171–74
  clinical/organizational ethics, 174–77